Handbook of

Mechanical Ventilatory Support

2nd Edition

Handbook of
Mechanical Ventilatory Support

2nd Edition

M. Christine Stock, MD
Associate Professor of Anesthesiology
Emory University School of Medicine
Atlanta, Georgia

Azriel Perel, MD
Chairman, Department of Anesthesiology and Critical Care
The Chaim Sheba Medical Center
Tel Aviv University
Tel Hashomer
ISRAEL

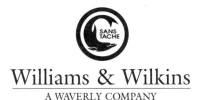

Williams & Wilkins
A WAVERLY COMPANY

BALTIMORE • PHILADELPHIA • LONDON • PARIS • BANGKOK
BUENOS AIRES • HONG KONG • MUNICH • SYDNEY • TOKYO • WROCLAW

Editor: Sharon R. Zinner
Managing Editor: Tanya Lazar
Marketing Manager: Diane M. Harnish
Production Coordinator: Peter J. Carley
Project Editor: Bill Cady
Copy Editor: Joann Nash
Designer: Mario Fernandez
Illustration Planner: Ray Lowman
Cover Designer: Circa 86
Typesetter: Maryland Composition Co., Inc.
Printer: Mack Printing Group
Digitized Illustrations: Maryland Composition Co., Inc.
Binder: Mack Printing Group

Copyright © 1997 Williams & Wilkins

351 West Camden Street
Baltimore, Maryland 21201-2436 USA

Rose Tree Corporate Center
1400 North Providence Road
Building II, Suite 5025
Media, Pennsylvania 19063-2043 USA

Accurate indications, adverse reactions, and dosage schedules for drugs are provided in this book, but it is possible that they may change. The reader is urged to review the package information data of the manufacturers of the medications mentioned.

Printed in the United States of America

First Edition, 1992

Library of Congress Cataloging-in-Publication Data
Handbook of Mechanical Ventilatory support / [edited by] M. Christine
    Stock, Azriel Perel. — 2nd ed.
        p.   cm.
    Includes bibliographical references and index.
    ISBN 0-683-30261-2
    1. Respiratory therapy.   2. Artificial respiration.
3. Respirators.
    [DNLM: 1. Respiration, Artificial.   WF 26 H236 1997]
    RC735.I5H36   1997
    615.8′36—dc21
    DNLM/DLC
    for Library of Congress   97-3786
                                                              CIP

The publishers have made every effort to trace the copyright holders for borrowed material. If they have inadvertently overlooked any, they will be pleased to make the necessary arrangements at the first opportunity.

To purchase additional copies of this book, call our customer service department at **(800) 638-0672** or fax orders to **(800) 447-8438.** For other book services, including chapter reprints and large quantity sales, ask for the Special Sales department.

Canadian customers should call **(800) 665-1148** or fax **(800) 665-0103.** For all other calls originating outside of the United States, please call **(410) 528-4223** or fax us at **(410) 528-8550.**

Visit Williams & Wilkins on the Internet: **http://www.wwilkins.com** or contact our customer service department at **custserv@wwilkins.com.** Williams & Wilkins customer service representatives are available from 8:30 am to 6:00 pm, EST, Monday through Friday, for telephone access.

98 99 00
2 3 4 5 6 7 8 9 10

For my husband, Stuart, and our wonderful children,
Michala, Sebastian, and Meredith,
who color my life with their love.
M.C.S.

To my wife, Taliah, my children,
Dana, Ronnie, Oriel, and Eliya,
and my grandson, Benjamin-Aharon.
A.P.

Foreword to First Edition

Mechanical ventilation has long been part of critical care medicine. In fact, early intensive care units were primarily devoted to the care of patients requiring various forms of respiratory support. In the ensuing years, much has been learned and many advances have taken place. Today, it is uncommon for the critically ill patient to die directly due to respiratory failure. All this has come about because of increased understanding of lung disease and the appropriate application of these various interventions.

Currently, we have a whole spectrum of sophisticated devices, all designed to fill particular needs. It is clear that one ventilatory mode or device will not meet all clinical situations. We are into the era of "niche" ventilatory modes. Today, we can care for sicker patients with more advanced pulmonary disease. Continuous advances in technology combined with meticulous care of the critically ill patient have combined to reduce the overall incidence of death in the ICU.

Drs. Perel and Stock have edited a volume that addresses both the technical and physiologic aspects of respiratory support. The clinician should find this exceedingly useful as an aid to understanding the various modalities currently available. This book belongs on every critical care physician's book shelf and should provide many years of useful information.

T. James Gallager, MD
Gainesville, Florida

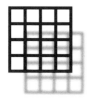 # Preface

We designed this book in its first edition to fulfill three purposes: to serve as a primer for those who have had limited exposure to mechanical ventilatory support; to provide the physiologic, pathophysiologic, and technical basis for the rational application of mechanical ventilatory support in a handbook format; and to serve as a review for those seeking intellectual refreshment.

The science and technology associated with mechanical ventilatory support grow and vary concomitantly with changes in microprocessor technology, changing disease patterns, and the development of entirely new ways to promote gas exchange. To accommodate the changes that we observe in the practice of critical care medicine, we designed this second edition to serve its three purposes by adding new information to all of the chapters, and by adding new chapters or sections of chapters that reflect the evolution of care since our last edition; "Noninvasive Ventilation in Acute Respiratory Failure" and "Ventilation of the Neurologically Injured" are but two examples.

The individual authors who contributed chapters to this book are clinical scientists with true expertise and extensive clinical acumen; they are all engaged in active clinical practice. Their ability to relate clearly the basis of technology and disease, and how to apply one to the other made this practical, practice-based book possible.

Finally, we thank Ms. Dianne Byrd for her unflagging editorial assistance, organization, patience, and persistence.

M. Christine Stock, MD
Atlanta, Georgia
Azriel Perel, MD
Tel Hashomer, Israel

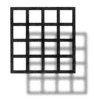 # Contributors

Michael Banner, RRT, PhD
Associate Professor of Anesthesiology
   and Physiology
Department of Anesthesiology
University of Florida College of
   Medicine
Gainesville, FL

Howard B. Bennett, MD
Instructor of Medicine
Department of Anesthesia
Northwestern University School of
   Medicine
Chicago, IL

M. Bombino, MD
Servizio di Anestesia e Rianimazione
Ospedale San Gerardo
Monza, MI, Italy

Richard D. Branson, RRT
Assistant Professor of Surgery
Department of Surgery
Division of Trauma/Critical Care
University of Cincinnati College of
   Medicine
Cincinnati, OH

Laurent Brochard, MD
Medical Intensive Care Unit
Henri Mondor Hospital
Assistance Publique-Hopitaux de
   Paris
Paris XII University, Creteil, France

Roy D. Cane, MBBch, FFA(SA)
Professor of Anesthesiology and
   Surgery
Director, Critical Care Medicine
Department of Anesthesiology
University of South Florida College
   of Medicine
Tampa, FL

James A. Colombo, MD
Instructor, Rush Medical College
Department of Anesthesiology
Asst, Attending Rush Presbyterian
   St. Luke's Medical Center
Chicago, IL

L. Gattinoni, MD
Istituto di Anestesia e Rianimazione
Università di Milano
Ospedale Maggiore
Milan, Italy

Carrie L. Gill-Murdoch, MD
Anesthesiologist and Medical Staff
   Member
Shriner's Hospital for Children
Tampa, FL

Stewart B. Gottfried, MD
Associate Professor Medicine
The Montreal General Hospital
Montreal, Quebec, Canada

Michael Joel Gurevitch, MD, FCCP
Assistant Clinical Professor of Medicine
Department of Pulmonary and Critical Care Medicine
University of Southern California School of Medicine
Los Angeles, CA
Director ICU Huntington Memorial Hospital
Pasadena, CA

Ashvini H. Gursahaney, MD, FRCP(C)
Assistant Professor
McGill University
Divisions of Pulmonary and Critical Care Medicine
Director-Medical Intensive Care
Montreal General Hospital
Montreal, Canada

Eric G. Honig, MD
Associate Professor of Medicine
Assistant Professor of Anesthesiology
Emory University School of Medicine
Pulmonary Medicine
Grady Memorial Hospital
Atlanta, GA

James J. Hurst, MD, FACS
Professor of Surgery and Anesthesia
Department of Surgery
University of Cincinnati College of Medicine
Cincinnati, OH

Robert R. Kirby, MD
Professor of Anesthesiology
University of Florida College of Medicine
Chief of Anesthesia
Veterans Affairs Medical Center
Gainesville, FL

Theodor Kolobow, MD
Chief, Section of Pulmonary and Cardiac Assist Devices
Laboratory of Cell Biology
National Heart, Lung and Blood Institute
National Institutes of Health
Bethesda, MD

Neil R. MacIntyre, MD
Professor of Medicine
Duke University Medical Center
Medical Director, Respiratory Services
Duke University Medical Center
Durham, NC

Robert C. Mackersie, MD, FACS
Associate Professor of Surgery
University of California San Francisco Medical Center
San Francisco General Hospital
San Francisco, CA

R. Marcolin, MD
Servizio di Anestesia e Rianimazione
Ospedale San Gerardo
Monza, MI, Italy

Theodore W. Marcy, MD
Associate Professor of Medicine
University of Vermont Medical
  College
Burlington, VT

John J. Marini, MD
Professor of Medicine
University of Minnesota
Director, Section of Pulmonary/
  Critical Care
St. Paul-Ramsey Medical Center
St. Paul, MN

Azriel Perel, MD
Associate Professor
Department of Anesthesiology
Sheba Medical Center
Tel Hashomer, Israel

William T. Peruzzi, MD
Associate Professor of Anesthesiology
Associate Chair, Perioperative
  Services
Chief, Section of Critical Care
  Medicine
Northwestern University Medical
  School
Chicago, IL

A. Pesenti, MD
Servizio di Anestesia e Rianimazione
Ospedale San Gerardo
Monza, MI, Italy

Reuven Pizov, MD
Department of Anesthesiology
Hebrew University
Hadassah Medical School
Hadassah Medical Center
Jerusalem, Israel

Jukka Räsänen, MD
Department of Anesthesiology
Helsinki University Children's
  Hospital
Helsinki, Finland

Jean-Jacques Rouby, PhD, MD
Professor of Anesthesiology
Clinical Director, Department of
  Anesthesiology
Surgical Intensive Care Unit
Hopital de la Pitié-Salpêtrieré
  Université
Paris, France

Hans Schweiger, MD
Assistant Professor of
  Anesthesiology &
  Critical Care Medicine
Director of Trauma Anesthesia
  Services
University of South Florida College
  of Medicine
Tampa, FL

R. Brian Smith, MD
Professor and Chairman
Department of Anesthesiology
University of Texas Health Science
  Center at San Antonio
San Antonio, TX

Robert A. Smith, MS, RRT
Assistant Professor
Department of Anesthesiology
University of South Florida
Tampa General Hospital
Department of Anesthesiology
Tampa, FL

M. Christine Stock, MD
Associate Professor of Anesthesiology
Assistant Professor of Internal
  Medicine
Emory University Medical School
Associate Chief of Anesthesiology
Emory University Hospital
Atlanta, GA

Jeffrey S. Vender, MD
Professor/Associate Chairman
Department of Anesthesiology
Northwestern University Medical
  School
Chicago, IL
Chief, Division of Anesthesia
Director Medical/Surgical ICU
Vice Chairman Department of
  Surgery
Evanston Hospital
Evanston, IL

Contents

Section I. General Aspects of Ventilatory Support

1/ Introduction to Ventilatory Support 3
  M. Christine Stock
  Azriel Perel
2/ Mechanical Ventilators—Fundamentals 7
  Michael J. Banner
3/ Monitoring During Ventilatory Support 35
  John (Hans) W. Schweiger
  Jukka Räsänen
4/ Pulmonary Effects of Mechanical Ventilation 49
  Theodor Kolobow
5/ Cardiovascular Effects of Mechanical Ventilation 57
  Azriel Perel
  Reuven Pizov
6/ Positive-pressure Ventilation: Renal, Hepatic, and Gastrointestinal
  Function 75
  Howard B. Bennett
  Jeffrey S. Vender

Section II. Ventilatory Modes

7/ Control Mode Ventilation and Assist/Control Ventilation 89
  Theodore W. Marcy
  John J. Marini
8/ Breathing Circuits for Spontaneous Ventilation and the Work
  of Breathing 111
  Robert A. Smith
9/ Intermittent Mandatory Ventilation 123
  Robert R. Kirby

10/ Positive End-Expiratory Pressure (PEEP) and
Continuous Positive Airway Pressure (CPAP) 139
Robert A. Smith

11/ Pressure Support Ventilation 155
Neil R. MacIntyre

12/ Inverse Ratio Ventilation and the Inspiratory/Expiratory Ratio 165
Michael Joel Gurevitch

13/ Differential Lung Ventilation 173
Richard D. Branson
James M. Hurst

14/ Airway Pressure Release Ventilation 183
M. Christine Stock

15/ Noninvasive Ventilation in Acute Respiratory Failure 193
Laurent Brochard

16/ Continuous Flow Apneic Ventilation and Other Techniques
of Intratracheal Gas Insufflation 205
R. Brian Smith

17/ High Frequency Ventilation 221
Jean-Jacques Rouby

18/ Extracorporeal Techniques to Support Ventilation 233
A. Pesenti
M. Bombino
R. Marcolin
L. Gattinoni

Section III. Disease-Oriented Ventilatory Support

19/ Adult Respiratory Distress Syndrome 249
Roy D. Cane
Carrie L. Gill-Murdoch

20/ Chronic Obstructive Pulmonary Disease and Asthma 273
Eric G. Honig

21/ Ventilatory Support Following Major Trauma 303
Robert C. Mackersie

22/ Ventilation of the Neurologically Injured 317
William T. Peruzzi
James A. Colombo

23/ Weaning from Mechanical Ventilation 339

Ashvini H. Gursahaney

Stewart B. Gottfried

24/ Ventilatory Support: Temptations and Pitfalls 359

Azriel Perel

M. Christine Stock

INDEX 373

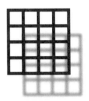

Glossary

ARDS: adult respiratory distress syndrome
ALI: acute lung injury
ABG: arterial blood gas
BAL: bronchoalveolar lavage
CMV: control mode ventilation
COPD: chronic obstructive pulmonary disease
CPAP: continuous positive airway pressure
cmH$_2$O: centimeters of water pressure
CNS: central nervous system
ECCO$_2$R: extracorporeal CO$_2$ removal
ECG: electrocardiogram
ECMO: extracorporeal membrane oxygenation
EMG: electromyogram
EPAP: expiratory positive airway pressure
f: frequency of mechanical ventilation (or, mechanical ventilatory rate)
F$_I$O$_2$: fraction of inspired oxygen
FRC: functional residual capacity
I/E: inspiratory-to-expiratory time ratio
ICU: intensive care unit
ICP: intracranial pressure
IPPB: intermittent positive pressure breathing

IMV: intermittent mandatory ventilation
IPAP: inspiratory positive airway pressure
IRV: inverse ratio ventilation
mmHg: millimeters mercury pressure
NO: nitric oxide
PaCO$_2$: partial pressure of CO$_2$ in arterial blood
PaO$_2$: partial pressure of O$_2$ in arterial blood
Palv: intra alveolar pressure
PC-IRV: pressure-controlled inverse ratio ventilation
PEEP: positive end-expiratory pressure
Pes: esophageal pressure
P$_{ET}$CO$_2$: partial pressure of CO$_2$ in end-tidal gas
pHa: pH of arterial blood
PIP: peak inflation pressure
P$_L$: transpulmonary pressure
Ppl: intrapleural pressure
P$_{O.1}$: pressure generated during the first 100 msec of an occluded inspiratory effort
PS, PSV: pressure support, pressure support ventilation
PtcCO$_2$: partial pressure of transcutaneously measured CO$_2$
Q̇sp/Q̇t: physiologic shunt fraction

RAM: random access memory
Raw: airway resistance
ROM: read-only memory
RQ: respiratory quotient
TNF: tissue necrosis factor
SIMV: synchronized intermittent mandatory ventilation
SaO$_2$: oxygen saturation of hemoglobin in arterial blood
SpO$_2$: saturation of hemoglobin in arterial blood obtained from pulse oximeter

S$\bar{v}$O$_2$: oxygen saturation of hemoglobin in mixed-venous blood
SVR: systemic vascular resistance
$\dot{V}_E$: expired minute ventilation
$\dot{V}_A/\dot{Q}$: ventilation-perfusion ratio
$\dot{V}CO_2$: rate of CO_2 production
V$_D$/V$_T$: dead space-to-tidal volume ratio
VQI: ventilation-perfusion index
V$_T$: tidal volume
$\dot{V}O_2$: rate of O_2 consumption
W: work

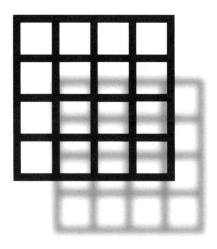

Section I
General Aspects
of Ventilatory Support

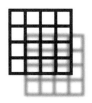

1
Introduction to Ventilatory Support

M. Christine Stock • Azriel Perel

Mechanical ventilatory support is one of the major supportive modalities used in critical care. An essential element of cardiopulmonary resuscitation, it can be life-saving during a variety of acute and chronic diseases, when respiratory drive is depressed, or when the patient lacks the neuromuscular ability to breathe. Further, the lung is usually one of the major organs involved in multiorgan failure. Thus, delivering appropriate ventilatory care can be challenging and may influence patient outcome.

The early generation of mechanical ventilators, used prior to the mid-1960s, was designed to support alveolar ventilation and to provide supplemental oxygen for those patients who were unable to breathe owing to neuromuscular impairment. As our collective understanding of lung pathophysiology increased and as the design of mechanical ventilators improved, ventilatory support became more specialized and complicated. Interestingly, the necessity for complicated modes of ventilation is confined to a small proportion of patients who require ventilatory support.

Larger tidal volumes (10–15 ml/kg), an occasional "sigh breath," and low levels of positive end-expiratory pressure ("physiologic" PEEP) were developed to overcome the gradual decrease in functional residual capacity (FRC)—the amount of gas in the lungs at end-expiration—that occurs during positive-pressure ventilation with lower tidal volumes and ambient expiratory airway pressure. These efforts help to overcome the most common complication of positive pressure ventilatory support: atelectasis. Further, the primary pulmonary defect during acute lung injury is a severely reduced FRC; thus, continuous positive airway pressure (CPAP) and PEEP became the primary supportive modes of mechanical support during acute lung injury.

The desire to improve the patient's tolerance of mechanical ventilation led to the development of assisted or patient-triggered ventilation. Unfortunately, the work required to trigger these ventilators to deliver a breath is no different from that required for the patient to inspire the entire breath spontaneously through the ventilator circuit. During partial ventilatory support, mechanical support supplements spontaneous ventilation. The advent of intermittent mandatory ventilation (IMV) in the early 1970s made partial ventilatory support feasible for adults outside the operating room.

As patients with increasingly impaired pulmonary physiology survived while receiving mechanical ventilatory support, more attention was devoted to weaning criteria and techniques. Additionally, alternate ventilatory modes emerged in the mid-1980s that were designed to meet the special needs of patients with the most severe pulmonary compromise. Most of these modes are still being developed.

Ideally, one should tailor ventilatory support to each patient's pathophysiology rather than employ a single technique for all patients with ventilatory failure. Current ventilatory support ranges from controlled mechanical ventilation (no opportunity for the patient to breathe spontaneously) to total *spontaneous* ventilation with CPAP for support of oxygenation and the elastic work of breathing. Partial ventilatory support bridges the gap for patients who are able to provide some ventilation but cannot entirely support their own alveolar ventilation. Decisions regarding the modes and level of ventilatory support are further complicated by our increasing awareness of the effect of mechanical ventilation on other organ systems.

Intense technologic research and development accompanied the evolution of ventilatory support. The second generation of ventilators included better electronics, but frequently fewer desirable mechanics. This generation of ventilators controlled the fraction of inspired oxygen (F_IO_2) better. Unfortunately, many of these ventilators also replaced the IMV inspiratory valve and high flow system with demand valves (valves that deliver a high flow of gas in response to the patient's inspiratory effort) that had high resistance and inertia. This "advance" forced patients to perform excessive work to inspire through the machine. Other mechanical factors that still needed improvement were excessively compliant circuitry, expiratory valves that allowed the development of dangerously high airway pressure, and inefficient alarms.

In recent years, we witnessed a surge of new ventilatory modes. This revolution stems from the imperfection of existing ventilatory options, the continuing challenge of treating various forms of ventilatory failure, the eagerness of physicians, and the market competition for ventilator manufacturers. The primary factor influencing the development of the most recent generation of ventilators is the introduction of microprocessors into the ventilators. Micro-processed ventilators are equipped typically with sensors that monitor breath-by-breath flow, pressure, and volume. Their ability to sense and transduce accurately, combined with computer technology, makes the interaction between the patient and ventilator more sophisticated. Whether this information, increased sophistication, and potentially more complicated system will change outcome or influence patient care has yet to be demonstrated. However, it seems as though these advances may be helpful in only a small percentage of patients.

New ventilatory modes may be aimed at improving one or more aspects of ventilatory assistance; for example, those that improve ventilation-perfusion imbalance, minimize positive pressure-related cardiovascular compromise, decrease the work of breathing, or facilitate the weaning process. Unfortunately, several of these new modes were incorporated into ventilators and released onto the market without sufficient information concerning their use. In recent years, clinical scientists are beginning to fill the knowledge void, especially with respect to pressure support ventilation.

The serious gap between the wide variety of options for ventilatory support and clinical knowledge of how to apply those options optimally prompted the creation of this book's first edition. As ventilators become more complicated and offer more options, the number of potentially dangerous decisions increases as well. Physicians, nurses, and respiratory therapists who care for the critically ill are faced with expensive, complicated machines with few clear guidelines for their use. Moreover, the unique characteristics of each ventilatory mode are publicized highly, although their potential pitfalls are frequently less well known.

Written by experts in ventilatory care, this book is intended to be clinically oriented and to inform the reader about the major clinical considerations in the administration of ventilatory support. The book contains three sections: Section I, which is introductory, covers general topics, such as the physical principles associated with mechanical ventilatory support and monitoring during ventilatory assistance, as well as the effects of mechanical ventilation on various organ systems. This basic knowledge is the foundation for decision-making in the care of patients requiring ventilatory support. Section II describes most of the ventilatory modes that are available today. Some of these modes have been in use for more than 20 years, whereas others are still considered experimental. Section III describes the common ventilatory problems encountered in the care of patients with specific problems (e.g., acute lung injury, chronic lung disease, and chest trauma). Problems associated with weaning ventilatory support also are discussed in this section. The last chapter of this section summarizes and highlights the important clinical considerations and possible pitfalls during the use of ventilatory support. We hope that this book will contribute to a better understanding and use of the excellent ventilatory equipment that is available today, and to an overall improvement in the care of critically ill patients.

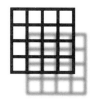

2
Mechanical Ventilators—Fundamentals

Michael J. Banner

Designed to facilitate the movement of gas into the lungs, mechanical ventilators have evolved from simple pressure-cycled devices to sophisticated microprocessor-controlled systems used for the treatment of critically ill patients with respiratory failure. Understanding fundamental concepts, such as the variety of ventilatory modes that are used and the classification and operation of mechanical life-support ventilators, is essential for the practice of respiratory care. Thus, the purposes of this chapter are to (*a*) define the various forms of mechanical and spontaneous positive-pressure breathing; (*b*) review ventilator cycling processes as a means of classifying ventilators; and (*c*) describe the new generation of microprocessor-controlled ventilators.

PEAK INFLATION PRESSURE

During mechanical inhalation, positive pressure (pressure greater than atmospheric pressure) is generated at the airway opening. The peak inflation pressure (PIP) generated is influenced by at least five variables: (*a*) the lung-thorax compliance (C_{LT}) and (*b*) airway resistance (Raw) of the patient, and the delivered (*c*) tidal volume V_T, (*d*) inspiratory flow rate ($\dot{V}_I$) and (*e*) baseline pressure (i.e., level of continuous positive airway pressure) from the mechanical ventilator. PIP varies inversely with C_{LT} and directly with V_T, Raw, and $\dot{V}_I$. These factors may be represented mathematically by the following equation:

$$PIP = V_T/C_{LT} + (Raw \times \dot{V}_I) + \text{Baseline Pressure}$$

Demonstrated in this fundamental equation are the interrelationships of respiratory mechanics and ventilator variables affecting airway pressure during mechanical ventilation. For example, consider an adult patient with *normal* C_{LT} (0.1 L/cmH_2O) and Raw (3 cmH_2O /L·sec) and receiving a V_T of 1 L with a constant $\dot{V}_I$ of 1 L/second and a baseline pressure of 5 cmH_2O, i.e.,

$$PIP + \frac{1\,L}{0.1\,L/cmH_2O} + (3\,cmH_2O/L\cdot sec^{-1} \times 1\,L/sec) + 5\,cmH_2O = 18\,cmH_2O$$

If the patient's C_{LT} suddenly decreased to 0.02 L/cmH$_2$O and all other variables were essentially unchanged, then the PIP would increase to ~58 cmH$_2$O, i.e.,

$$PIP = \frac{1\ L}{0.02\ L/cmH_2O} + (3\ cm\ H_2O/L\cdot sec^{-1} \times 1\ L/sec) + 5\ cmH_2O$$

$$= 58\ cmH_2O$$

Similarly, a marked increase in Raw or in the delivered V_T and $\dot{V}_I$ from the mechanical ventilator would result in proportional increases in PIP.

CLASSIFICATION OF VENTILATORY SUPPORT

Controlled Mechanical Ventilation

Controlled mechanical ventilation (CMV) (see Chapter 7, Controlled Mechanical Ventilation and Assist/Control ventilation) delivers a preselected ventilatory rate, tidal volume, and inspiratory flow rate, which are independent of spontaneous effort on the part of the patient (Fig. 2.1). The peak inflation pressure generated varies inversely with C_{LT} and directly with airway resistance (if the ventilator is volume- or time-cycled). Indications for CMV include apnea, secondary to central nervous system depression (brain trauma, spinal cord trauma, or both); drug overdose; or neuromuscular paralysis (either drug-induced or the result of pathology (e.g., Guillain-Barré syndrome, myasthenia gravis, poliomyelitis). Because many patients treated with CMV are sedated, paralyzed, or hyperventilated below their apneic thresholds, accidental disconnection or a mechanical malfunction represents a life-threatening situation. Therefore, a "disconnect" or "failure-to-cycle" alarm is crucial.

Continuous Positive-Pressure Ventilation

Continuous positive-pressure ventilation (CPPV), like CMV, delivers a positive-pressure breath followed by a fall in airway pressure to a previously selected positive-pressure plateau; airway pressure never returns to zero (see Fig. 2.1). This form of ventilation was popularized by Ashbaugh et al. (1) for treatment of adult respiratory distress syndrome (ARDS) to prevent alveolar collapse during the ventilator's expiratory phase and, thereby, to improve and to maintain overall alveolar ventilation-to-perfusion $\dot{V}_A/\dot{Q}$ relationships.

Patient-Initiated or Triggered Mechanical Ventilation

With patient-initiated or -triggered mechanical ventilation (see Chapter 7 and Fig. 2.1), if the patient does not initiate a spontaneous breathing effort, the ventila-

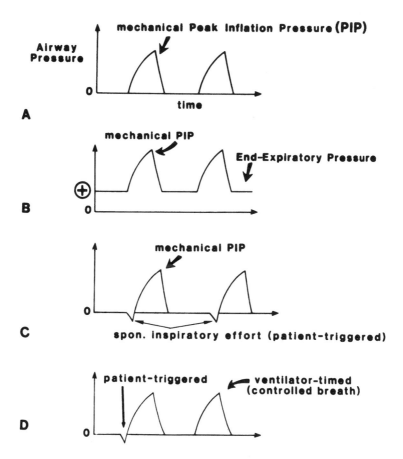

Figure 2.1. **A.** Mechanical ventilatory airway pressure patterns. Controlled mechanical ventilation (CMV). Mechanical ventilator rate, V_T, and inspiratory flow rate are preset and cannot be affected by the patient's respiratory efforts. **B.** CMV with end-expiratory pressure. When mechanical inhalation ends, pressure drops to a set positive-pressure plateau, i.e., the end-expiratory pressure level. **C.** Patient-initiated or -triggered mechanical ventilation. Patient-triggered mechanical inhalation; V_T is preset and cannot be affected by the patient. If the patient does not initiate inhalation, the ventilator does not switch "ON." **D.** Patient triggered—controlled mechanical ventilation. The ventilator may be triggered to mechanical inhalation by the patient's inspiratory efforts or by a timing device, whichever comes first. The patient may trigger the ventilator as often as desired, and the timing device determines the minimum ventilator cycling rate. (Reprinted with permission from Banner MJ, Gallagher TJ. Respiratory failure in the adult: Ventilatory support. In: Kirby RR, Desautels DA, Smith RA (eds). Mechanical ventilation. New York, Churchill Livingstone, Inc. 1985, p 221.)

tor *will not* deliver a mechanical breath; thus, apnea can be fatal with this mode of ventilation. This technique has been employed as intermittent positive-pressure breathing for short-term delivery of gases and therapeutic aerosols to patients with pulmonary parenchymal or airway disease. It is also used (infrequently now) for support of patients with acute or chronic respiratory failure. Some practitioners also use assisted mechanical ventilation to wean patients from CMV and to promote spontaneous breathing.

The greatest operational difficulty with assisted mechanical ventilation is that many of the assist mechanisms, which trigger the inhalation phase, may be unreliable (2). Response sensitivity must be preset and, as the patient's condition changes, his or her ability to generate an appropriate effort (usually a decrease in the breathing circuit pressure associated with spontaneous inspiratory effort) varies. The ventilator sensitivity may then be too great (resulting in repetitive cycles or autocycling) or too slight, so that the ventilator fails to cycle.

Patient-Triggered Control Ventilation

This technique combines patient-triggered mechanical ventilation and CMV (see Chapter 7); the ventilator may be triggered by the patient's spontaneous inspiratory efforts or by a timing device, whichever comes first (see Fig. 2.1). The patient may trigger the ventilator "ON" at any time, but the timer determines a *minimal* preselected rate. Hence, CMV acts as a backup should the patient become apneic or attempt to breathe at a lower rate than that set by the timer.

Intermittent Mandatory Ventilation

Originally proposed by Kirby et al. (3) as a method to ventilate infants with hyaline membrane disease and by Downs et al. (4) for use with adults, IMV (see Chapter 9, Intermittent Mandatory Ventilation) allows the patient to breathe spontaneously with a mechanical inflation provided at preset intervals (Fig. 2.2). The mechanical ventilatory rate, like CMV, cannot be influenced by the patient. Between sequential mechanical breaths, an unrestricted gas flow rate is provided that is equal to or greater than the patient's peak spontaneous inspiratory flow rate demand.

Intermittent mandatory ventilation was introduced initially as a method to wean patients from mechanical ventilation by permitting a smooth transition from mechanical ventilation to spontaneous breathing as the rate of cycling was gradually decreased and spontaneous effort increased. With increased clinical experience in its use, IMV has evolved as a primary ventilatory technique.

The IMV rate should be titrated to deliver only that support which, in conjunction with spontaneous breathing, maintains normal alveolar ventilation and $PaCO_2$. When used in patients with antecedent pulmonary disease (e.g., emphy-

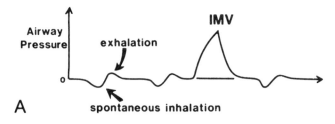

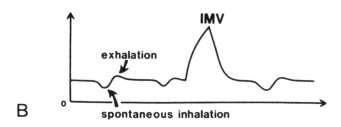

Figure 2.2. **A**. IMV airway pressure patterns. With IMV, the patient is allowed to breathe spontaneously as desired; however, at set intervals, a mechanical inflation is provided (the ventilator rate is the IMV rate). IMV V_T is set and cannot be affected by the patient. **B**. With IMV and CPAP, the patient breathes spontaneously with CPAP between IMV breaths. (Reprinted with permission from Banner MJ, Gallagher TJ. Respiratory failure in the adult: ventilatory support. In: Kirby RR, Desautels DA, Smith RA (eds). Mechanical ventilation. New York, Churchill Livingstone, Inc., 1985, p 223.)

sema, chronic bronchitis), IMV is extremely useful in regulating $PaCO_2$ and pHa compared with either CMV or assisted mechanical ventilation.

Synchronized Intermittent Mandatory Ventilation

Synchronized intermittent mandatory ventilation (SIMV) (see Chapter 9), like IMV, allows the patient to breathe spontaneously between mechanical breaths. At regular intervals, the mandatory breath is synchronized to begin with the next spontaneous inhalation in a manner analogous to assisted mechanical ventilation. This technique was introduced because of concern that a mechanical breath might be superimposed on a spontaneous breath ("breath stacking"), which might predispose to increases of peak inflation, mean airway, and mean intrapleural pressures. Similar fears were expressed if the mechanically delivered volume was added at the peak of spontaneous exhalation.

Subsequently, investigations were conducted to examine the clinical efficacy of SIMV. Hasten et al. (5) compared SIMV with IMV in 25 critically ill patients and found that, although PIP was greater with IMV than with SIMV, cardiovascular variables (blood pressure, cardiac output, stroke volume, central venous pressure, and pulmonary artery pressure) in the two groups did not differ significantly. In another study, Heenan et al. (6) obtained baseline data from spontaneously breathing, anesthetized dogs that were subsequently near-drowned and ventilated with IMV or SIMV. Again, no differences between the two modes were noted with respect to cardiac output, stroke volume, intrapleural pressure, and intrapulmonary shunting ($\dot{Q}sp/\dot{Q}$). Peak inflation and mean airway pressures were significantly increased with IMV, and breath stacking occurred but without demonstrable adverse effects. Based on these data, SIMV does not seem to offer any physiologic advantage compared with IMV and may be an expensive solution to a problem that has not been shown to exist.

Mandatory Minute Volume

Hewlett et al. (7) described a technique called mandatory minute volume in which the patient is guaranteed a preselected minute volume, either through spontaneous ventilation or as positive-pressure breaths from the ventilator. If the desired minute volume is breathed spontaneously, then no mandatory ventilation is provided by the ventilator. If not, that portion of the preselected minute volume that is not breathed spontaneously, is then provided by the ventilator and delivered automatically. Theoretically, weaning with mandatory minute volume is simplified because the clinician is not required to make periodic adjustments to the ventilator rate as spontaneous ventilation changes.

Because it ensures a minimal level of support, mandatory minute volume has been advocated for weaning patients from mechanical ventilation (7). However, it is not without potential problems. Patients may become tachypneic and breathe with a small V_T; under these conditions, the spontaneous minute volume can equal or even exceed the preselected mandatory minute volume. Consider an adult at a preselected mandatory minute volume of 8 L/minute; if the spontaneous breathing frequency and V_T were 40/minute and 225 ml, respectively, the spontaneous minute volume would equal 9 L/minute and, thus, exceed the level of mandatory minute volume. Although indicated, *no* mechanical ventilation would be provided by the ventilator. Hence, it would be inappropriate to allow this pattern of ventilation to continue because the patient could become even more tachypneic and, eventually, fatigued, followed by deterioration of his or her pulmonary function.

Continuous Positive Airway Pressure and Expiratory Positive Airway Pressure

CPAP (see Chapters 8 and 10) and expiratory positive airway pressure are positive-pressure modes used with spontaneous breathing, and can be employed

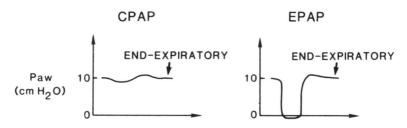

Figure 2.3. Airway pressure (*Paw*) tracing for *CPAP* and expiratory positive airway pressure (*EPAP*), e.g., 10 cm$_2$O. CPAP and EPAP are positive-pressure modes of *spontaneous* breathing that can be employed individually or in conjunction with mechanical ventilation (e.g., IMV).

individually or in conjunction with mechanical ventilation (e.g., IMV, see Fig. 2.2*B*). With CPAP, both inspiratory and expiratory pressures are positive, although the inspiratory level is less than that of the expiratory. With expiratory positive airway pressure, airway pressure is zero or negative (subambient) during inhalation but increases at the end of exhalation to a predetermined positive pressure (Fig. 2.3). The level of CPAP or expiratory positive airway pressure used is designated by the value measured at end-exhalation. Both are designed to increase expiratory transpulmonary pressure and lung volume (FRC).

The relationship between the rate of gas inflow provided to the breathing system and the rate of the patient's inspiratory flow determines whether the system provides CPAP or expiratory positive airway pressure. If the rate of gas inflow is greater than the patient's spontaneous inspiratory flow rate, CPAP results (i.e., airway pressure is positive during inhalation). Conversely, when the inflow rate to the breathing system is less than the patient's inspiratory flow rate, expiratory positive airway pressure results (i.e., airway pressure is zero or subambient during inhalation). The latter situation is associated with increased inspiratory work of breathing.

Site of Airway Pressure Measurement and the Imposed Work of Breathing

The breathing apparatus, which may be defined as the endotracheal tube, breathing circuit tubing and valves, and ventilator, represents a series of resistors over which a pressure decrease must be overcome by the patient to spontaneously inhale. The *endotracheal* tube is the primary resistor in the breathing apparatus (8–11).

Accurate measurement and assessment of airway pressure changes during spontaneous breathing with CPAP should be done at the tracheal or carinal end of the endotracheal tube (Fig. 2.4). Measuring pressure inside the ventilator or at

A. <u>PRESSURE MEASURING SITE: EXHALATION LIMB OF VENTILATOR</u>

<u>SMALLER</u> **CHANGE IN AIRWAY PRESSURE**

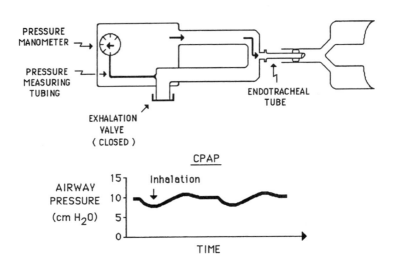

B. <u>PRESSURE MEASURING SITE: TRACHEAL END OF ENDOTRACHEAL TUBE</u>

<u>LARGER</u> **CHANGE IN AIRWAY PRESSURE**

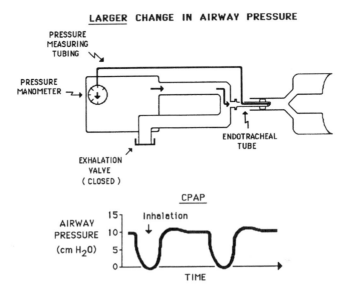

the Y-piece of the breathing circuit (commonly used pressure measuring sites), results in significant *underestimations* of pressure compared with measuring at the carinal end of the endotracheal tube (12). This is especially true when narrow internal diameter endotracheal tubes are used and peak inspiratory flow rate demands are high. The narrower the tube and the greater the flow rate demand, the greater the discrepancy in measured pressure inside the ventilator or at the Y-piece compared with the carinal end of the endotracheal tube (13,14).

The further from the trachea that the pressure is measured, the smaller the deviations in pressure that occur during spontaneous breathing with CPAP and thus, the more spurious the value in imposed work of breathing (i.e., resistive work performed by the patient to breathe spontaneously through the breathing apparatus, which is calculated by integrating the change in pressure measured at the *carinal* end of the endotracheal tube and tidal volume) (13). For example, smaller deviations in pressure and, thus, imposed work are measured at the Y-piece of the breathing circuit compared with the carinal end of the endotracheal tube. Small deviations in pressure during spontaneous inhalation may lead the clinician to conclude, erroneously, that the flow rate provided on demand by the ventilator is sufficient and that the imposed work of breathing is minimal, when, in fact, large deviations in pressure and a high work load may be occurring. The clinician is "blinded" to this situation because of the inappropriate site used for pressure measurement.

The pressure measurement site also influences the peak inflation pressure measure during *mechanical* ventilation (14). During volume cycled ventilation, for example, peak inflation pressure varies directly with total resistance (breathing apparatus plus physiologic airways) and inversely with total compliance (lungs plus chest wall). When pressure is measured inside the ventilator during mechanical inflation, it is generated as a result of the series resistance of the breathing circuit, endotracheal tube, and the patient's airways, as well as the patient's total compliance. Pressure measured at the carinal end of the endotracheal tube is the result of the patient's airway resistance and compliance only. Consequently, the peak inflation pressure measured inside the ventilator will always be greater than at the carinal end of the endotracheal tube. The narrower the internal diameter of the

◄───

Figure 2.4. Effect of the *site* of pressure measurement on changes in airway pressure are illustrated. Pressure changes during spontaneous inhalation with CPAP are measured inside the ventilator on the exhalation limb of the breathing circuit (**A**) (an approach used on many ventilators) and in the endotracheal tube at the carinal or tracheal end of the tube (**B**). Under similar peak inspiratory flow rate demands, larger changes in pressure are measured at the carinal site because of the resistance of the endotracheal tube. The *true* change in pressure on the airways is at the carinal site, not inside the ventilator. Spuriously smaller changes in pressure are measured inside the ventilator and, thus, should *not* be used.

endotracheal tube and the greater the mechanical inspiratory flow rate, the greater the discrepancy in peak inflation pressure measured inside the ventilator compared with the carinal end of the endotracheal tube.

During spontaneous and mechanical ventilation, the *true* pressure generated on airways and lungs is at the carinal end of the endotracheal tube. Measuring pressure inside the ventilator or at the Y-piece leads to inaccuracy (i.e., airway pressure measurements are spuriously low during spontaneous ventilation and high during mechanical ventilation).

Two approaches for measuring airway pressure at the carinal end of the endotracheal tube have been described (15). Endotracheal tubes with a pressure-measuring lumen embedded in the sidewall and opening at the carinal end of the tube are commercially available (e.g., NCC Malinkrodt, Argyle, NY). This approach has been successfully employed with the Bunnell infant ventilator (Bunnell, Inc., Salt Lake City, UT) for several years with no complications. The other approach is to insert a 1-mm outside diameter catheter into the endotracheal tube (e.g., Bicore Monitoring Inc., Irvine, CA). We have successfully used this approach on adults (15).

Occlusion of the pressure lumen with both measuring approaches is of concern. Microprocessor-controlled ventilators can be programmed appropriately to assess the patency of the lumen. As in the Bunnell ventilator, the microprocessor directs air pulses at regular intervals from the ventilator through the pressure-sensing lumen to keep it patent. Another approach is to employ a "watch dog" subroutine that provides continuous surveillance of the pressure-measuring lumen patency. If an occlusion is detected, then audible and visual alarms are activated, and a default mode is entered, so that pressure is temporarily measured at an alternative site within the breathing circuit (e.g., inside the ventilator). After the sensing lumen is cleared, the microprocessor can verify that the lumen is patent and then resume pressure monitoring. Pressure measurement from the carinal end of the endotracheal tube can be obtained consistently and *safely* by using the above approaches only if clinicians and manufacturers are willing to understand the issues and to change their attitudes. Accuracy in pressure monitoring is the issue; conservative and obsolete thinking, attitudes that paralyze progress, must be overcome.

Pressure Support Ventilation

Newer microprocessor-driven mechanical ventilators include pressure support ventilation (see Chapter 11) that operates in conjunction with demand flow valve systems. The airway pressure, flow, and lung volume changes during pressure support ventilation are more akin to assisted mechanical ventilation than to breathing spontaneously with CPAP. Work of breathing appears to be decreased by pressure support ventilation; however, the technique is based on an entirely different concept than CPAP. In the pressure support ventilation mode, the ventilator is patient-triggered "ON" and continues in the inhalation phase to a preselected positive-pressure limit (8). *As long as the patient's inspiratory effort is maintained, the preselected airway pressure stays constant, with a variable flow rate of gas from the ventilator.* Inhalation cycles "OFF" when the patient's inspiratory flow demand decreases to a predetermined percentage of the initial peak mechanical inspiratory flow rate (Fig. 2.5). The ventilator, thus, is *flow-cycled,* following which passive exhalation occurs. With pressure support ventilation, the peak inspiratory flow rate, flow wave form, inspiratory time, V_T, mean airway pressure, and airway pres-

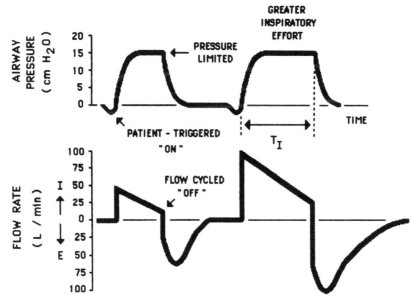

Figure 2.5. Pressure support ventilation (*PSV*). The ventilator is patient-triggered "ON" and, as long as inspiratory effort is maintained, airway pressure stays constant with a variable flow rate of gas from the ventilator. The ventilator cycles "OFF" when the patient's inspiratory flow rate demand decreases to a predetermined percentage of the peak inspiratory flow rate (i.e., the ventilator is flow-cycled "OFF"). In the PSV mode, the airway pressure level is preselected, while the patient retains control over inspiratory time and flow rate, tidal and minute volume, and ventilator rate. On the right, the patient increases inspiratory effort and generates a longer inspiratory time compared with the PSV breath on the left. Because tidal volume equals inspiratory time times inspiratory flow rate, a greater tidal volume is delivered than the previous breath. Even though peak inflation pressure is constant from breath to breath, tidal volume is thus variable with patient effort.

sure contour depend on the patient's breathing pattern. V_T is determined by patient effort, C_{LT}, airway resistance, and the level of pressure support ventilation.

Two approaches to using pressure support ventilation have been described: (*a*) Low-level pressure support ventilation (5–20 cmH$_2$O) to assist spontaneous breathing to decrease patient work of breathing by *partially* unloading the respiratory muscles; and (*b*) high-level pressure support ventilation (20–50 cmH$_2$O) as an independent or stand-alone mechanical ventilatory mode to unload *totally* the respiratory muscles (16,17).

Partial unloading of the respiratory muscles results when, after the initial decreases in intrapleural pressure at the onset of inhalation, the ventilatory is patient-triggered "ON" and airway pressure rises abruptly to the preselected positive-pressure level. (Integration of airway pressure with respect to V_T represents work performed by the ventilator.) A further decrease in intrapleural pressure is indicative of work performed by the patient, who thus interacts with the positive-pressure assisted breath to regulate V_T. (Integration of intrapleural pressure with respect to V_T represents work performed by the patient to inflate the lungs.) Total work, thus, is performed in part by the ventilator and in part by the patient (i.e., a work sharing effect).

Alternatively, the level of pressure support ventilation may be set high enough to unload the ventilatory muscles completely, to provide essentially all the work of breathing, and to allow the patient to rest. A negligible amount of work is performed by the patient to trigger the ventilator "ON." Pressure levels >40 cmH$_2$O have been used in patients with large minute ventilation demands and severely impaired pulmonary mechanics. Used in this manner, pressure support ventilation is similar to conventional patient-triggered positive-pressure ventilation, but with a pressure limit.

CYCLING MECHANISMS—VENTILATOR CLASSIFICATION

Time, volume, pressure, and flow rate are interrelated variables that are used to describe spontaneous and mechanical positive-pressure ventilation (Table 2.1). The changeover from the mechanical inhalation to the exhalation phase (i.e., the process used to cycle the ventilator "OFF") is a means of classifying mechanical ventilators. Time, volume, pressure, or flow-cycling mechanisms are employed on most conventional, as well as microprocessor-controlled, ventilators.

Time-Cycled Mechanical Inhalation

Time-cycled mechanical inhalation is terminated after a preselected inspiratory time elapses. The timing mechanism can be pneumatic (e.g., IMV Bird, Bird

Table 2.1. Parameters Used to Describe Ventilation

Time
- May be divided into inspiratory (I) and expiratory (E) periods and is expressed in seconds or by the relation of inspiratory time to expiratory time expressed as an I/E ratio
- Used to define the number of respiratory cycles within a given period of time

Volume
- A measure of the V_T delivered by the ventilator to the patient
- Reflects the volume of gas the patient breathes
- Is usually expressed in ml for V_T and in L for minute volume

Pressure
- A measure of the impedance to gas flow rate encountered in the ventilator breathing circuit and the patient's airways and lungs
- Refers to the amount of back pressure generated as a result of airway resistance and lung-thorax compliance
- Is expressed in cmH_2O, mmHg, or Kilopascals (kPa) (1 mmHg = 1.36 cmH_2O, 7.6 mmHg = 1 kPa)

Flow rate
- A measure of the rate at which the gas volume is delivered to the patient
- Refers to the volume change per unit time
- Is expressed as L/sec or L/min

Products Co., Palm Springs, CA) or electronic (e.g., Hamilton Veolar, Hamilton Medical, Inc., Reno, NV). The key concept is that the duration of the inhalation phase is controlled by the operator and not influenced by the peak inflation pressure generated or by the patient's C_{LT} and airway resistance. The V_T delivered is the product of inspiratory time (sec) and inspiratory flow (ml/sec) (Fig. 2.6). Peak inflation pressure generated is inversely proportional to C_{LT} and directly proportional to airway resistance and the V_T delivered (Table 2.2). Thus, when C_{LT} decreases, for example, inspiratory time is unaffected, but peak inflation pressure increases. Under these conditions, inspiratory flow rate may decrease as a result of increased back pressure and, thus, V_T decreases. V_T can be restored to the initial value by increasing either inspiratory time or inspiratory flow rate.

Pressure-Limited, Time-Cycled Mechanical Ventilation

A pressure limit is preselected to a specific value with pressure-limited, time-cycled mechanical ventilation. Once the pressure limit is reached, airway pressure is held at that level until the ventilator time-cycles "OFF" (Fig. 2.7). Gas actively flows from the ventilator during the pressure limit or the inspiratory pressure plateau period. This is in contrast to an end-inspiratory pause; when flow from the ventilator is interrupted during the hold period, gas is redistributed throughout the ventilator circuit and the patient's airways, and a characteristic decrease occurs

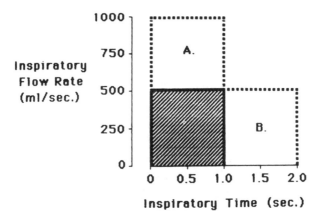

Inspiratory
Flow Rate
(ml/sec.)

Inspiratory Time (sec.)

Figure 2.6. With a time-cycled ventilator, mechanical inhalation is terminated after a preselected inspiratory time elapses. V_T is the product of inspiratory flow rate and inspiratory time, and is represented as the area under the curve. The *shaded curve* represents a V_T of 500 ml. V_T may be increased to 1000 ml either by increasing flow rate as shown in *A*, or by increasing inspiratory time as shown in *B*.

Table 2.2. Time-Cycled Ventilators[a]

Definition: Mechanical inhalation terminates after a preselected
inspiratory time T_I elapses

$$V_T = T_I \times \dot{V}_I$$

Where: V_T is measured in ml; $\dot{V}_I$ is measured in ml/sec;

$$PIP = \frac{T_I \times \dot{V}_I}{C_{LT}}$$

Where: PIP is measured in cmH_2O; C_{LT} is measured in ml/cmH_2O; e.g.,

Normal adult C_{LT}:

$$10 \ cmH_2O = \frac{(2 \ sec) \times (500 \ ml/sec)}{100 \ ml/cmH_2O}$$

Decreased C_{LT}:

$$100 \ cmH_2O = \frac{(2 \ sec) \times (500 \ ml/sec)}{10 \ ml/cmH_2O}$$

[a] Abbreviations used in this table: T_I, inspiratory time; V_T, tidal volume; $\dot{V}_I$, inspiratory flow rate; PIP, peak inflation pressure; C_{LT}, lung-thorax compliance.

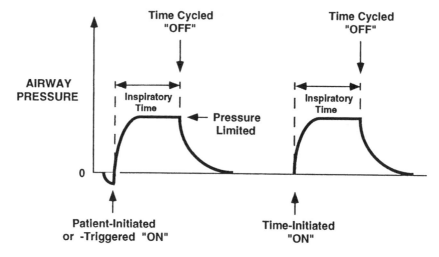

Figure 2.7. Airway pressure waveform for pressure controlled ventilation (*PCV*) is depicted. The ventilator may be patient initiated or triggered "ON" or time initiated "ON," whichever occurs first. The ventilator cycles "OFF" after a preselected inspiratory time lapses. The clinician preselects the pressure limit, inspiratory time, and minimum ventilator rate.

in airway pressure from PIP to the elastic recoil or plateau pressure. The decrease in pressure is directly related to airway resistance.

Pressure support ventilation (PSV) or pressure-limited, time-cycled mechanical ventilation is used for adults and infants diagnosed with acute respiratory distress syndrome. Limiting peak inflation pressure can also reduce the risk of barotrauma. Pressure-limited, time-cycled ventilation has been advocated by Reynolds (18), who has posited that one factor in the pathogenesis of bronchopulmonary dysplasia in infants is mechanical trauma to the lung caused by high airway pressures during mechanical ventilation. In terms of gas exchange, it is suggested that arterial oxygenation and distribution of ventilation may be improved if alveoli are held open longer with mechanical inhalation (10).

Volume-Cycled Mechanical Inhalation

Volume-cycled mechanical inhalation is terminated after a preselected V_T has been ejected from the ventilator, irrespective of the peak inflation pressure, inspiratory time, and inspiratory flow rate, (e.g., Puritan-Bennett MA-1, Puritan-Bennett Co., Carlsbad, CA) (Table 2.3). A common misconception is that V_T delivered to the patient is always constant despite increases in peak inflation pressure as a result of decreases in C_{LT} or increases in airway resistance. During mechanical

Table 2.3. Volume-Cycled Ventilator[a]

Definition: Mechanical inhalation terminates after a preselected volume (V_T) has been ejected from the ventilator.

$$PIP = \frac{V_T}{C_{LT}}$$

Where: PIP is measured in cmH_2O; C_{LT} is measured in ml/cmH_2O; e.g.,

Normal adult C_{LT}:

$$10 \ cmH_2O = \frac{1000 \ ml}{100 \ ml/cmH_2O}$$

Decreased C_{LT}:

$$100 \ cmH_2O = \frac{1000 \ ml}{10 \ ml/cmH_2O}$$

[a] *Abbreviations used in this table: V_T, tidal volume; PIP, peak inflation pressure; C_{LT}, lung-thorax compliance.*

inhalation, ejected V_T is distributed in the ventilator breathing circuit tubing and in the patient's lungs. The greater the peak inflation pressure, the greater the fraction of V_T compressed or "left behind" in the breathing circuit, and the less volume delivered to the patient (Fig. 2.8). The more compliant the breathing circuit tubing, the more volume remains in the tubing and the less volume the patient receives. When high peak inflation pressures are required, noncompliant and nondistensible tubing should be used, and the humidifier should be full to minimize gas compression. Thus, the so-called "volume-constant ventilator" is a myth. No ventilator currently available delivers constant V_T as alterations in pulmonary mechanics occur! Thus, exhaled V_T should be measured between the Y-piece of the breathing circuit and the endotracheal tube to ascertain the actual, delivered V_T that the patient receives.

Pressure-Cycled Mechanical Inhalation

Pressure-cycled mechanical inhalation is terminated when a preselected peak inflation pressure is achieved within the ventilator breathing circuit, irrespective of the V_T, inspiratory time, or inspiratory flow rate (e.g., Bird Mark 7, Bird Products). When the preselected peak inflation pressure is reached, inspiratory flow rate ceases and the exhalation valve opens to allow passive exhalation. Delivered V_T and inspiratory time are related directly to C_{LT} and inversely to airway resistance. V_T may be expressed as the product of the change in airway pressure and C_{LT} (Table 2.4). Therefore, with a pressure-cycled ventilator, a decrease in C_{LT} or increase in airway resistance predispose to a decrease in inspiratory time, and because V_T = inspiratory time $\times$ inspiratory flow rate, V_T decreases.

Substantial leaks in the breathing circuit tubing or at the airway (e.g., improperly inflated endotracheal tube cuff) may preclude the requisite inspiratory cycling pressure from being generated. Most of the ventilators formerly used for intermittent positive pressure-breathing therapy were pressure-cycled.

Flow-Cycled Mechanical Inhalation

Flow-cycled mechanical inhalation is terminated when the inspiratory flow rate delivered by the ventilator decreases to a critical value, irrespective of inspiratory time and V_T. Flow-cycling is employed by microprocessor-controlled mechanical ventilators operating in the pressure-support ventilation mode. For example, in the pressure support ventilation mode, when the ventilator is patient-triggered "ON" (as in patient-triggered mechanical ventilation), an abrupt increase in airway pressure and a high peak inspiratory flow rate are delivered immediately to the patient. The inhalation phase continues until the inspiratory flow rate decays

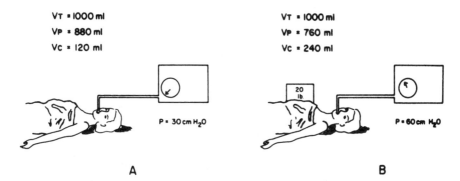

V_T = 1000 ml
V_P = 880 ml
V_C = 120 ml

V_T = 1000 ml
V_P = 760 ml
V_C = 240 ml

P = 30 cm H_2O

P = 60 cm H_2O

A

B

Figure 2.8. Effect of changing compliance (simulated by a weight on the chest) on patient ventilation. **A.** The volume-cycled ventilator is set to deliver a V_T of 1000 ml, of which 880 ml reaches the patient and 120 ml is compressed within the ventilator circuit. Note that the peak inflation pressure (P) is 30 cmH_2O. **B.** A 20-lb weight is placed on the patient's chest to simulate a decrease in lung-thorax compliance. The ventilator again delivers the 1000-ml V_T, but, because of the patient's decreased compliance, a pressure of 60 cm H_2O is required and only 760 ml reaches the patient, while 240 ml is compressed or "left behind" in the breathing circuit tubing. In this example, the compression factor is 4 ml/cmH_2O, i.e., 4 ml/cmH_2O $\times$ 60 cmH_2O = 240 ml, (V_T = set tidal volume; V_P = patient tidal volume; V_C = compression volume). (Reprinted with permission from Kirby RR, Desautels DA, Smith RA. Mechanical ventilation. In: Burton GG, Hodgkin JE (eds). Respiratory care, 2nd ed. Philadelphia, JB Lippincott Co., 1984, p 556.)

Table 2.4. Pressure-Cycled Ventilators[a]

Definition: Mechanical inhalation terminates when a preselected PIP is achieved within the breathing circuit tubing

$$V_T = PIP \times C_{LT}$$

Where: PIP is measured in cmH_2O; C_{LT} is measured in ml/cmH_2O; e.g.,

Normal adult C_{LT}:

1000 ml = 10 cmH_2O × 100 ml/cmH_2O

Decreased C_{LT}:

100 ml = 10 cmH_2O × 10 ml/cmH_2O

[a] *Abbreviations used in this table: PIP, peak inflation pressure; V_T, tidal volume; C_{LT}, lung-thorax compliance.*

to a predetermined percentage of the initial peak value; at this critical value, flow rate ceases (i.e., the ventilator flow cycles "OFF"), and the exhalation valve opens, allowing passive exhalation (see Fig. 2.5).

CONSTANT AND NONCONSTANT FLOW GENERATORS

Inspiratory Flow Wave Forms

Constant, sinusoidal, decelerating, or accelerating inspiratory flow wave forms available on many newer microprocessor-controlled mechanical ventilators may be another means of classifying mechanical ventilators (Fig. 2.9)(i.e., ventilators may be classified as either constant or nonconstant flow generators). Constant flow generators require a high driving pressure to maintain a large pressure gradient between the ventilator and the patient. A constant or square inspiratory flow wave form is delivered with this type of ventilator (Fig. 2.9, *column 1*). Ideally, the inspiratory flow wave form and volume should not be affected by alterations in C_{LT} and airway resistance.

An eccentric cam and piston mechanism (e.g., IMV Emerson Ventilator, J. H. Emerson, Co., Cambridge, MA) generates flow rate that varies over the inspiratory time and is, therefore, a nonconstant flow generator. A sinusoidal inspiratory flow wave form is delivered with this type of ventilator (Fig. 2.9, *column 2*). The inspiratory flow wave form should remain essentially the same from breath to breath as changes in lung mechanics occur. Decelerating and accelerating inspiratory flow wave forms are obviously nonconstant flow rate profiles; therefore, ventilators delivering these wave forms may be considered nonconstant flow generators (Fig. 2.9, *columns 3* and *4*).

Whether a particular type of inspiratory flow wave form can improve the distribution of ventilation, $\dot{V}_A/\dot{Q}$ matching, and gas exchange is controversial. The discrepancy among some reports relates to a host of confounding variables. In some studies, altering the inspiratory flow wave form may have affected inspiratory time, inhalation-to-exhalation time ratio (I/E), peak inspiratory flow rate, V_T, and minute ventilation. Some investigators, using an end-inspiratory pause, have compared various inspiratory flow wave forms and have found little difference in distribution of ventilation. However, inspiratory time duration is increased by the presence of an end-inspiratory pause, which suggests that it is as important, if not more so, than the type of flow wave form in influencing the distribution of ventilation and gas exchange (19).

MICROPROCESSOR-CONTROLLED VENTILATORS

Microprocessor and pneumatic technologies have combined to produce a new generation of mechanical ventilators—microprocessor-controlled ventilators.

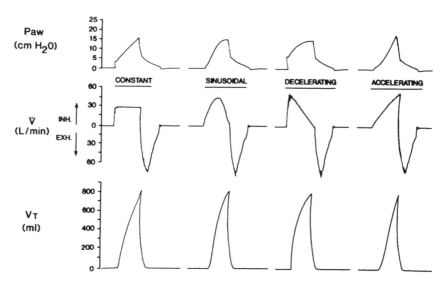

Figure 2.9. Airway pressure (*Paw*), flow rate ($\dot{V}$) and tidal volume (V_T) are shown for constant, sinusoidal, accelerating, and decelerating inspiratory flow wave forms. Inspiratory time, V_T, lung compliance, and airway resistance were held constant. Peak inflation pressure was highest with the accelerating wave form and lowest with the decelerating one; however, mean airway pressure was highest with the latter inspiratory flow wave form.

Such ventilators (e.g., Puritan-Bennett 7200a, Puritan-Bennett, Co., Carlsbad, CA; Bird 6400 ST, Bird Products, Co., Palm Springs, CA; Hamilton Veolar and Amadeus, Hamilton Medical Inc., Reno, NV; Bear V, Bear Medical Systems, Riverside, CA; and Ohmeda CPU-1, Ohmeda, Madison, WI) differ in several respects from the more traditional, nonmicroprocessor ventilator designs (e.g., Puritan-Bennett MA-1) (20). Capable of multiple ventilation and computerized monitoring modes, microprocessor-controlled ventilators also can acquire, process, store, and retrieve data. Potential advantages of microprocessor-controlled ventilators are summarized in Table 2.5.

The microprocessor, also known as a central processing unit (CPU), is the

Table 2.5. Potential Advantages of Microprocessor-Controlled Ventilators

General versatility
- Capable of providing various modalities of mechanical and spontaneous PPV
- Ability to ventilate with a variety of inspiratory flow wave forms
- Choice of cycling mechanisms (e.g., time-, volume-, or pressure-cycled)
- Capability of being easily reprogrammed and upgraded to prevent premature obsolescence
- Ability to ventilate adult and pediatric patients

Monitoring capability
- Real-time monitoring of a variety of ventilatory parameters
- Ability to calculate and monitor: lung-thorax compliance, airway resistance, minute exhaled ventilation, mean airway pressure, respiratory work, etc.
- Each microprocessor self-checks and cross-checks to ensure proper functioning of computer and pneumatic operation
- Computer memory permits the storage and retrieval of ventilation data for trend analyses

Computer correction capability
- Allegedly, the microprocessor should be able to perform automatic corrections to maintain the inspiratory flow rate and wave form and V_T as peak inflation pressure increases due to changes in lung-thorax compliance and airway resistance
- Measured tidal and minute volumes corrected to BTPS
- Allegedly, volume losses in the ventilator breathing circuit secondary to compression may be calculated and/or compensated

Display and communications capability
- Computer-controlled displays indicate all current ventilatory parameters, alarms, and limits
- Communication with other microcomputers or mainframe computers is available for the monitoring and storage of data

Repairs and maintenance
- System down-time should be reduced due to the relative ease of diagnosing and troubleshooting ventilation programs and the moving components in a microprocessor-controlled ventilator
- Modulator components facilitate repair

BTPS = *Body temperature, pressure, saturated*

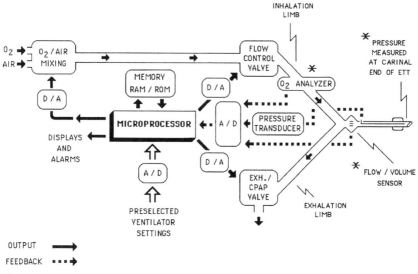

Figure 2.10. Diagrammatic representation showing the operation of a microprocessor-controlled ventilator. Preselected ventilator settings entered as analog signals via knobs on the front panel are converted to digital data via an analog-to-digital converter (A/D) and then directed to the **microprocessor** which controls the overall operation of the ventilator. The data are, in turn, directed to random access memory (RAM). The general ventilator control program can be stored on read only memory (ROM). **Output** control data (*solid lines*), via digital-to-analog conversion (D/A), are then directed from the microprocessor to the oxygen/air mixing system, inspiratory flow control valve, and exhalation/continuous positive airway pressure (CPAP) valve. **Feedback** data (*dashed lines*), via A/D conversion, are directed back to the microprocessor from the oxygen analyzer, airway pressure transducer, and flow/volume sensor. Ideally, the ventilator should function as a closed-loop feedback control system. On most ventilators the sites of pressure and flow/volume measurement are either inside the ventilator on the exhalation limb of the breathing circuit or at the Y piece. For greater accuracy it is recommended to measure airway pressure at the *carinal* end of the endotracheal tube (ETT) and a flow/volume at the *Y* piece of the breathing circuit (see Fig 2.4).

"brain" of a microprocessor-controlled mechanical ventilator; it is where the processing and decisions actually occur (21) (Fig 2.10). Microprocessors are integrated circuit chips programmed for specific tasks using appropriate software. The miniature electrical circuits integrated into the microprocessor enable it to perform arithmetic (addition, subtraction, multiplication, and division), relational, and logical operations, as well as to control the processing and flow of information (21). Microprocessors are used in a variety of equipment that requires extensive control, such as complex instrumentation devices and mechanical ventilator life-support systems. Personal microcomputers consist of microprocessors, memory modules, and input/output interfaces. Similarly, microprocessor-controlled mechanical ventilators have the same hardware, in addition to the requisite mechanical components, to provide mechanical ventilation. Thus, microprocessor-controlled ventilators may be thought of as a mechanical ventilator coupled with the computing power of a microcomputer.

Open- and Closed-Loop Systems

Control systems in mechanical ventilators may be either open- or closed-loop in design (21). An open-loop control system *does not* use feedback (process by which the output of a system is directed back and used as additional input data to modulate the system output) for its operations. Open-loop control systems are typical of many nonmicroprocessor-designed mechanical ventilators. For example, an open-loop control system is employed in the Puritan-Bennett MA-1 nonmicroprocessor mechanical ventilator. With this ventilator, there is no feedback of airway pressure, flow rate, and V_T (system output) to the control mechanism of the ventilator.

In contrast, closed-loop control systems, as found in many microprocessor-equipped mechanical ventilators, feed output data back to the microprocessor control mechanism to drive the ventilator (i.e., the difference [error] between the reference input [preselected ventilator parameters] and the measured output [actually delivered parameters] drive the system to the desired output). As a result, it is alleged that inspiratory flow rate, for example, can be maintained at or near the preselected value as changes in respiratory mechanics occur (22). However, when the airway pressure, flow rate, and V_T characteristics of microprocessor-controlled ventilators were compared, it was noted that, as lung compliance decreased and airway resistance increased, thereby causing peak inflation pressure to increase, decreases in the preselected inspiratory flow rate and V_T resulted (20). These observations are disappointing, to say the least. Two possible explanations for these observations are that the response time (time for a system to react and respond to an input or instruction) of the closed-loop control system is too slow or that the location of the airway pressure and flow transducers may be inappropriate (21). Further, the performance of a closed-loop control system is dependent on the accuracy of the feedback transducers. Inaccurate or improperly placed transducers will degrade closed-loop performance. It is recommended that these transducers be located at the airway opening, not inside the ventilator or on the expiratory limb of the breathing circuit.

Several components arranged in series constitute the closed-loop control system of a microprocessor-controlled ventilator (Fig. 2.10). A microprocessor receives *digital* data (data that are encoded in the form of binary digit or "bit" patterns) input from a keypad on the ventilator's control panel (i.e., the preselected ventilator parameters). Because digital data from a microprocessor are meaningless to the outside world, they are converted to *analog* signals (a continuous signal that can have an infinite number of values) via a digital-to-analog converter. These analog voltage signals are the instructions governing the flow control valve operation during the ventilator's inspiratory and expiratory phases. Output from the flow control valve is monitored by flow and pressure transducers. Because microprocessors work only with digital data, analog signals from these transducers must be transformed to appropriate digital data by an analog-to-digital converter. These digital data, in turn, are directed back to the microprocessor as additional input data, thus constituting a feedback loop as described.

Random Access Memory and Read Only Memory

Memory is essential for the operation of a microprocessor-controlled ventilator. Random access memory (RAM) and read only memory (ROM) are two types of memory modules found in microprocessor-controlled ventilators. For example, to display a trend in C_{LT}, the ventilator must be capable of acquiring and then "remembering" or storing the changes in C_{LT} over time. In this example, RAM is where data are stored for later retrieval. A disadvantage of RAM is that when the electrical power is discontinued, all stored data are lost. RAM, therefore, would be unsuitable for storing a ventilator control program, for example. In contrast, with ROM or permanent memory, data are not lost when the electrical power is discontinued. Thus, ROM is used to store the routines or algorithms that control ventilator operation (see Fig. 2.10). The ventilator control program is written into ROM and cannot be accidentally deleted or written over during ventilator operation.

Operating Algorithms

The microprocessor, combined with appropriate software, performs specific routines or algorithms to operate and to monitor a variety of ventilator functions. Algorithms are used to control the operation of the ventilator's flow control valve to deliver the preselected inspiratory flow wave form, peak inspiratory flow rate, and V_T, for example. Preprogrammed routines are also used to check the input of preselected ventilation parameters and then monitor the ventilator's output (Fig. 2.11). Other algorithms are used to check preselected alarm limits (e.g., peak inflation and mean airway pressures). Still other algorithms are used to calculate, monitor, and display data in a real-time fashion (a signal that is processed and displayed as fast as it is physically generated; e.g., an ECG display), such as V_T, inspiratory flow rate, the levels of CPAP, and pressure support ventilation, C_{LT}, airway resistance, and respiratory work.

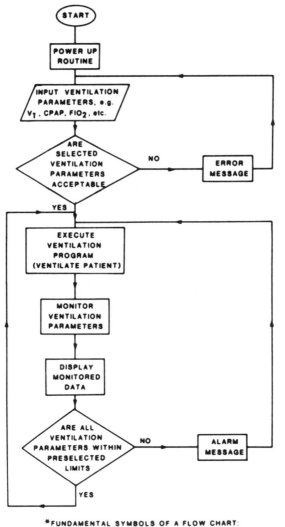

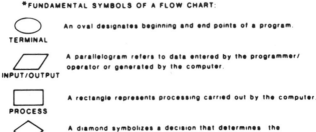

*FUNDAMENTAL SYMBOLS OF A FLOW CHART:

An oval designates beginning and end points of a program.
TERMINAL

A parallelogram refers to data entered by the programmer/operator or generated by the computer.
INPUT/OUTPUT

A rectangle represents processing carried out by the computer.
PROCESS

A diamond symbolizes a decision that determines the computer's next action.
DECISION

Clinical Application

A challenge to respiratory care practitioners is patients with severe forms of respiratory failure (i.e., those with a marked decrease in lung-chest wall compliance and increases in airway resistance, $\dot{Q}sp/\dot{Q}t$, and physiologic dead space, as well as those with a labile cardiovascular system). Such patients are difficult to manage and may benefit from the variety of ventilatory approaches as well as the monitoring capabilities of microprocessor-controlled ventilators (23). For example, consider a patient with severe chronic obstructive pulmonary disease with ventilation maldistribution and marked increases in airways resistance and work of breathing. Pressure-limited, time-cycled IMV could be applied. To improve ventilation distribution, inspiratory time could be increased and a decelerating inspiratory flow wave form used. Real-time monitoring of lung-chest wall compliance and airway resistance may be useful for appropriately setting inspiratory time vis-à-vis the patient's total inspiratory time constant (time constant = lung-chest wall compliance × airway resistance (19)), as well as for assessing the effects of therapy. To reduce the work of breathing to more tolerable levels during spontaneous ventilation, real-time measurement of work of breathing is useful for titrating appropriate levels of pressure support ventilation (16,17,24).

VENTILATOR EVALUATION/SAFETY

Evaluation of mechanical ventilators has been described in detail (25). Specific procedures for evaluating mechanical ventilators are necessary to ensure proper operation, as well as patient safety (see Chapter 3, Monitoring During Ventilatory Support). An evaluation form or checklist to document a ventilator's capabilities, as well as its alarm monitoring characteristics, is advocated. Such an evaluation prior to purchasing and using a mechanical ventilator would address specific questions, such as:

1. Does the ventilator operate in accordance with the manufacturer's design specifications?
2. Does the ventilator possess the pressure, flow rate, and volume capabilities, and other characteristics needed for the types of patients at my institution?

◄――――――――――――――――――――――――――――――――――――

Figure 2.11. This flowchart is a generic ventilator control program for a microprocessor-controlled ventilator. It depicts a preprogrammed routine that might be used to check the input of preselected ventilation parameters and then monitor the ventilator's output. (Reprinted with permission from Lampotang S. Microprocessor-controlled ventilation, systems and concepts. In: Kirby RR, Banner MJ, Downs JB (eds). Clinical applications of ventilatory support. New York, Churchill Livingstone, Inc., 1990, p. 107.)

3. Is the patient's work of breathing excessive when CPAP is applied?
4. Is the ventilator too simple or too sophisticated for my needs?
5. Is the ventilator too difficult to operate?
6. Does the ventilator have a comprehensive alarm and monitoring package?
7. Are the monitoring capabilities such that too much or not enough data are displayed?
8. Can the ventilator be upgraded easily as improvements and innovations occur, or will the ventilator become obsolete in a short period of time?
9. What is the cost of the ventilator?

Finally, regarding alarms and monitors, many of the newer generation of mechanical ventilators have factory-installed alarm-monitoring packages that can be adjusted to the patient's ventilatory requirements. Pressure and flow transducers are employed to monitor airway pressures (e.g., peak inflation pressure, mean airway pressure), CPAP, and gas flow rate (e.g., expiratory flow rate, V_T and minute volume). Calculated from these data are lung-chest wall compliance, airway resistance, and work of breathing. Audible and visual alarms are used to indicate such things as sudden changes in the F_1O_2, apnea, loss of CPAP, leak in the ventilator breathing circuit, and peak inflation pressure limit. Used to assess the adequacy of ventilation, capnographs monitor continuously end-tidal carbon dioxide tension ($P_{ET}CO_2$). Alarm limits for $P_{ET}CO_2$ are set to indicate ventilatory abnormalities.

References

1. Ashbaugh D, Bigelow D, Petty T, et al. Acute respiratory distress in adults. Lancet 2:319, 1967.
2. Kirby RR. Mechanical ventilation in acute respiratory failure: facts, fiction, and fallacies. In: Gallagher TJ (ed). Advances in anesthesia. Chicago, Year Book Medical Publishers, 1984, pp 51–88.
3. Kirby RR, Robison E, Schulz J. A new pediatric volume ventilator. Anesth Analg 50:553, 1971.
4. Downs JB, Klein EF, Desautels DA, et al. Intermittent mandatory ventilation, a new approach to weaning patients from mechanical ventilators. Chest 64:331, 1973.
5. Hasten RW, Downs JB, Heenan TJ. A comparison of synchronized and nonsynchronized intermittent mandatory ventilation. Respir Care 25:554, 1980.
6. Heenan TJ, Downs JB, Douglas ME. Intermittent mandatory ventilation—is synchronization important? Chest 77:598, 1980.
7. Hewlett AM, Platt AS, Terry VG. Mandatory minute volume. A new concept in weaning from mechanical ventilators. Anesth Analg 32:163, 1977.
8. Bolder PM, Healy EJ, Bolder AR, et al. The extra work of breathing through adult endotracheal tubes. Anesth Analg 65:853–859, 1986.
9. Fiastro JF, Habib MP, Quan SF. Pressure support compensation for inspiratory work due to endotracheal tubes and demand continuous positive airway pressure. Chest 93:499–505, 1988.
10. Bersten AD, Rutten AJ, Vedig AE, et al. Additional work of breathing imposed by endotracheal tubes, breathing circuits, and intensive care ventilators. Crit Care Med 17:671–677, 1989.
11. Shapiro M, Wilson RK, Casar G, et al. Work of breathing through different sized endotracheal tubes. Crit Care Med 14:1028–1031, 1986.

12. Banner MJ, Kirby RR, Blanch PB. Site of pressure measurement during spontaneous breathing with continuous positive airway pressure: effect on calculating imposed work of breathing. Crit Care Med 20(4):528, 1992.

13. Banner MJ, Blanch PB, Kirby RR. Imposed work of breathing and methods of triggering demand-flow, continuous positive airway pressure system. Crit Care Med 1993;21(2):183, 1993.

14. Saqer JG, Banner MJ, Blanch PB, Goodwin SR, Berman LS. Effect of pressure measuring *SITE* on change in airway pressure during spontaneous and mechanical ventilation. Crit Care Med 23 (Suppl. 1):A18, 1995.

15. Banner MJ, Kirby RR, Blanch PB, Layon AJ. Decreasing imposed work of the breathing apparatus to zero using pressure-support ventilation. Crit Care Med 21(9):1333, 1993.

16. MacIntyre N. Respiratory function during pressure support ventilation. Chest 89:677, 1986.

17. Banner MJ, Kirbyu RR, Gabrielli A, Blanch PB, Layon AJ. Partially and totally unloading respiratory muscles based on real time measurements of work of breathing. Chest 106: 1835–1842, 1994.

18. Reynolds EOR. Pressure waveform and ventilator settings for mechanical ventilation in severe hyaline membrane disease. Bourns Educational Series ES1. Boston, Little, Brown and Co, 1977, p 1.

19. Banner MJ, Lampotang S. Clinical use of inspiratory and expiratory flow waveforms. In: Kacmarek RM, Stoller JK (eds). Current respiratory care. Philadelphia, BC Decker, 1988, pp 137–143.

20. Banner MJ, Blanch P, Desautels DA. Mechanical ventilators. In: Kirby RR, Banner MJ, Downs JB (eds). Clinical applications of ventilatory support. New York. Churchill Livingstone, Inc, 1990, pp 401–503.

21. Lampotang S. Microprocessor-controlled ventilation, systems and concepts . In: Kirby RR, Banner MJ, Downs JB (eds). Clinical applications of ventilatory support. New York, Churchill Livingstone, Inc., 1990, pp 105–120.

22. Bear 5 Ventilator Instruction Manual. Bear Medical Systems Inc, Riverside, CA, 1986, pp 11.17–11.18.

23. Spearman CB. Appropriate ventilator selection. In: Kacmarek RM, Stoller JK (eds). Current respiratory care. Philadelphia, BC Decker, Inc, 1988, pp 123–127.

24. Fiastro JF, Habib MP, Quan SF. Pressure support compensation for inspiratory work due to endotracheal tubes and demand continuous positive airway pressure. Chest 93:499, 1988.

25. Desautels DA. Ventilator performance evaluation. In: Kirby RR, Smith RA, Desautels DA (eds). Mechanical ventilation. New York, Churchill Livingstone, Inc, 1985, pp 115–135.

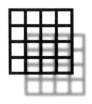

3
Monitoring During Ventilatory Support

John (Hans) W. Schweiger • Jukka Räsänen

The initiation of mechanical ventilation to support a patient with pending acute or chronic ventilatory failure results in major alterations in that individual's cardiopulmonary physiology. The normal transpulmonary pressure gradient, which is usually generated by a decrease in intrathoracic pressure, is functionally reversed because an elevation in airway pressure is used to inflate the lungs during inspiration. Mechanical ventilatory support, thereby, not only results in the efficient pulmonary excretion of carbon dioxide (CO_2) and the adequate oxygenation of the pulmonary capillary blood, but concomitantly causes perturbations in the central hemodynamics and peripheral blood flow (1). Moreover, critically ill patients dependent on mechanical ventilation are at high risk for a number of complications secondary to the natural progression of their diseases or as a consequence of receiving ventilatory support itself (2). Therefore, to distinguish the favorable from the adverse cardiopulmonary effects, adequate monitoring of ventilation, oxygenation, and circulation must be employed whenever mechanical ventilatory support is instituted and used in patient care.

MONITORING OF VENTILATION

When providing any form of respiratory support it is essential that ventilatory function is monitored with vigilance, even in those circumstances when artificial ventilation per se is not being used. A classic example would be in patients with chronic obstructive pulmonary disease, where even supplemental oxygen therapy requires periodic assessment of ventilation to detect respiratory depression resulting from abolition of the individual's central, hypoxic respiratory drive. Monitoring of ventilatory function must account for both the adequacy of alveolar ventilation and the amount of respiratory work required to sustain it.

When evaluating ventilatory function, it must be understood that both the acceptability of a patient's respiratory workload and the adequacy of alveolar ventilation may vary depending on changes in the clinical circumstances or pathophysiology of the disease. A previously healthy patient with an isolated, acute lung infection may well be able to tolerate a level of respiratory muscle work much higher than he or she could after the infection has progressed to multisystem organ failure with adult respiratory distress syndrome. Similarly, a patient may be able to sustain adequate spontaneous ventilation under normal conditions, but might develop ventilatory failure when CO_2 output rises as a result of coexisting infection or iatrogenic administration of an excessive carbohydrate load. It is extremely difficult to quantify respiratory work clinically and no "gold standard" or universally accepted endpoint has been identified to which monitoring efforts can easily be directed (3). Therefore, the practitioner usually monitors the work of breathing at the patient's bedside by careful, repeated clinical assessments (4). In contrast, the matching of alveolar ventilation and carbon dioxide production, under routine circumstances, is accurately reflected by the arterial blood's carbon dioxide tension ($PaCO_2$), and can easily be monitored through arterial blood gas (ABG) analysis.

The quickest and simplest way to assess ventilatory function is by direct observation of the patient's breathing pattern and by auscultation of breath sounds. No currently available mechanical monitor provides information concerning respiratory mechanics as accurately and as cost-efficiently as that provided by the trained eyes and ears of the seasoned practitioner. Because timely correction of ventilation and oxygenation derangements is often lifesaving, initial decisions regarding respiratory therapy frequently must depend on clinical assessment alone. Observation of the symmetry and amount of volume change in the chest, inspiratory and expiratory time, and the quality of breath sounds in the different lung fields gives an estimate of the tidal volume (V_T), amount and location of any airway obstruction, and the distribution of ventilation within the chest. Additionally, respiratory rate measurement; observation of any suprasternal, intercostal, and subcostal retractions; and assessment for use of any accessory inspiratory and expiratory muscles provide an estimate of the patient's minute ventilation and current respiratory workload. The appearance of any sudden or erratic alterations in the individual's respiratory depth or frequency indicates impending respiratory fatigue and necessitates the immediate availability of ventilatory support to avoid potential respiratory arrest.

Although clinical examination of the respiratory system by a trained practitioner is reasonably reliable and perhaps the only readily available method for evaluating a patient's respiratory workload, it is, however, notoriously inaccurate in estimating the adequacy of alveolar ventilation with regard to CO_2 output (5). Hence, the diagnosis of ventilatory failure usually requires the careful analysis of $PaCO_2$ and pH from an arterial blood sample. Modern respiratory care practices, as well as the medicolegal environment in the United States, have fostered the evolution of automated means of continuously monitoring for alterations of a patient's vital signs and physiological functions during the course of treatment (6,7). Hence, repetitive clinical assessment has been supplemented by devices that continuously monitor one or several variables essential to ventilatory function (8). Some are based on sensing respiratory movements and changes in airway pressure or gas flow, whereas others provide direct or indirect estimates of the patient's $PaCO_2$.

Respiratory Movements

Several methods of detecting respiratory movements have been devised for application under a variety of clinical situations. Probes are available for sensing movements of the body or chest wall, as well as for detecting changes in thoracic electrical impedance. This type of monitoring is most commonly used with premature infants or infants at risk for apnea due to functional immaturity of the respiratory center. They have become popular in this setting, because they are convenient, noninvasive, and relatively reliable. However, these devices are unable to detect partial or total airway obstruction if respiratory movements continue at a relatively normal frequency. Under these circumstances, the infant may already have been severely hypoxemic for a considerable period of time before the catastrophic respiratory arrest ultimately triggers an alarm from the apnea monitor. Therefore, patients at risk for ventilatory problems other than arrest or dysfunction of the respiratory center may best be monitored using standard pulse oximetry.

Airway Pressure

Airway pressure is the most commonly measured variable during continuous ventilatory function monitoring of patients requiring support. Alterations in the phasic pressure pattern during spontaneous or mechanical respiratory cycles warn of several potentially deleterious events related to the patient or to malfunction of the ventilator itself. Airway pressure measurements should, therefore, always be displayed while mechanical ventilatory support is being administered (9). In some ventilators, a low airway pressure alarm limit may be set to sense the presence or absence of positive-pressure breaths and to calculate the ventilator's frequency rate. The alarm trigger level is then set between the patient's peak airway pressure and end-expiratory pressure. Failure of the airway pressure to reach this predetermined level usually indicates inadequate delivery of volume into the patient's lungs. This may be caused by insufficient gas supply to the ventilator unit, inadvertent changes in the ventilator's settings, failure of the ventilator to initiate a breath, a leak in the breathing circuit, or a disconnection between the patient-ventilator interface. Theoretically, large increases in lung-thorax compliance or a decrease in airway flow resistance can result in a substantial decrease in peak airway pressure. However, in clinical practice this change is rarely large enough to trigger an alarm, assuming that the "low" pressure limit is appropriately set.

If a separate low tidal volume indicator is used to monitor for the presence of ventilation, then the "low" pressure alarm may be dedicated to detect loss of circuit pressure during continuous positive-pressure therapy. Under these conditions, the sensor level should be set below the positive end-expiratory airway pressure. It is, however, vital to remember that regardless of the monitoring system in use, once a ventilator's "low" pressure alarm has been triggered, it should always be considered to indicate inadequate ventilatory support, not merely a system malfunction. This approach will help minimize potentially catastrophic airway disasters, because an alarm system malfunction should only be considered in the differential diagnosis after immediate life-threatening causes have been thoroughly ruled out by the clinician.

A "high" pressure limit in the breathing circuit serves a dual safety function. It not only provides an indication of elevated peak airway pressures, but when high simultaneously triggers a release of excess circuit pressure, thereby protecting the airway from over distension and barotrauma. The ventilator's "high" pressure limit should always be preset before connecting a patient to the breathing circuit. The appropriate level can be estimated at ~10 mmHg above the patient's expected peak airway pressure.

The peak pressure generated during inflation of a patient's lungs, given constant volume and flow, is dependent on that individual's lung compliance and airway resistance. Therefore, either a decrease in lung compliance, an increase in airway pressure, or a combination of both may produce an increase in the measured peak airway pressure. Common causes of abruptly elevated peak airway pressure include airway occlusion secondary to accumulated secretions or a kinked endotracheal tube, undetected endobronchial intubation, acute bronchoconstriction, and pneumothorax. A more gradual rise can be seen following the deterioration of a patient's pulmonary parenchymal function (e.g., pulmonary edema), causing lung compliance to decrease progressively and airway resistance to increase.

Differentiating between the effects of compliance and resistance on airway pressure requires the practitioner to measure both the peak airway pressure and the airway pressure during an end-inspiratory pause. Peak airway pressure is a function of both lung compliance and airway resistance, whereas plateau pressure only reflects compliance parameters. A fall in lung-thorax compliance simultaneously elevates the peak airway pressure and the plateau pressure. In contrast, an increase in airway resistance increases only the peak pressure, thereby widening the difference between peak and plateau pressures. Some ventilators are equipped with volume and flow meters that, in addition to displaying both peak and plateau pressures, calculate lung-thorax compliance and airway resistance on line.

Airway pressure monitoring may also be used to detect the presence or absence of spontaneously initiated respiratory cycles. The triggering event is identified as a drop in the circuit pressure during spontaneous inspiration. Such a sudden fall in airway pressure occurs when the patient's inspiratory flow approaches the maximal flow capacity of the breathing circuit and requires the patient to perform active respiratory muscle work. The trigger sensitivity must, therefore, be meticulously set to assure error-free detection of spontaneous breaths with a minimal increase in the patient's work of breathing. Although continuous monitoring for alterations in airway pressure is a simple and useful tool in patients receiving respiratory therapy, it should be noted that airway pressure monitoring provides more information about the functioning of the breathing circuit than it does about the patient's ventilatory pattern. Hence, a seemingly "normal" airway pressure tracing does not, in and of itself, guarantee that gases are flowing into and out of the patient's lungs.

Expiratory Volume and Flow

To provide the clinician with a better estimate of a patient's effective pulmonary ventilation, many ventilators are now equipped with a flow probe or a volume gauge located in the expiratory limb of the breathing circuit. These devices can range from simple, manually operated mechanical spirometers to electronic devices with sophisticated averaging and alarm capabilities. Expiratory volume measurements provide useful information regarding the patient's ventilatory status as well as the functioning of the breathing circuit. By comparing the preset inspiratory tidal volume and minute ventilation with the readings from the expiratory spirometer, the practitioner can indirectly evaluate the volume delivered into the patient's lungs. Breathing circuit leaks and loss of ventilation through bronchopleural fistulas could, for example, result in a significant discrepancy between the inspiratory and expiratory tidal volumes. It is particularly useful to monitor the expiratory minute ventilation when considering adjustments in ventilators for pediatric patients because they may have significant obligatory gas leaks around their uncuffed endotracheal tubes. Moreover, careful monitoring also allows for estimation of the effectiveness of spontaneous respiratory efforts during intermittent mandatory ventilation and unassisted spontaneous breathing. The expiratory volumes measured during assisted ventilation or pressure support ventilation are, in fact, a combination of the patient's spontaneous respiratory effort along with the mechanical support in a proportion that cannot be accurately or easily determined at the bedside.

In most cases, the airway pressure pattern and the expiratory tidal volume, which correspond to a given patient's size and underlying pulmonary function, are associated with adequate alveolar ventilation. However, these variables measure the mechanical function of the respiratory apparatus and do not necessarily reflect "effective" gas exchange in the lung. Inadvertent ventilation of the stomach, as well as atelectatic or poorly perfused lung units, may at times produce airway pressures and expiratory volumes that are not readily distinguishable from normal ventilatory patterns. Thus, when respiratory or mechanical ventilatory support is administered, it is advisable to monitor its endpoints intermittently; that is, removal of CO_2 and oxygenation of the arterial blood through ABG analysis.

End-tidal Carbon Dioxide

Capnography seeks to measure and display expiratory CO_2 concentrations to assess alveolar ventilation adequacy (10). End-tidal CO_2 is intended to reflect $PaCO_2$ in the patient's arterial blood at that particular moment in time. Because CO_2 diffuses so rapidly through the alveolar-capillary membrane, the alveolar and end-capillary partial pressures should approach functional equilibrium given an ideally ventilated and perfused lung unit (ventilation-to-perfusion ratio approaches). When the lung is forced to empty during exhalation, the exhaled gas composition changes from predominately dead-space gas at the onset of exhalation toward that of primarily alveolar gas later in the cycle. The carbon dioxide concentration at end-exhalation ($P_{ET}CO_2$), therefore, is physiologically the best reflection of the concentration within the alveoli and the end-capillary blood. Unfortunately, end-tidal expired gas is normally contaminated by a small contribution from poorly perfused alveoli that constitute the alveolar dead space. This accounts for the 5 mmHg average gradient which exists between $PaCO_2$ and $P_{ET}CO_2$, making $P_{ET}CO_2$ a slight underestimate of $PaCO_2$. The extent of the gradient naturally depends on the amount of the patient's alveolar dead space relative to alveolar ventilation. Furthermore, such factors as the patient's age, position, volume status, ventilatory modality, and coexisting pulmonary disease may change the relationship between $PaCO_2$ and $P_{ET}CO_2$, thereby increasing the amount of the normal gradient.

Capnography, the on-line measurement of $P_{ET}CO_2$, allows for breath-by-breath, noninvasive assessment of ventilation adequacy. It has, therefore, been established as an integral part of the routine, perioperative monitoring during the delivery of a general anesthetic. Standard ventilatory monitoring of airway pressures and noninvasive $P_{ET}CO_2$ can be considered sufficient if the patient's underlying illness or surgical procedures are not expected to cause additional cardiopulmonary instability. In those patients with significant pre-existing cardiac or pulmonary disease, or when the surgery itself is likely to adversely effect underlying cardiopulmonary function, preoperative ABG analysis is required to determine the extent of the gradient between the $PaCO_2$ and $P_{ET}CO_2$. If the $P_{ET}CO_2$ changes suddenly after the initial blood gas analysis, then factors which might possibly affect the "$PaCO_2$—$P_{ET}CO_2$" gradient need to be systematically investigated before additional changes are made in the ventilatory settings.

The use of monitoring $P_{ET}CO_2$ to assess ventilatory function in patients who require chronic, long-term ventilator therapy presents several problems (11). First, as per the aforementioned comments, ventilatory modalities used in the intensive care unit (ICU) frequently employ variable combinations of spontaneous and mechanical ventilation in proportions that are not readily identifiable. This results in a constantly changing dead space-to-tidal volume ratio, which may subsequently alter the relationship between $PaCO_2$ and $P_{ET}CO_2$. Moreover, any significant changes in the patient's pulmonary pathophysiology might have a similar effect. Second, long-term ventilator therapy is frequently administered by using "continuous-flow" breathing circuits. If expiratory gas is sampled to close to the continuously flowing fresh gas source, then dilution of the exhaled CO_2 may give falsely low $P_{ET}CO_2$ readings. Third, in situations when the ventilator rate needs to be high and the tidal volume small (e.g., in infants and small children), it may be difficult to get an appropriate end-tidal gas sample. Consequently, $P_{ET}CO_2$ may considerably underestimate the true $PaCO_2$ values. Despite these potential shortcomings, capnography has become more prevalent in the ICU, particularly in patients who are largely dependent on "full" mechanical ventilatory support. Even though the end-tidal values need to be compared with arterial blood gas values intermittently, they provide a noninvasive, on-line method of quickly detecting changes in a patient's ventilatory status. The fact that $P_{ET}CO_2$ monitoring is affected by the volume of respiratory dead space makes it useful in diagnosing conditions that lead to an increase in inefficient or wasted ventilation. Examples that might be commonly encountered in the operating room and in the ICU are acute pulmonary hypertension, air embolus, and pulmonary embolus. All of these conditions result in a sudden, pronounced decrease in $P_{ET}CO_2$ relative to $PaCO_2$. A similar, although more gradual, fall in $P_{ET}CO_2$ is observed when systemic and pulmonary blood flows are diminished by developing hypovolemia or heart failure. The dependence of expiratory CO_2 measurements on ventilation-perfusion relationships in the lung has led investigators to attempt to estimate $PaCO_2$ directly. Currently available techniques predicated on this principle include transcutaneous carbon dioxide ($PtcCO_2$) measurement and the use of indwelling arterial lines for continuous, on-line monitoring of ABG values.

Transcutaneous Carbon Dioxide

The partial pressures of O_2 and CO_2 can be measured transcutaneously using heated electrodes attached to the skin. Transcutaneous monitoring provides a continuous, noninvasive, real-time estimate of arterialized blood $PaCO_2$ that could prove useful in monitoring ventilation. However, this technique has not found widespread acceptance in operating rooms or ICUs (12). The relatively complex preparation process and calibration of electrodes, as well as the need for cutaneous monitoring and periodic changes of the measurement site to prevent thermal skin burns, are some of the practical reasons why transcutaneous monitoring has been infrequently used. Additionally, transcutaneously derived gas values may be significantly affected by the blood flow directly underneath and around the electrode. Thus, it may prove difficult to interpret the data in situations when the patient's cardiac output is low or the cutaneous blood flow is diminished by vasoconstriction or peripheral vascular disease states (13).

Arterial Blood Gas Analysis

The universally accepted standard for monitoring ventilation is the direct measurement of $PaCO_2$ and pH in the patient's arterial blood sample. The partial gas pressures and pH values are usually measured off line using a blood gas analyzer, but devices that monitor these variables continuously from an indwelling arterial line have been developed for clinical application. $PaCO_2$ content reflects the balance between alveolar ventilation and the CO_2 output of the patient's body. Accurate evaluation of ventilatory function, however, requires simultaneous consideration of the blood pH. Ventilatory failure is commonly defined to be present when a patient's ABG has a combination of $PaCO_2$ >50 mmHg *and* an arterial pH <7.30 (acidemia). However, the concomitant clinical situation must always be carefully considered. For example, in a spontaneously breathing patient inadequate ventilatory compensation for metabolic acidosis may indicate limited ventilatory reserve even though $PaCO_2$ is in the normal range. In patients with chronic obstructive pulmonary disease and a concurrent hypoxic ventilatory drive, appropriate respiratory therapy is very difficult to administer without a full blood gas analysis. Because the respiratory center has lost its responsiveness to CO_2, it is essential to monitor arterial blood oxyhemoglobin saturation and pH, whereas CO_2 values, although still important, are relegated to secondary importance.

As was mentioned, clinical assessment of the patient should never be overlooked, even when ABG analysis is readily available to the practitioner (14). Some patients with impending respiratory failure are capable of maintaining their ABG values within a surprisingly normal range for quite sometime. In such cases, laboratory evidence of ventilatory failure ultimately appears rapidly and commensurate with overt exhaustion and respiratory failure. Nevertheless, careful, serial physical examinations can often warn the clinician of the impending respiratory collapse long before the ABG values ultimately prove conclusive. Moreover, in patients suffering from cardiogenic respiratory failure, the adverse effects of the increased respiratory workload and cardiopulmonary dysfunction may become significant long before any overt signs of ventilatory failure or impaired oxygenation can be seen in an ABG analysis. Therefore, monitoring during ventilatory support should not be limited to ventilatory function, but must also include assessment of both the patient's oxygenation status and cardiovascular performance.

MONITORING OF OXYGENATION

The institution of mechanical ventilatory support frequently has profound effects, either favorably or unfavorably, on the oxygenation status of the patient's arterial blood. Mechanical ventilation per se will correct hypoxemia when it is secondary to hypoventilation or to increased tissue oxygen extraction. Under certain circumstances, however, mechanical ventilation may impair arterial blood oxygenation by depressing cardiac output and/or by inducing ventilation-perfusion abnormalities within the lung itself. These potentially adverse consequences, coupled with the inherent perturbations in underlying cardiopulmonary function, warrant close monitoring of the oxygenation status in all patients receiving respiratory or ventilatory therapy. Clinical assessment of oxygenation depends on the detection of cyanosis, tachypnea, and secondary cardiovascular changes (e.g., hypertension and tachycardia). Because clinical evaluation is not entirely sensitive or specific, the presence or absence of hypoxemia should always be confirmed by using pulse oximetry or ABG analysis.

Pulse oximetry is, by far, the most clinically useful method for monitoring oxygenation during mechanical ventilatory support (15). It continuously provides a noninvasive estimate of arterial blood oxyhemoglobin saturation in on-line fashion, by combining the principles of spectrophotometry and impedance plethysmography. The advent of pulse oximetry has virtually eliminated the routine use of $PtcO_2$ monitoring in adults, and on-line arterial PaO_2 in the operating room. It has also diminished the excessive number of PaO_2 measurements in the ICU setting. Reliable pulse oximeter monitoring requires that saturation values be read only when an acceptable plethysmographic pulse contour is observed. The probe's shape and size should be appropriate for the measurement site. Probes that exert excessive pressure on the capillary bed may give inaccurate readings and cause pressure sores by reducing blood flow to the appendage. Inappropriately large probes may also give erroneous saturation values by allowing pulsatile shunting of light in the probe. The sensor surface needs to be shielded from any external light source to prevent disturbing interference. When these factors are carefully addressed, the modern pulse oximetry units allow for an accurate estimation of arterial blood oxyhemoglobin saturations (SpO_2) in a range between 60% and 100%. However, if the clinician suspects that the pulse oximeter saturation values are incompatible with the patient's clinical status, then the values should be confirmed by arterial blood gas analysis or co-oximetry. Arterial blood oximetry is also required in patients with known or suspected methemoglobinemia or carboxyhemoglobinemia, because these abnormal hemoglobin molecules are partially interpreted as oxyhemoglobin and result in inaccurate readings by all pulse oximeters currently available on the market.

Arterial blood oxygenation monitoring seeks to assure adequate oxyhemoglobin saturation on the "delivery" side of the cardiopulmonary system. Unfortunately, clinically significant hypoxemia may be caused by either pulmonary gas exchange defects or by an imbalance between systemic oxygen supply and concomitant demand in the central and peripheral tissues. The adequacy of the interrelationship between oxygen supply and oxygen demand can be estimated through the simultaneous use of mixed-venous oxyhemoglobin saturation ($S\bar{v}O_2$) monitoring (16). Pulmonary artery catheters equipped with internalized fiberoptic bundles necessary to measure venous oxygenation are now commercially available and are frequently utilized in high-risk, critically ill patients. Whereas pulse oximetry can only detect clinical hypoxemia, integrated monitoring of arterial and mixed venous oxygen saturation allows for the evaluation of its etiology. Therefore, intermittent sampling and analysis of mixed-venous blood, coupled with continuous mixed-venous oximetry, has gradually become an essential part of the monitoring armamentarium for patients with unstable cardiopulmonary systems.

Simple manipulation of the Fick equation allows the clinician to appreciate the possible causes of changes in SO_2 measurements; that is oxygen consumption $=$ cardiac output $\times$ the difference in arterial $-$ venous O_2 content, or $\langle \dot{V}O_2 = \dot{Q}t \times (CaO_2 - C\bar{v}O_2) \rangle$, may be modified to reflect $(CaO_2 - C\bar{v}O_2) = (\dot{V}O_2 / \dot{Q}t)$. If we can assume that oxygen consumption, hemoglobin concentration, and arterial saturation (SaO_2) remain constant, and that distribution of systemic blood flow remains relatively constant, then changes in $S\bar{v}O_2$ should reflect alterations in the patient's cardiac output in a curvilinear relationship. The major causes of an abnormally low or falling $S\bar{v}O_2$ measurement include the following: (*a*) anemia or abnormal hemoglobin species; (*b*) a decrease in cardiac output or a significant increase in systemic vascular resistance (SVR) with subsequent decrease in O_2 delivery to peripheral tissues; (*c*) hypoxemia or a decrease in arterial oxygen saturation; and (*d*) increased metabolic rate or cellular oxygen consumption.

In contrast, an increase in $S\bar{v}O_2$ readings may be attributed to several causes including: (*a*) an increase in hemoglobin concentration; (*b*) an increase in cardiac output or a decrease in SVR with a subsequent increase in O_2 delivery to peripheral tissues; (*c*) hyperoxia or an increase in the arterial oxygen saturation; (*d*) decreased metabolic rate or impaired ability of cells to extract O_2; (*e*) permanently occluded or "over-wedged" PA catheter tracing; (*f*) significant left-to-right intracardiac shunt; and (*g*) severe mitral regurgitation. Controversy exists whether or not the additional expense and effort associated with continuous $S\bar{v}O_2$ monitoring improves patient outcome and cost-effectiveness. Nevertheless, when used in selective populations of critically ill patients, it can provide the clinician with a tremendous amount of real-time information about the pathophysiology of the disease state and the patient's subsequent response to therapeutic interventions that would otherwise be unavailable (17). Moreover, the continuous measurement of arterial (SpO_2) and mixed-venous oxygen $(S\bar{v}O_2)$ saturations, often referred to as dual oximetry, can be used to accurately estimate the amount of right-to-left intrapulmonary shunt (18). This has been described as the ventilation-perfusion index (VQI), which is derived from the relationship between $\dot{Q}sp/\dot{Q}t$ as follows:

$$VQI = \frac{\dot{Q}sp}{\dot{Q}t} = \frac{Sc'O_2 - SaO_2}{Sc'O_2 - S\bar{v}O_2} = \frac{1 - SaO_2}{1 - S\bar{v}O_2} = \frac{1 - SpO_2}{1 - S\bar{v}O_2}$$

where $Sc'O_2$ is the oxyhemoglobin saturation of pulmonary end-capillary blood. Hence, calculation of the VQI provides a near linear estimate of $\dot{Q}sp/\dot{Q}t$ at arterial saturations <100%, because the effect of the oxyhemoglobin dissociation curve is no longer present.

In addition to monitoring the oxygenation status of the patients, ventilators themselves must be equipped with a method of monitoring the oxygen supply to the breathing circuit. In most modern ventilators, the oxygen supply alarm is set to respond to a sudden fall in the oxygen line pressure beneath a predetermined threshold. In addition, some breathing circuits have had an in-line oxygen concentration monitor and alarm placed for added safety. Oxygen analyzers can also be added as separate, freestanding monitors to the patient's breathing circuit. An erroneously low inspired oxygen concentration must always be considered, and carefully ruled out, when encountering a patient with clinical signs of hypoxemia. The possibility that a faulty gas other than oxygen has been supplied or that an accidental supply-line "switch-over" has occurred must be included in the differential diagnosis when encountering a hypoxemic patient receiving mechanical ventilatory support. Moreover, this danger emphasizes the need for continuously monitoring in-line oxygen supply with an appropriate oxygen analyzer in all patients who receive respiratory support.

MONITORING OF CIRCULATION

Almost all currently available forms of artificial mechanical ventilation have pronounced direct and/or indirect effects on a patient's circulatory function and cardiopulmonary reserve. Biphasic fluctuations in airway and intrathoracic pressures change the preload conditions on the right side of the heart by altering venous return, transmural pressure gradients, and pulmonary vascular resistance. Coexisting pulmonary parenchymal disease modifies these effects by modulating transmission of airway pressure into the intrathoracic space. These complex cardiopulmonary interactions warrant circulatory function monitoring during ventilatory support. In normovolemic patients who have no evidence of cardiopulmonary disease, airway and intrathoracic pressure elevation during mechanical ventilation will result in a slight, usually well-tolerated decrease in mean arterial blood pressure and cardiac output. Circulatory function in these patients is adequately monitored by using continuous electrocardiography and intermittent measurement of noninvasive blood pressure.

In hypovolemic patients with otherwise normal cardiopulmonary status, hypotension and hypoperfusion are exacerbated by the simultaneous administration of positive-pressure ventilation or continuous positive-pressure breathing. This phenomenon occurs because the sharp increase in intrathoracic pressure tends to impair venous return back to the right side of the heart. In these patients, continuous, invasive arterial pressure and central venous pressure monitoring would seem prudent. Furthermore, adequate large-bore peripheral intravenous access for the rapid infusion of large volumes of fluid is recommended both on initiation and during administration of positive-pressure ventilatory support to such hypovolemic patients.

Patients with significant cardiac or pulmonary disease may have an unpredictable response to mechanical ventilatory support. Those patients with relatively low lung compliance and congestive, afterload-dependent heart failure are usually not significantly affected by the adverse circulatory sequelae attendant with sustained elevations in airway pressure. On the other hand, individuals with compliant, emphysematous lungs, a stiff chest, and a relatively low blood volume may experience exaggerated circulatory effects of positive-pressure ventilation. Therefore, the risks of these potentially devastating cardiopulmonary derangements constitute an additional factor favoring invasive monitoring of the circulatory system. Continuous arterial pressure monitoring with measurement of systemic blood flow and pulmonary artery catheterization with mixed venous oxyhemoglobin saturation monitoring usually proves valuable in such vulnerable patients. Techniques are now available for continuous monitoring of cardiac output using bioimpedance or Doppler ultrasound. These devices have not yet established their place in routine monitoring because data concerning their accuracy during low and high output states are inconclusive, and because they have not been shown to be cost-effective. In addition to creating a need for monitoring, mechanical ventilatory support also modifies data obtained by these commonly used devices. Alterations in airway and intrathoracic pressure should always be taken into account when recording intrathoracic vascular pressures. A widely accepted practice is to consistently measure these pressures at the end-expiratory phase of spontaneously or mechanically generated respiratory cycles. Expiratory airway pressure is then taken into consideration by subtracting from this end-expiratory value the fraction of positive expiratory airway pressure that is theoretically transmitted into the intrathoracic space. If lung compliance and chest wall compliance are both within normal limits, then this transmitted fraction is estimated to approach 50% of the measured value. The low extreme of pressure transmission is 20% to 30% under situations when lung compliance is low and chest wall compliance is high. In contrast, the high end of the spectrum approaches 60% to 70% when lung compliance is high and chest wall compliance is low. If the clinician does not take pressure transmission from the airway into account, then serious misinterpretation of the hemodynamic profiles of patients with positive end-expiratory airway pressures >10 cmH_2O may occur. Circulatory assessment should always be performed at the onset and thereafter at repetitive intervals during the prescribed respiratory therapy. Intermittently disconnecting a patient from the ventilator to measure hemodynamic profiles is not a wise practice. It not only invalidates the significance of any of these measured assessments to the mechanically ventilated state, but also subjects the patient to potentially serious derangements in cardiopulmonary function.

SUMMARY

All modern mechanical ventilators should be equipped with an airway pressure gauge and gas-supply alarm that indicates loss of oxygen supply, and should have a method for detecting loss of circuit pressure. In-line measurement of inspired oxygen concentration is strongly recommended for optimal patient safety. A continuous estimate of $PaCO_2$ should be made available by using $P_{ET}CO_2$ or $PtcCO_2$ monitoring unless an arterial line is in place and a blood gas analyzer is readily available. Arterial blood oxygenation monitoring through use of a pulse oximetry or a $PtcCO_2$ sensor is mandatory if immediate analysis of arterial blood samples is not feasible. All patients receiving ventilatory therapy should have continuous monitoring of their ECG and they should have their arterial blood pressure measured intermittently by noninvasive sphygmomanometry. Moreover, a person specifically trained in airway management and artificial ventilation techniques should be available at all times in the operating room or in the ICU where mechanical ventilatory therapy is being administered to patients. These monitoring requirements constitute a minimal standard and should be enhanced or expanded on by the clinician in specific clinical situations, or in direct relationship to the unique needs of individual, critically ill patients.

References

1. Räsänen J. Respiratory support in patients with heart failure. Bull Eur Physiopathol Respir 23: 183–195, 1987.
2. Kirby RR. The respiratory system. In: Gravenstein N (ed). Manual of Complications During Anesthesia. Philadelphia: J.B. Lippincott, 1991, pp 303–352.
3. Blanch PB, Banner MJ. A new respiratory monitor that enables accurate measurement of work of breathing: A validation study. Resp Care 34:897–905, 1994.
4. Marini JJ, Rodriguez RM, Lamb VJ. Bedside estimation of the inspiratory work of breathing during mechanical ventilation. Chest 89:56–60, 1986.
5. Thorson SH, Marini JJ, Pierson DJ, Hudson LD. Variability of arterial blood gas values in stable patients in the ICU. Chest 84:14–18, 1983.
6. Cheney FW, et al. Standard of care and anesthesia liability. JAMA 261:1599–1603, 1989.
7. Tinker JH, et al. Role of monitoring devices in prevention of anesthetic mishaps: A closed claims analysis. Anesthesiology 71:535–540, 1989.
8. Caplan RA, et al. Adverse respiratory events in anesthesia: A closed claims analysis. Anesthesiology 72:828–833, 1990.
9. Marini JJ, Truwit J. Monitoring the respiratory system. In Hall JB, et al. Principles of Critical Care. New York: McGraw-Hill, Inc. 1992, p. 211.
10. Hess D. Capnometry and capnography: Technical aspects, physiologic aspects, and clinical applications. Respir Care 35:557–576, 1990.

11. Hoffman RA, Krieger BP, Kramer MR, Segel S, Bizousky F, Gazeroglu H, Sackner MA. End-tidal carbon dioxide in critically ill patients during changes in mechanical ventilation. Am Rev Respir Dis 140:1265–1268, 1989.
12. Martin RJ. Transcutaneous monitoring: Instrumentation and clinical applications. Respir Care 35:577–583, 1990.
13. Tremper KK, Shoemaker WC. Transcutaneous oxygen monitoring of critically ill adults, with and without low flow shock. Crit Care Med 9:706–709, 1981.
14. Thorson SH, Marini JJ, Pierson DJ, Hudson LD. Variability of arterial blood gas values in stable patients in the ICU. Chest 84:14–18, 1983.
15. Severinghaus JW, Kelleher JF. Recent developments in pulse oximetry. Anesthesiology 76:1018–1038, 1992.
16. Vaughn S, Purl VK. Cardiac output changes and continuous mixed venous oxygen saturation measurement in the critically ill. Crit Care Med 16:495–498, 1988.
17. Kraft P, Steltzer H, Heismayr M, Klimscha W, Hammerle AF. Mixed venous oxygen saturation in critically ill septic shock patients: The role of defined events. Chest 103:900–906, 1993.
18. Räsänen J, Downs JB, Malec DJ, et al. Real-time continuous estimation of gas exchange by dual oximetry. Intensive Care Med 14:118–122, 1988.

Suggested Readings

Eichhorn JH, Cooper JB, Cullen DJ, et al. Anesthesia practice standards at Harvard: A review. J Clin Anesth 1:55–65, 1988.

Lysal SZ, Prough DS. Monitoring for patients receiving airway pressure therapy. Anesth Clin North Am 5:821–841, 1987.

Pinsky MR. The hemodynamic effects of artificial ventilation.In: Vincent JL (ed). Update in Intensive Care and Emergency Medicine, 5th ed. Heidelberg, Springer Verlag, 1988, pp 187–201.

Räsänen J, Downs JB, Malec J, et al. Oxygen tensions and oxyhemoglobin saturations in the assessment of pulmonary gas exchange. Crit Care Med 15:598–602, 1987.

Reinhart K, Schafer M, Specht M. Indications and limitations of $S\bar{v}O_2$ and $ScvO_2$ monitoring. In: Vincent JL (ed). Update in Intensive Care and Emergency Medicine, 5th ed. Heidelberg, Springer Verlag, 1988, pp 428–435.

Shapiro BA, Harrison RA, Walton JR. Clinical application of blood gases, 2nd ed. Chicago, Year Book Medical, 1977.

Swedlow DB. Capnometry and capnography: The anesthesia disaster early warning system. Semin Anesth 4:194–205, 1986.

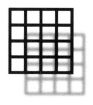

4
Pulmonary Effects of Mechanical Ventilation

Theodor Kolobow

"We define mechanical ventilatory support as positive airway pressure therapy that is applied primarily to enhance carbon dioxide secretion."
—R. D. Cane and B. A. Shapiro (1).

Healthy volunteers placed on mechanical ventilation on room air evidence negligible changes in pulmonary function or structure. Patients with neuromuscular disorders alone, when placed on mechanical ventilation, similarly show no impairment in pulmonary function or structure attributable to mechanical ventilation; problems while on mechanical ventilation can be largely attributed to intubation or decreased mobility while receiving mechanical ventilation. In both of these examples, lungs are ventilated with normal tidal volumes (V_T), low peak airway (inflation) pressures, and at normal respiratory rates. Not surprisingly, the functional residual capacity (FRC), lung compliance, alveolar ventilation-to-perfusion ($\dot{V}_A/\dot{Q}$) ratio, and arterial blood gases remain within normal range.

Such may not be the case when the amount of healthy lung is reduced by 50%, or even 75%, for example, through surgical removal of one or more lobes of the lungs (Fig. 4.1). The pulmonary circulation usually adapts readily to this change. However, to sustain adequate alveolar ventilation and, hence, $PaCO_2$, the ventilation of the remaining lung will have to be increased by nearly 100% and 300%, respectively. This increase in minute ventilation can be achieved with a substantial increase in V_T and/or an increase in respiratory rate, and will result in a rise in peak inflation pressure. This process may exceed the physiologic tolerance of the lungs following hours or days of mechanical ventilation. Additionally, the overexpansion of the remaining lung tissue to fit the thoracic cage may pose an additional pathophysiologic stress.

On the other hand, experimentally induced, spontaneous hyperventilation-hyperinflation produced by injecting sodium salicylate into the cisterna magna in an animal model, will cause substantial deterioration of pulmonary function within 24 hours. In some animals, death from hypoxia resulted (2).

These observations suggest that the physiologic limit to hyperinflation and to hyperventilation of healthy lungs may be narrower than previously assumed. These

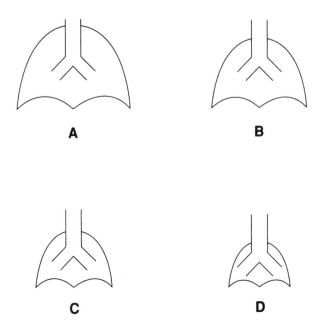

Figure 4.1. The normal pulmonary parenchyma (**A**) is gradually reduced through, for example, surgical means (**B,C,D**). The alveolar ventilation of such decreased small lung must be increased in proportion, resulting in unphysiologic pulmonary ventilation.

same factors are likely to play a role in patients who are now considered candidates for mechanical ventilation.

Patients with lungs impaired by disease processes face a potentially insurmountable problem. On one hand, the total fraction of pulmonary parenchyma partaking in gas exchange will be reduced to varying degrees by the underlying disease (Fig. 4.2), while ventilation per unit lung volume will be greatly increased. On the other hand, the higher metabolic load in sick patients may require increased alveolar ventilation to accommodate higher CO_2 production. This combination invariably leads to high airway pressures, biochemical alterations in pulmonary cellular functions, and barotrauma affecting mostly the healthiest and, hence, the most compliant regions of the lungs.

Barotrauma is an all-inclusive term that ranges from pulmonary interstitial emphysema, pneumomediastinum, pneumoperitoneum, and subcutaneous emphysema to such life-threatening complications as pneumothorax and tension pneumothorax. Most agree that the primary causative factor is high peak inflation pressure. Peak inflation pressures >40 cmH$_2$O are associated with a high incidence of barotrauma. The apparent site of pulmonary disruption occurs at the common border of the alveolar base and the vascular sheath. An early indicator of barotrauma is pulmonary interstitial emphysema, which may manifest as linear air streaking toward the hilum, parenchymal air cysts, pneumatocele, subpleural air, or perivascular air blebs. Although pneumothorax can be drained through placement of chest tubes, its presence complicates patient management and greatly increases the risk of morbidity and mortality.

The onset of air leaks alone would not be of such great consequence were it not also a marker of underlying cellular dysfunction. Experimental animals, following mechanical ventilation at pressures >30 cmH$_2$O, manifest a substantial rise in minimal surface tension of saline lung lavage fluid, indicative of type II alveolar cellular dysfunction (3). Those lungs become atelectatic as a result of surfactant depletion and require high airway pressures and positive end-expiratory pressure (PEEP) to maintain lung volume.

The lungs are a unique metabolic organ. The pulmonary parenchyma hosts more than 100 distinct cell lines ranging from ciliated epithelial cells to goblet cells, mucous glands, endocrine-like cells, brush cells, "special type cells" of various kinds, Clara cells, alveolar type I and type II cells, alveolar macrophages, lymphatic endothelium, many types of blood vascular endothelium, myelinated and unmyelinated nerve endings, parasympathetic ganglion cells, visceral mesothelium, and

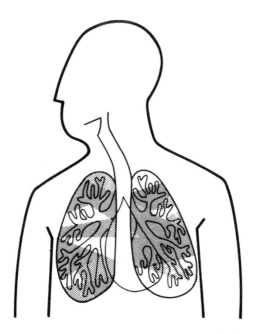

Figure 4.2. Diseased lungs evidence regions with different $\dot{V}_A/\dot{Q}$ ratios. As in Figure 4.1, only a small part of such lungs may participate in alveolar ventilation, resulting in unphysiologic pulmonary ventilation.

so forth. Because of their close proximity, nearly all of the cell lines unavoidably become involved in the disease process precipitated by barotrauma.

As stated, the efficacy and safety of mechanical ventilators has only been demonstrated in patients with neuromuscular disorders when used on those with healthy lungs at normal V_T and respiratory rates and pressures. Extrapolation of these observations to patients with pre-existing pulmonary pathology is unwise. In patients with normal lungs, ventilation proceeded at safe rates and volumes, while maintaining excellent gas exchange during room air ventilation. In those with ventilatory failure due to pulmonary pathology, lung mechanics are grossly abnormal and adequate alveolar ventilation is usually accomplished in a "small" lung at greatly elevated peak airway pressures.

Greenfield et al. (4) in 1964 first showed that 2 hours of mechanical ventilation in previously healthy dogs at a peak inflation pressure of 26–32 cmH$_2$O resulted in significant bilateral pulmonary atelectasis 24 hours later. The minimal surface tension of saline lung lavage fluid in these dogs was greatly elevated, showing that such a brief period of mechanical ventilation could evoke significant injury to alveolar cellular function. Importantly, these changes, which were not immediate while the animals were on mechanical ventilation, were delayed. Similar studies were conducted in 1970 by Barsch et al. (5) in dogs surviving for 22–70 hours at a peak inspiratory pressure of 34 cmH$_2$O. Their lungs demonstrated vascular injury, hyaline membranes, alveolar edema, atelectasis, and hemorrhage. More recently, we (6) ventilated healthy sheep with peak inflation pressures of 50 cmH$_2$O over several days. Depending on respiratory rate, there was progressive deterioration in pulmonary mechanics and gas exchange, leading to such severe lung damage that no form of mechanical ventilation could effect gas exchange. Control animals ventilated at normal V_T and respiratory rates and low peak inflation pressures showed no alterations in lung function.

Hernandez et al. (7) studied the effect of mechanical ventilation at a peak inflation pressure of 45 cmH$_2$O in a rabbit model and measured pulmonary microvascular permeability. They found a fourfold rise in microvascular permeability after 45 minutes of mechanical ventilation. When other rabbits were similarly ventilated, except that they were encased in a full body plaster cast to limit the V_T delivered to normal range, there was no significant rise in microvascular permeability. They concluded that pulmonary injury from high-pressure mechanical ventilation was the result of over distension of airway structures rather than the result of high peak inflation pressures themselves. Studies on microvascular permeability edema and other studies on extravascular lung water content were short-term studies, at relatively high peak inflation pressures for this animal model. It is likely that changes in permeability and lung water content also could occur at lower pressures if time on mechanical ventilation were extended.

As stated, mechanical ventilation in a clinical setting generally presupposes the existence of an underlying parenchymal disease process. Conversely, we assume the existence of some remaining, reasonably healthy pulmonary parenchyma that participates in gas exchange (see Fig. 4.2). These healthy regions are well ventilated and well perfused, while the remaining regions of the lungs are ventilated and perfused at abnormal $\dot{V}_A/\dot{Q}$ ratios. Mechanical ventilation at above normal peak inspiratory pressures preferentially directs most of the gas flow to the most compliant regions of the lungs, subjecting those parts of the lungs to the majority of the volume, and flow, and leads to over expansion well beyond the normal.

Mueller et al. (8) explored how much healthy lung was needed to sustain normal gas exchange in an anesthetized sheep. After surgically removing the left lung (43% of total lung), they had little difficulty ventilating the right lung with conventional mechanical ventilation, at normal peak inspiratory pressure, taking care to use low volumes, and high respiratory rates. It was also possible to sustain ventilation when both the left lung and the right lower lobe had been surgically removed, relying only on the right upper lobe and the right middle lobe (19% of total lung) for pulmonary ventilation. When all lung had been surgically removed except for the right upper lobe ($12\frac{1}{2}$% of total lung), good gas exchange was maintained for the first few hours, while the right upper lobe was ventilated at a respiratory rate up to 120 per minute and at the smallest V_T to sustain eucapnia. After 2 to 3 hours, PaO_2 progressively declined, $PaCO_2$ rose, and peak inspiratory pressure rose, with death occurring within 8 hours. The histologic findings in the right upper lobe showed extensive hyaline membrane formation and other features commonly found in hyaline membrane disease. Thus, although gas exchange was initially normal, prolonged hyperexpansion of normal lung resulted in parenchymal injury due to the mechanical ventilation itself.

In the same sheep model with only the right upper lobe remaining, this same group then applied intratracheal pulmonary ventilation (9), during which fresh gas was introduced directly at the level of the carina through a small catheter. Using this gas flow to reduce dead space ventilation allowed ventilation of the right upper lobe with a tidal volume of 2.5 ml/kg and respiratory rate of 120 per minute. The resultant peak inspiratory pressure was <17 cmH$_2$O. Within 2 hours, those sheep could be weaned to room air ventilation and had peak inspiratory pressures of 12 cmH$_2$O. Therefore, by limiting V_T and minimizing alveolar distension, gas exchange and lung parenchymal integrity were maintained, and mechanical ventilation did not injure normal lungs.

The cardinal step to prevent mechanical ventilation-induced lung injury is to lower the peak inflation pressure. One can choose an appropriately low peak airway pressure by (*a*) using a low V_T (<10–12 ml/kg), (*b*) determining optimal V_T through the construction of a compliance curve, (*c*) avoiding short inspiratory times (or very low inspiratory-to-expiratory time ratios), (*d*) reducing peak flow, (*e*) choosing appropriate ventilatory mode, (*f*) using paralysis and sedation judiciously, (*g*) using only necessary PEEP levels, and (*h*) changing body position. In addition, minimizing CO$_2$ production by controlling body temperature and providing appropriate nutritional support minimizes the minute ventilation required to eliminate CO_2. Permissive hypercapnia (tolerating a mildly elevated $PaCO_2$) also allows reduction of minute ventilation. Finally, limiting F_IO_2 to <0.50 helps prevent cellular damage to the lungs. Experimental strategies, such as pulmonary surfactant administration, may join our armamentarium in several years.

In neonates with severe respiratory distress syndrome and an expected mortality rate of >80% (e.g., patients for whom mechanical ventilation failed in meconium aspiration syndrome or those with congenital diaphragmatic hernia), "resting the lungs" and providing total to near-total gas exchange with an extracorporeal membrane artificial lung, resulted in 80% survival. Those neonates' lungs were ventilated with normal respiratory rates, low peak inflation pressures of 20 cmH_2O and PEEP 3–5 cmH_2O. With these peak airway pressures, V_T was as low as 1–4 ml/kg and aeration was limited to the most compliant parts of the lungs. This experience in the newborn population suggests that adult patients with severe respiratory distress syndrome, who are managed in a similar manner, and provided with total or near-total extracorporeal blood gas exchange, might benefit similarly. Such treatment, if successful, might then be applied to alveolar ventilation control to reduce or to eliminate pulmonary injury from the effects of mechanical ventilation at high peak inflation pressure.

The Consensus Conference on Mechanical Ventilation (10) convened in January 1993 in Northbrook, Illinois. Prior to this conference, laboratory studies had shown persuasively that mechanical ventilation at a peak inspiratory pressure of 40–50 cmH_2O, and even those as low as 30 cmH_2O, was injurious (3–6). Based primarily on animal data, the Consensus Committee recommended that the plateau airway pressure should be maintained <35 cmH_2O, even if the $PaCO_2$ was allowed to remain slightly elevated (permissive hypercapnia). In addition, the Committee recommended that PEEP be used to sustain SaO_2 >90%. The suitability of various treatment modalities is extensively discussed in the proceedings of the Consensus Committee Summary.

Based primarily on laboratory data and some clinical data, we recently questioned accepted views on lung management in acute respiratory failure. Studies by Raszynski et al. (11) and Wilson et al. (12) showed that using intratracheal oxygen insufflation and V_T of 2.5 ml/kg can sustain pulmonary ventilation in patients who otherwise could not be weaned from extracorporeal membrane oxygenation (ECMO). This technique, which used low peak inspiratory pressures, avoided hypercapnia. Our recent laboratory studies showed that normocapnic pulmonary ventilation can be sustained in a lethal adult respiratory distress syndrome (ARDS) model by using intratracheal oxygen and insufflation at normal peak area pressures, V_T of 2–5 ml/kg. The animals in this study recovered over a 2-day period (13). In a follow-up study, continuous positive airway pressure (CPAP) was combined with intratracheal oxygen and insufflation and similar results were obtained (14). In both studies, there was immediate and massive diuresis when converting to intratracheal oxygen and insufflation. In none of the studies was any attempt made to aggressively recruit the lungs with positive area pressure.

There is wide consensus that adverse effects from mechanical ventilation with high peak inspiratory pressures have worsened pulmonary function of ARDS patients. It stands to reason that early efforts at greatly reducing dead space ventilation and maintaining peak airway pressures <30–35 cmH$_2$O, may be the preferred route with respect to the ultimate recovery of the patient.

SUMMARY

Mechanical ventilation of the normal lung at normal airway pressure is well tolerated, save for the discomfort from tracheal intubation and reduced mobility. Adverse effects due to mechanical pulmonary ventilation relate primarily to ventilating healthy parts of the diseased lungs, and lungs still recruitable, at pressures, volumes, and PEEP settings required to sustain adequate alveolar ventilation and required blood oxygenation. Beyond a certain point, mechanical ventilation, itself, may lead to impairment of lung function. Those adverse changes manifest in worsening in lung compliance, barotrauma, changes in microvascular permeability and in a rise in extravascular lung water content, in addition to alterations in the biochemical function of the lung and the resulting systemic effects.

The current trend is to restrict peak inspiratory pressure to <35 cmH$_2$O, and resort to "permissive hypercapnia." Tracheal gas insufflation techniques promise to enhance alveolar ventilation and blood oxygenation and open the possibility to sustain mechanical ventilation at normal or near normal peak inspiratory pressure and with low to very low V$_T$, below what is now considered possible.

References

1. Cane RD, Choppier BA. Mechanical ventilatory support. JAMA 254:87–92, 1985.
2. Mascheroni M, Kolobow T, Fumagalli R. et al. Acute respiratory failure following pharmacologically induced hyperventilation: an experimental animal study. Intensive Care Med 15:8–14, 1988.
3. Tsuno K, Prato P, Kolobow T. Acute lung injury from mechanical ventilation at moderately high airway pressures. J Appl Physiol 69:956–961, 1990.
4. Greenfield LJ, Ebert PA, Benson DW. Effect of positive pressure ventilation on surface tension properties of lung extracts. Anesthesiology 25:312–316, 1984.
5. Barsch J, Birbara C, Eggers GWN, et al. Positive pressure as a cause of respiratory induced lung disease [abstract]. Ann Intern Med 72:810, 1970.
6. Kolobow T, Moretti MP, Fumagalli R, et al. Severe impairment in lung function induced by high peak airway pressure during mechanical ventilation. Am Rev Respir Dis 135:312–315, 1987.

7. Hernandez LA, Peevy KJ, Moise AA, et al. Chest wall restriction limits high airway pressure-induced lung injury in young rabbits. J Appl Physiol 66:2364–2368, 1989.
8. Muller EE, Kolobow T, Mandava S, Jones M, Vitale G, Aprigliano M, Yamada K. How to ventilate lungs as small as $12\frac{1}{2}$% of normal: the new technique of intratracheal pulmonary ventilation. Pediatr Res 34:606–610, 1993.
9. Kolobow T, Powers T, Mandava S, Aprigliano M, Kawaguchi A, Tsuno K, Mueller E. Intratracheal pulmonary ventilation (ITPV): control of positive end-expiratory pressure at the level of the carina through the use of a novel ITPV catheter design. Anest Analg 78:455–461, 1994.
10. Slutsky AS. Consensus conference on mechanical ventilation—January 28–30, 1993 at Northbrook, Illinois, USA. Part 1. Intensive Care Med 20:64–79, 1994.
11. Raszynski A, Hyltquist KA, Lativ H, Susmane J, Soler M, Alam A, Brao J, Amor J, Kilheeney D, Kolobow T, Wolfsdorf J. Rescue from pediatric ECMO with prolonged hybrid intratracheal pulmonary ventilation: a technique for reducing dead space ventilation and preventing ventilator induced lung injury. ASAIO J 39:681–685, 1993.
12. Wilson JM, Thompson JR, Schnitzer JJ, Bower LK, Lillehei CV, Perlman ND, Kolobow T. Intratracheal pulmonary ventilation and congenital diaphragmatic hernia: a report of two cases. J Pediatr Surg 28:484–487, 1993.
13. Rossi N, Kolobow T, Aprigliano M, Tsuno K, Giacomini M. Mechanical ventilation at normal airway pressures in a model of severe ARF using intratracheal pulmonary ventilation (ITPV). Crit Care Med 149:A70, 1994.
14. Giacomini M, Kolobow T, Reali-Forster C. CPAP-intratracheal pulmonary ventilation (CPAP-ITPV) in a model of severe acute respiratory failure (ARF). Crit Care Med 151:A445, 1995.

Suggested Readings

Bakhle YS, Vane JR (eds). Metabolic functions of the lung. New York and Basel, Marcel Dekker, Inc. 1977.

Haake R, Schlichtig R, Ulstad DR, et al. Barotrauma. Pathophysiology, risk factors and prevention. Chest 91:608–613, 1987.

Ryan US (ed). Pulmonary endothelium in health and disease. New York and Basel, Marcel Dekker, Inc., 1987.

Yung JF. Applied respiratory physiology, 3rd ed. London, Boston, Butterworths, 1987.

5
Cardiovascular Effects of Mechanical Ventilation

Azriel Perel • Reuven Pizov

The heart, the great vessels, and the pulmonary vascular bed lie within the chest and are, therefore, directly affected by changes in the intrathoracic pressure that are associated with mechanical ventilation. In addition to changing pressures, the cardiovascular system may also be affected by changes in lung volume, by neuroreflexes, and by the release of neurohumoral substances from the lung tissue. Nevertheless, the substantial change that occurs in the pressure within the chest is the most important determinant of the cardiovascular effects of mechanical ventilation. As mechanical respiratory support often is instituted to increase oxygen transport, an associated decrease in cardiac output may defeat this purpose. Therefore, physicians who administer respiratory support should be well aware of the possible effects of mechanical ventilation on cardiovascular function.

In this chapter, we describe the factors that affect the transmission of airway pressure to the heart and great vessels, the effects of this transmitted pressure on the cardiovascular system under different clinical conditions, and the possible cardiovascular effects of different ventilatory modes. Finally, we describe the respiratory variations in the arterial pressure wave form and explain how these variations can help in assessing cardiovascular function.

TRANSMISSION OF AIRWAY PRESSURE TO THE INTRATHORACIC CARDIOVASCULAR SYSTEM

During spontaneous breathing, both airway pressure and pleural pressure fall with each inspiration, whereas during positive-pressure ventilation both of them increase. Their difference, which is termed the transpulmonary pressure, determines the tidal volume (V_T). During mechanical ventilation, the degree by which the increase in airway pressure is transmitted to the pleural space is determined by the lung and chest wall compliance. Lung compliance equals V_T divided by the change in transpulmonary pressure, whereas chest wall compliance equals V_T divided by the change in pleural pressure. Because compliance of both lung and chest wall are normally about equal, the transpulmonary pressure equals the change in pleural pressure. As the transpulmonary pressure also equals the difference between the changes in the airway and pleural pressures, in normal lungs it is obvious that about one-half of the increase in airway pressure is transmitted to the pleural space, the heart, and the great vessels within the chest.

The change in the pleural pressure during a mechanical breath, thus, depends on the V_T itself and on the lung and chest wall compliance. In the presence of high V_T, high lung compliance, or low chest wall compliance, the increases in pleural pressure will be exaggerated. Low V_T, or low lung or high chest wall compliance minimizes changes in pleural pressure (1).

The dominant cardiovascular effect from mechanical ventilation is a decrease in venous return, which, in turn, depends greatly on the magnitude of the change in pleural pressure. Thus, it is clear why patients with emphysema (high lung compliance), circular bandages around the chest, or large chest burns (low chest wall compliance) are more likely to develop cardiovascular depression, whereas the cardiovascular system of patients with adult respiratory distress syndrome (ARDS), congestive heart failure (low lung compliance), or an open chest after median sternotomy (high chest wall compliance), are relatively more resistant to the effects of mechanical ventilation.

The change in pleural pressure can be directly measured through a catheter introduced into the pleural space (clinically difficult in most cases) or through an existing chest drain. Otherwise, it can be measured by a catheter or a balloon placed in the esophagus, which is clinically practical, although the esophageal pressure tends to underestimate positive-pressure swings. This measurement technique may also underestimate the direct pressure that the lungs exert on the heart during inspiration, which is better measured in experimental models by a pericardial balloon.

A more practical but rarely used technique for assessing change in pleural pressure is the measurement of changes in the central venous pressure (CVP) wave form with each inspiration, as the change in CVP closely approximates the change in pleural pressure (Fig. 5.1). The continuous monitoring of the CVP wave form, thus, gives immediate information to the degree by which airway pressure is transmitted to the pleural space and, in the presence of excessively high airway pressures, enables the observer to differentiate between low lung and low chest wall compliance (Fig. 5.2).

When the pleural pressure is subtracted from intravascular pressures measured within the chest, the resulting transmural or filling pressures are a true measure of intravascular pressure changes during mechanical ventilation. When transmural pressures are not available, intrathoracic vascular pressures, such as CVP, pulmonary artery, pulmonary capillary wedge, and left atrial, should at least be read directly from the monitor at end-expiration to eliminate the negative fluctuations of spontaneous breathing or the positive fluctuations of mechanical ventilation on these pressures. Reading pressures from the digital readout of monitors may be misleading in the presence of large swings in pleural pressure.

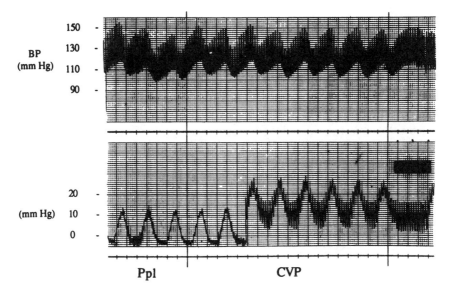

Figure 5.1. The wave forms of central venous pressure (CVP) and directly measured pleural pressure. Note that the inspiratory increases in CVP and pleural pressure (Ppl) are equal.

When measuring CVP or pulmonary capillary wedge pressure, one should not disconnect the patient from the ventilator or flatten the bed. Such maneuvers may cause acute hemodynamic changes, induce stress, and promote pulmonary edema, especially in patients whose extravascular lung water content is high and whose positive end-expiratory pressure (PEEP) level is >10 cmH$_2$O. From the considerations mentioned, it is clear that a PEEP level of 10 cmH$_2$O will cause intrathoracic vascular pressures to increase by ~5 cmH$_2$O when lung compliance is normal. In edematous noncompliant lungs, this PEEP effect on intrathoracic vascular pressures will be much smaller, whereas in emphysematous patients it will be exaggerated.

Because mechanical ventilation exerts its cardiovascular effects through changes in the airway pressure and because the airway pressure wave form is very variable depending on the mode of ventilation used, it is useful to quantify airway pressure as a mean value.

HOW DOES MECHANICAL VENTILATION AFFECT CARDIAC OUTPUT?

The best known and, indeed, most important circulatory effect of mechanical ventilation is to reduce venous return as intrathoracic pressure rises during a me-

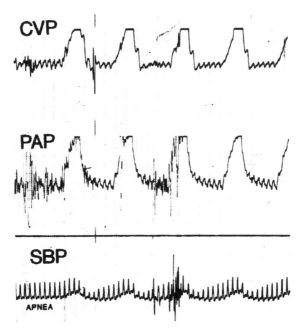

Figure 5.2. Central venous pressure (CVP), pulmonary artery pressure (PAP), and systemic arterial blood pressure (SBP) wave forms of a patient following massive resuscitation for ruptured aortic aneurysm. The extreme inspiratory increases of the CVP wave form are indicative of the increases in the pleural pressure due to the reduction in the compliance of the very edematous chest wall. Note also the severe depression of arterial pressure with each mechanical breath.

chanical breath. However, its effects on the circulation are more complex because it may affect, to varying degrees, all the factors that determine the cardiac output (i.e., preload, afterload, contractility, and heart rate).

The direct effects of mechanical ventilation on cardiac contractility are often associated with changes in preload and afterload, and are probably of little clinical significance in most cases. The heart rate also is not significantly affected by mechanical ventilation per se under normal conditions, even though a vagally mediated vasodepressor reflex may be associated with lung hyperinflation. However, when mechanical ventilation improves hypoxemia or hypercarbia, or when it significantly reduces the work of breathing, it may also normalize associated changes in heart rate. In this respect, it is important to note that when cardiac output is increased due to increased work of breathing and the stress associated with it, instituting mechanical ventilation may beneficially lower the cardiac output simply due to the decrease in oxygen demand. Thus, reduction of cardiac output with institution of mechanical ventilation is not necessarily a bad sign.

The main circulatory effects of mechanical ventilation are on the preload and afterload of the right and left ventricles. The preload, which is the length of the cardiac muscle fibers at the beginning of contraction, is estimated by the amount of blood present in the ventricle at end-diastole. The afterload is the myocardial tension that develops during systole, usually equated with the vascular resistance that the ventricle must overcome to eject blood.

The increase in intrathoracic pressure during a mechanical breath has two major effects on preload: (*a*) The preload of the right ventricle (i.e., the venous return) decreases as vena caval and right atrial pressures increase and blood is hindered from entering the chest. (*b*) The preload of the left ventricle increases as blood is squeezed from the pulmonary vascular bed through the pulmonary veins into the left atrium and ventricle. Thus, with the initiation of a positive-pressure breath, there is a growing disparity between the outputs of both ventricles, that of the right ventricle decreases and that of the left ventricle increases (2). Later, when the intrathoracic pressure returns to its end-expiratory value, the preload of the right side increases as the venous blood eventually enters the chest without difficulty, while the preload to the left side diminishes as the relatively smaller right ventricular stroke outputs of the preceding inspiration traverse the pulmonary circulation and reach the left ventricle. Thus, during late inspiration and early expiration, right ventricular output becomes greater than that of the left ventricle (2). The cyclic changes in the left ventricular stroke output are reflected by the arterial pressure wave form (Fig. 5.3), which is discussed below. These changes account also for the significant variability of random measurements of cardiac output using the thermodilution technique in ventilated patients (3). Cardiac output thermodilution measurement variability in ventilated patients may also be due to the surprisingly high incidence of tricuspid regurgitation and vena caval backward flow also found in mechanically ventilated patients (4).

The increase in intrathoracic pressure also affects right and left ventricular afterloads. Normally, the right ventricular afterload (i.e., pulmonary vascular resistance) is minimal at resting lung volume, functional residual capacity (FRC). As lung volume increases, major pulmonary vessels dilate and their resistance falls, while juxta-alveolar vessels are compressed by the inflating alveoli and their resistance increases. The overall change in pulmonary vascular resistance during mechanical ventilation of normal lungs is, therefore, not significant. However, in patients with hyperinflated lungs due to chronic obstructive lung disease, asthma, or high levels of PEEP, additional increase in lung volume may significantly increase right ventricular afterload. The introduction of the thermodilution pulmonary artery catheter with rapid response thermistor enables a better estimation of right heart function under different clinical conditions. Several studies undertaken in patients ventilated with different PEEP levels have shown that pulmonary vascular resistance increases gradually with increasing airway pressures. Right ventricular

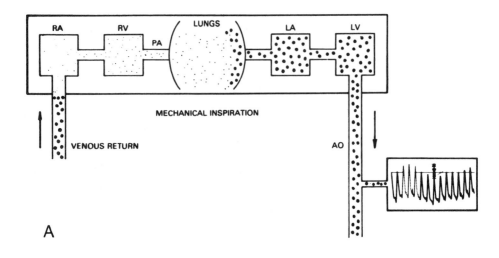

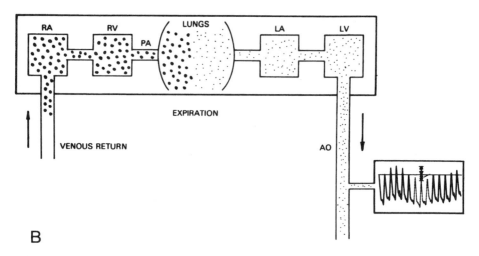

Figure 5.3. Schematic diagram of the circulation showing the effect of a positive-pressure breath on the preloads of the right (RV) and left (LV) ventricles. The changes in left ventricular stroke output are reflected in the arterial pressure, which increases during early inspiration and later decreases as a result of the inspiratory decrease in venous return. AO, aorta; LA, left atrial.

contractility, however, remained preserved until pulmonary artery pressure rose to critical levels (5).

The effect of increased airway pressure on left ventricular afterload has been the subject of much interest in recent years. When airway pressure increases, the associated increase in pleural pressure is transmitted to the left ventricle and the thoracic aorta. Thus, their pressures are transiently increased relative to the extra-thoracic aorta, and the tension that the left ventricle has to develop to eject blood is decreased (i.e., afterload) (6). In contrast, the significant decreases in pleural pressure associated with spontaneous ventilation during upper airway obstruction, severe bronchospasm, or severely decreased lung compliance, have been shown to increase left ventricular afterload and influence cardiac performance considerably (7).

We have hitherto described the various effects of a mechanical breath on the preload and afterload of the right and left ventricles. The ultimate result of these effects on the cardiac output depend on the baseline cardiovascular function. In the presence of hypovolemia, cardiac output is greatly influenced by any further change in the inadequate venous return. Thus, the decrease in venous return that is associated with mechanical ventilation may dramatically decrease cardiac output, especially when high mean airway pressure is applied. During hypervolemia, however, the decrease in venous return associated with the mechanical breath will not affect cardiac output to any great extent and, indeed, volume loading has been repeatedly shown to negate the depressive cardiovascular effects of mechanical ventilation. During hypervolemia, the increase in left ventricular preload during inspiration is much more significant than during hypovolemia due to the large quantity of blood that enters the left ventricle from the congested pulmonary vasculature. The resulting cardiac output depends on the ability of the left ventricle to cope with this additional preload. The simultaneous decrease in left ventricular afterload can be of significance under these circumstances.

Controlled mechanical ventilation (CMV) also has been shown to have beneficial effects on the cardiovascular system. CMV prevented ischemia in patients with acute myocardial infarction (8). It also augmented cardiac output when phasic high intrathoracic pressure was applied to patients in congestive heart failure (9). The most extreme example of the beneficial effects of increased airway pressure on cardiac output is that arterial pressure and consciousness could be maintained during ventricular fibrillation by vigorous coughing (10). In addition, the decrease in the work of breathing, improved oxygenation, and reduction in both the preload of the right ventricle and the afterload of left ventricle make mechanical ventilation an especially important therapeutic intervention in patients with myocardial is-chemia, cariogenic shock, or pulmonary edema. The use of a continuous positive airway pressure (CPAP) mask in cardiogenic pulmonary edema can have strikingly beneficial hemodynamic effects: in addition to those mentioned, the patient senses an immediate relief of dyspnea as FRC increases and the pulmonary edema fluid gets flattened on the surface of the tracheobronchial tree. (See, also, Chapter 15, Noninvasive Ventilation.) This is another example wherein reduction in blood pressure and heart rate usually indicates that a beneficial decrease in the symentho-adrenal response has occurred.

To summarize, the cardiovascular effects of mechanical ventilation will be determined by the magnitude of airway pressure, the degree to which this pressure is transmitted to the pleural space and intrathoracic great vessels, and, above all, the baseline hemodynamic condition of the patient. All of these factors must be taken into account in selecting the appropriate ventilation mode.

EFFECTS OF VARIOUS VENTILATION MODES ON THE CARDIOVASCULAR SYSTEM

The choice of a ventilation mode and the ventilatory parameters should take into account not only the prospective changes in oxygenation and ventilation, but also the possible cardiovascular effects. In this section, we describe the most commonly encountered cardiovascular effects of various ventilation modes.

Spontaneous Ventilation

Spontaneous ventilation is, theoretically, the ventilatory mode which usually has the best hemodynamic effect because it enhances venous return. Its inclusion in the various modes of partial ventilatory support and during the application of PEEP partially offsets the often harmful effects of increased intrathoracic pressure on hemodynamics. Spontaneous ventilation should be the ventilation mode of choice in hypovolemic patients, although there are often overriding considerations for instituting CMV during hypovolemia (e.g., decreased consciousness, decreased ventilatory drive, and impending cardiovascular collapse). When the inspiratory negative swings in pleural pressure are exaggerated (e.g., in acute asthma, upper airway obstruction, or low lung compliance), cardiac output may decrease owing to the significant increase in left ventricular afterload (7). Also, significant inspiratory effort increases intra-abdominal pressure as a result of maximal diaphragmatic contraction. Such increase in intra-abdominal pressure may cause the inferior vena cava to collapse and decrease venous return. Significant inspiratory decreases in systolic blood pressure are a well-known sign of hypovolemia in spontaneously breathing (and mechanically ventilated) patients. In addition, very low pleural and, hence, pulmonary interstitial pressures, may also cause an increase in the extravascular lung water content, the extreme being postobstructive pulmonary edema. It is important to note, however, that spontaneously breathing patients who have increased lung water due to a microvascular permeability defect, may develop frank alveolar pulmonary edema following endotracheal intubation owing to the loss of the glottic mechanism that is responsible for creating intrinsic PEEP. Thus, in these patients, the introduction of an endotracheal tube may necessitate adding some form of ventilatory assistance as well as PEEP.

Spontaneous ventilation also may be associated with high cardiac output due to increased work of breathing. Therefore, the decrease in cardiac output that may follow the institution of mechanical ventilation does not necessarily reflect cardiovascular depression.

Controlled Mechanical Ventilation

Continuous mechanical ventilation is usually well tolerated by most normovolemic patients, and may actually support circulation in patients with congestive heart failure. Its cardiovascular effects will depend on the V_T, the respiratory rate, and the inspiratory/expiratory ratio, which ultimately determine the mean airway pressure. In order to minimize its hemodynamic effects in hypovolemic patients who have no respiratory problem, V_T of not more than 7–10 ml/kg, respiratory rate of 7–10/minute, and an inspiratory/expiratory ratio of 1:3 should be used. It is important to realize that the end-tidal CO_2 in these patients may greatly underestimate $PaCO_2$ due to the reduced pulmonary blood flow and increased dead space.

Special attention is needed in patients who are deliberately hyperventilated due to brain edema, as the resulting high mean airway pressure may reduce cardiac output even in seemingly normovolemic patients. The institution of hyperventilation for titration of blood pH in other circumstances is very rarely justified, and nearly always harmful to cardiovascular function. Deliberate hypoventilation, better known as permissive hypercapnia, is used nowadays as part of the management of severe ARDS and may cause pulmonary hypertension and lead to impaired left ventricular (LV) function (11). Such untoward response to hypercarbia may be prevented if the tidal volume is decreased gradually (12).

Assist/Controlled Mechanical Ventilation

Assist/controlled mechanical ventilation usually is associated with high mean airway pressure because each spontaneous breath triggers a mechanical one. This is especially true in patients with persistently increased ventilatory drive (e.g., some forms of head injury, severe metabolic acidosis, or pulmonary edema). In addition to the possible decrease in cardiac output, the resulting respiratory alkalosis may cause hypokalemia and hypocalcemia that may cause arrhythmias.

Intermittent Mandatory Ventilation/Synchronized Intermittent Mandatory Ventilation

Intermittent mandatory ventilation/synchronized intermittent mandatory ventilation (IMV/SIMV) supplements the patient's spontaneous breathing and usually supplies the minimal number of mechanical breaths necessary to maintain a normal pH. The negative pleural pressure during the spontaneous breaths and the reduction in the number of mechanical breaths compared with CMV produce a lower mean airway pressure that may be beneficial to the cardiovascular system. Indeed, the advocates of very high PEEP levels for the treatment of severe ARDS claim that IMV, combined with volume loading, prevented cardiovascular deterioration in their patients.

Before the introduction of SIMV, it was feared that the possible delivery of a mechanical breath on top of a spontaneous one ("stacking") might cause cardiovascular depression, as well as increase the danger of barotrauma. Although this theoretical effect of IMV was never demonstrated, most new ventilators incorporate SIMV as a standard feature. IMV may also affect the cardiovascular system by imposing excessive inspiratory resistance owing to insensitive demand valves, especially when a significant PEEP level is present. Such increased respiratory work may lead to unnecessary and possibly harmful increases in catecholamine secretion, cardiac output, and oxygen consumption, as well as respiratory fatigue and failure of weaning. Such significant loading of the respiratory muscles may already occur when the IMV rate is reduced by 50% during the weaning process.

Positive-End Expiratory Pressure/Continuous Positive Airway Pressure

Positive-end expiratory pressure/continuous positive airway pressure is associated with an increase in airway pressure that is continuous rather than transient. Thus, any increase in PEEP causes an identical increase in the mean airway pressure. Therefore, PEEP is notorious for decreasing cardiac output whenever the intravascular volume cannot sustain a considerable increase in airway pressure. Although the main mechanism in the decrease of cardiac output by PEEP is inadequate preload, it seems that high PEEP levels may also cause an increase in the size of the right ventricle and a leftward shift of the interventricular septum, resulting in a decrease in left ventricular size, compliance, and contractility. The detrimental cardiovascular effects of PEEP in ARDS patients may be minimized by gradually reducing the tidal volume to 5–8 ml/kg (12).

Positive-end expiratory pressure may be hemodynamically beneficial in the treatment of cardiogenic pulmonary edema because it reduces preload, improves oxygenation, ameliorates lung compliance, and reduces the work of breathing and the subjective feeling of breathlessness. Because the hemodynamic effects of PEEP may be more significant than its respiratory effects, its overall influence on oxygen delivery (cardiac output $\times$ arterial oxygen content) should always be considered or actually measured, especially when high PEEP levels are administered.

The actual PEEP level is not always fully appreciated by the ventilator pressure gauge and when expiration is not given adequate time, especially in the presence of bronchoconstriction, auto-PEEP is created (i.e., the end-expiratory pressure in the distal airways is more positive than that in the proximal airways). Because auto-PEEP can have detrimental effects on hemodynamics, its presence should be clinically recognized by observing the capnograph or the expiratory flow trace, both showing incomplete exhalation. External PEEP applied to counterbalance auto-PEEP has not caused any further hemodynamic effects in patients with chronic obstructive pulmonary disease (13).

Pressure Support Ventilation

Pressure support may cause a considerable increase in mean airway pressure as each spontaneous breath is augmented to a preset pressure level. When that level is in excess of 15–20 cmH$_2$O, pressure support should be considered to be a controlled mode of ventilation, although the patient is "breathing spontaneously." Typically, when the level of the pressure support is increased, the respiratory rate decreases, so that the overall effect on the mean airway pressure may vary. An increase in mean airway pressure may be associated with a decrease in peak airway pressure.

High Frequency Ventilation

High frequency ventilation is characterized by low volumes and pressures. It has therefore been advocated as a ventilatory mode of choice for hypovolemic patients. However, the mere use of high frequency ventilation does not guarantee low airway pressures as the V$_T$ necessary to provide adequate gas exchange may be considerable. In addition, the increase in FRC due to air-trapping may be significant and cause hemodynamic deterioration. Thus, high frequency ventilation is rarely practical in supporting the systemic circulation and careful measurement of airway pressures near the carina is necessary to avoid inadvertently high P$_{aw}$. High frequency jet ventilation has also been used to augment cardiac output by synchronizing jet delivery to early systole. This method, which is still considered experimental, aims to achieve maximal cardiac output by synchronizing the afterload reducing effect associated with the increased airway with left ventricular systole.

Inverse-Ratio Ventilation

Inverse-ratio ventilation is associated usually with high mean airway pressure as the intrathoracic pressure is elevated during most of the respiratory cycle. The degree of the increase in mean airway pressure depends on the inspiratory-to-expiratory time (I/E) ratio, as well as on the levels of the extrinsic and intrinsic PEEP. Thus, increasing the I/E ratio may lead to a considerable depression of the cardiac output. Limiting the peak airway pressure-controlled inverse ratio ventilation (PC-IRV) may limit the potential detrimental hemodynamic effect.

Large fluctuations in the cardiac output may occur during the inversed respiratory cycle so that thermodilution results may be more variable than usual.

Airway Pressure Release Ventilation

Airway pressure release ventilation is theoretically associated with lower mean airway pressure compared with CPAP, as gas exchange is achieved by intermittent CPAP release. Indeed, airway pressure release ventilation was shown to improve cardiac output considerably compared with conventional positive-pressure ventilation in patients who required CPAP. However, the users of this mode should be wary of those patients in whom CPAP release results in inadequate V_T. Increasing the CPAP level in order to increase the volume of gas that is released during each breath may eventually result in an inadvertently high mean airway pressure, which may be detrimental to the cardiovascular system.

CARDIOVASCULAR EFFECTS OF MECHANICAL VENTILATION AS REFLECTED BY THE ARTERIAL PRESSURE WAVE FORM

The systolic pressure variation is the difference between the maximal and minimal values of the systolic pressure during one respiratory cycle (14,15). It is com-

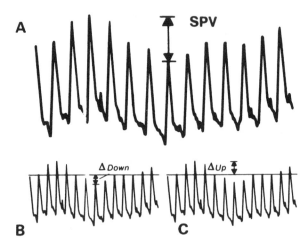

Figure 5.4. The systolic pressure variation (SPV) is the difference between the maximal and minimal values of the systolic pressure during one mechanical breath. It is composed of the Δup and Δdown, which are the respective increase and decrease in systolic pressure relative to its value during a short apnea.

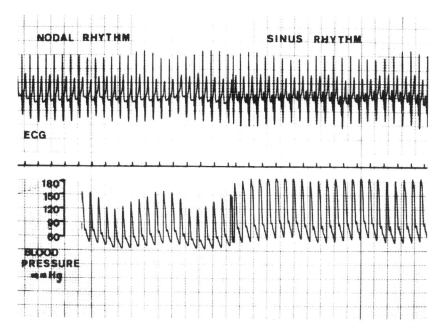

Figure 5.5. The significant respiratory variations in the arterial pressure wave form during nodal rhythm reflect a reduction in effective preload. Note the change in the systolic pressure variation when sinus rhythm is restored.

posed of the delta up (Δup) segment, which is the difference between the maximal systolic pressure and the systolic pressure during the preinspiratory period or during a short apnea, and the delta down (Δdown) segment, which is the difference between the systolic pressure at apnea and the minimal value of systolic pressure during the respiratory cycle (Fig. 5.4). Each of these segments has a distinct physiologic significance, the Δup being a measure of the inspiratory augmentation of cardiac output and the Δdown, which is a measure of the decrease in venous return (see Fig. 5.3).

In patients who were mechanically ventilated following vascular surgery, the mean systolic pressure variation, Δup and Δdown were found to be 8.6, 2.7, and 5.9 mmHg respectively (16). In another group of 226 intensive care unit (ICU) patients the mean systolic pressure variation was 9.2 mmHg and correlated significantly with the pulmonary artery occlusion pressure (17).

During hypovolemia, when the cardiac output is extremely dependent on venous return, each mechanical breath will cause a significant Δdown segment, creating the well-known "hypovolemic curve." Assessing the size of the Δdown is extremely useful in cases of latent hypovolemia, when a normal blood pressure is maintained by excessive systemic vascular resistance. In a model of graded hemorrhage in dogs, the Δdown and the cardiac output were equal in their ability to reflect latent hypovolemia, whereas other commonly measured hemodynamic variables did not change significantly (14). During active hemorrhage in patients it was found that the removal of 1000 ml of blood was associated with a systolic pressure variation of 19.6 mmHg, which decreased by about 8.6 mmHg on the first 500-ml volume replacement (18). A significant Δdown segment may also appear in other conditions that decrease preload. These include the use of large tidal volumes, the presence of a low chest wall compliance (see Fig. 5.2), and the development of a nodal rhythm (Fig. 5.5).

Although a significant Δdown segment reflects inadequate preload, its total disappearance is an important characteristic of congestive heart failure (19). This is a reflection of the fact that inspiratory decrease in venous return does not affect left ventricular stroke output. Thus, the arterial pressure wave form of a ventilated patient can differentiate between hypovolemia (large Δdown) and reduced contractility associated with increased preload (minimal Δdown).

As the role of mechanical ventilation in improving cardiac output in cardiac patients is gaining more recognition, the existence of a significant Δup segment

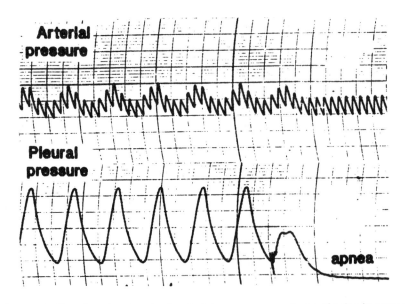

Figure 5.6. The pleural and systemic arterial pressure wave forms of a dog in congestive heart failure, during ventilation with positive-pressure ventilation combined with synchronized external chest compression, and during apnea. Note that the respiratory variations in systolic pressure are positive only (i.e., Δup is the dominant variability denoting a positive cardiovascular effect of mechanical ventilation).

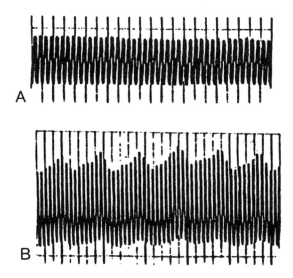

Figure 5.7. The arterial pressure wave form during separation from cardiopulmonary bypass: **A,** Arterial pressure during first unsuccessful attempt shows no Δup. The heart is enlarged and contracts poorly. **B,** Arterial pressure during second successful attempt, after repair and addition of coronary graft, shows restoration of left ventricular volume responsiveness.

should be sought as proof of such beneficial effect. Both during hypervolemia, as well as in a model of congestive heart failure in dogs, it was indeed shown that the Δup is the dominant variable of the arterial pressure wave form (19) (Fig. 5.6).

Another condition where the Δup is of extreme importance is during separation from cardiopulmonary bypass. Although the chest is open and mechanical ventilation has little effect on venous return, each breath normally creates a Δup segment owing to the increased pulmonary venous return to the left side of the heart. The absence of such Δup segment during the crucial period of separation from cardiopulmonary bypass is a sign of the nonresponsiveness of the left ventricle to increased volume. Such nonresponsiveness is due most commonly to ischemic left ventricular dysfunction and is a unique sign of inadequate or nonfunctioning coronary grafts (Fig. 5.7). Thus, arterial pressure wave form analysis is a simple, readily available monitoring technique in ventilated patients. The V_T serves as a repetitive challenge to the cardiovascular system, whereas the information derived from the systolic pressure variation, Δup, and Δdown is equal to a two-point Starling curve because it evaluates the response of left ventricular stroke output to a change in preload. We are currently examining the usefulness of the Respiratory Systolic Variation Test, which is a respiratory maneuver that includes four successive pressure-controlled breaths. The line of best fit that connects the four lowest respective systolic pressures after each breath should reflect volume responsiveness in a manner similar to the LV function Starling curve. Thus, pressure wave form analysis in ventilated patients can be used to assess baseline cardiovascular function, to follow up on the effects of volume therapy, and to assess the effects of mechanical ventilation on the circulation.

References

1. Chapin JC, Downs JB, Douglas ME, et al. Lung expansion, airway pressure transmission, and positive end-expiratory pressure. Arch Surg 114:1193–1197, 1979.
2. Jardin F, Farcot JC, Gueret P, et al. Cyclic changes in arterial pulse during respiratory support. Circulation 68:266–274, 1983.
3. Jansen JRC, Schreuder JJ, Settels JJ, et al. An adequate strategy for the thermodilution technique in patients during mechanical ventilation. Intensive Care Med 16:422–425, 1990.
4. JullienT, Valtier B, Hongnat JM, et al. Incidence of tricuspid regurgitation and vena caval backward flow in mechanically ventilated patients. Chest 107:488–493, 1995.
5. Biondi JW, Schulman DS, Soufer R, et al. The effect of incremental positive end-expiratory pressure on right ventricular hemodynamics and ejection fraction. Anesth Analg 67:144–151, 1988.
6. Robotham JL, Cherry D, Mitzner W, et al. A re-evaluation of the hemodynamic consequences of intermittent positive pressure ventilation. Crit Care Med 11:783–793, 1983.
7. Buda AG, Pinsky MR, Ingels NB, et al. Effect of intrathoracic pressure on left ventricular performance. N Engl J Med 301:453–459, 1979.
8. Rasanen J, Nikki P, Heikkila J. Acute myocardial infarction complicated by respiratory failure. The effects of mechanical ventilation. Chest 85:21–28, 1984.
9. Pinsky MR, Summer WR. Cardiac augmentation by phasic high intrathoracic pressure support in man. Chest 84:370–375, 1983.
10. Niemann JT, Rosborough J, Hausknecht M, et al. Cough-CPR. Documentation of systemic perfusion in man and in an experimental model: a "window" to the mechanism of blood flow in external CPR. Crit Care Med 8:141–146, 1980.
11. Feihl F, Peret C. Permissive hypercapnia. How permissive should it be? Am J Respir Crit Care Med 150:1722–1737, 1994.
12. Ranieri VM, Mascia L, Fiore T, et al. Cardiorespiratory effects of positive end-expiratory pressure during progressive tidal volume reduction (permissive hypercapnia) in patients with acute respiratory distress syndrome. Anesthesiology 83:710–720, 1995.
13. Baigorri F, De Monte A, Blanch L, et al. Hemodynamic responses to external counterbalancing of auto-positive end-expiratory pressure in mechanically ventilated patients with chronic obstructive pulmonary disease. Crit Care Med 22:1782–1791,1994.
14. Perel A, Pizov R, Cotev S. The systolic pressure variation is a sensitive indicator of hypovolemia in ventilated dogs subjected to graded hemorrhage. Anesthesiology 67:498–502, 1987.
15. Perel A, Segal E, Pizov R. Assessment of cardiovascular function by pressure wave form analysis. In Vincent JL. Update in Intensive Care and Emergency Medicine 1989. Heidelberg, Springer Verlag, 1989, pp 542–550.
16. Coriat P, Vrillon M, Perel A, et al. A comparison of systolic pressure variations and echocardiographic estimates of end-diastolic left ventricular size in patients after aortic surgery. Anesth Analg 78:46–53, 1994.

17. Marik PE. The systolic pressure variation as an indicator of pulmonary capillary wedge pressure in ventilated patients. Anaesth Intensive Care 21:405–408, 1993.
18. Rooke GA, Schwid HA, Shapira Y. The effect of graded hemorrhage and intravascular volume replacement on systolic pressure variations in humans during mechanical and spontaneous ventilation. Anesth Analg 80:925–932, 1995.
19. Pizov R, Ya'ari Y, Perel A. The arterial pressure waveform during acute ventricular failure and synchronized external chest compression. Anesth Analg 68:150–156, 1989.

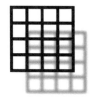

6
Positive-pressure Ventilation: Renal, Hepatic, and Gastrointestinal Function

Howard B. Bennett • Jeffery S. Vender

Critically ill patients are at risk of succumbing to their primary disease or to the undesired sequelae associated with their therapy. Although frequently lifesaving, airway pressure therapy has numerous undesired physiologic consequences. Positive-pressure ventilation (PPV) and positive end-expiratory pressure (PEEP), typically, are the most discussed forms of airway pressure therapy. Although not commonly recognized as important effects of PPV or PEEP, alterations in renal, hepatic, and gastrointestinal functions have been described. Although individual articles have addressed specific forms of airway pressure therapy, this chapter discusses PPV and PEEP interchangeably.

POSITIVE-PRESSURE VENTILATION: RENAL FUNCTION

The relationship between PPV and renal function has been studied by numerous investigators. In 1947, Drury et al. first reported a decrease in urine output in human subjects exposed to PPV (1). Despite a wide variation in experimental design, investigators have repeatedly concluded that PPV is responsible for an overall decline in renal function.

In animal studies, Hall et al. (2) and Gammanpila et al. (3) demonstrated a decline in urine output, glomerular filtration rate, and urinary sodium. In 1968, Sladen et al. (4) described a group of patients receiving PPV who retained water and developed a decrease in serum sodium concentration and hematocrit. Those studies inferred that PPV institution was responsible for the reported change. Geiger et al. (5) studied another group of patients receiving PPV who developed similar changes in renal function. In seven patients on positive-pressure ventilation, Annat et al. (6) demonstrated decreases in urinary output (34%), glomerular filtration rate (19%), renal blood flow (32%), and sodium excretion (33%). The mechanisms responsible for the decline in renal function induced by PPV are

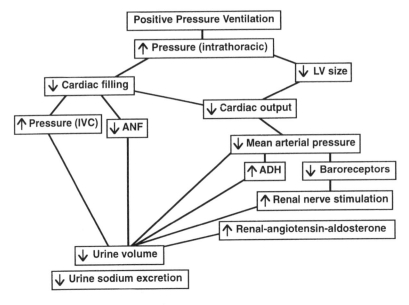

Figure 6.1. Schematic representation of the multiple effects of positive pressure ventilation on renal function. ADH, antidiuretic hormone; IVC, inferior vena cava; LV, left ventricular; ANF, atrial natriuretic factor.

not clearly understood, but they appear multifactorial (Fig. 6.1). The proposed mechanisms can be divided into two broad categories.

Direct:
  Decreased cardiac output
  Redistribution of renal blood flow
  Altered venous pressure
Indirect:
  Sympathetic stimulation
  Hormonal changes

Decreased Cardiac Output

The decline in cardiac output in response to PPV is attributable to at least three mechanisms (see, also Chapter 5, Cardiovascular Effects of Mechanical Ventilation):

1. Decreased venous return to the right side of the heart
2. Right ventricular dysfunction
3. Alterations in left ventricular distensibility

These mechanisms directly decrease cardiac output and, subsequently, renal blood flow. Ultimately, a decrease in urine output, glomerular filtration rate, and urine sodium excretion will result. Most studies demonstrating a decline in renal function during PPV have observed a simultaneous decrease in cardiac output. This would suggest a cause-and-effect relationship between reduced cardiac output and impaired renal function. A direct effect, however, of decreased cardiac output on renal function is difficult to establish because of simultaneous changes in arterial perfusion pressure, intravascular volume, and possible changes in intrarenal blood flow distribution. Priebe et al. (7) demonstrated that the restoration of intravascular volume by transfusion of 25 ml/kg of autologous blood, despite a continued decline in cardiac output, restored renal function to its pre-PPV status in dogs. Venus et al. (8) demonstrated that aggressive crystalloid administration likewise prevented the adverse renal effects of PPV, although in this study, cardiac output was maintained.

Redistribution of Renal Blood Flow

Changes in intrarenal blood flow distribution as a direct result of PPV also have been postulated to be responsible for the observed decline in renal function. As renal juxtamedullary perfusion increases, the fractional reabsorption of sodium increases and urinary sodium decreases. A study in dogs demonstrated a correlation between PPV and an increase in the percentage of renal blood flow perfusing the juxtamedullary zone as well as a slight decrease in perfusion of the outer renal cortex (2). No change in total renal blood flow was noted. This report that no change occurred in total renal blood flow despite a fall in cardiac output is in contrast to the work of other investigators (3). Redistribution of renal blood flow may directly contribute to changes in renal function associated with PPV, but its role, if any, is probably not significant.

Increased Venous Pressure

A third factor proposed as directly contributing to the decline in renal function associated with PPV relates to the fall in renal perfusion pressure due to an increase in renal venous pressure. This increase in renal venous pressure is secondary to an increase in intrathoracic pressure, thereby increasing the inferior vena caval pressure, and ultimately increasing renal venous pressure. It is unlikely that a rise in renal venous pressure alone is sufficient to explain any significant decline in renal function associated with PPV; however, it may have additive effects when a fall in systemic arterial pressure occurs.

Autonomic Innervation

Neurohormonal responses are reported to be indirectly responsible for the decline in renal function seen in association with PPV. The kidneys have autonomic innervation via the renal sympathetic nerves. These nerves are affected by changes in carotid sinus baroreceptor activity. A decrease in baroreceptor stimulation in response to a fall in mean arterial pressure results in an increase in renal sympathetic stimulation. Renal sympathetic nerve stimulation results in a decrease in both renal blood flow and renal sodium excretion. Katz and Shear (9) occluded the carotid arteries in dogs, eliminating baroreceptor stimulation, thus increasing renal sympathetic stimulation. Conversely, Berne (10) demonstrated an increase in renal function in dogs after renal denervation. In another study, Fewell and Bond (11) compared dogs with intact nervous systems to dogs with denervated carotid baroreceptors. As expected, dogs with intact nervous systems had the usual decline in renal function associated with PPV whereas denervated dogs had no changes in renal function. These studies demonstrate that renal sympathetic stimulation in response to decrease firing of carotid baroreceptors contributes to the decline in renal function associated with PPV.

Antidiuretic Hormone

Several researchers have investigated antidiuretic hormone (ADH) and have reached conflicting conclusions as to its role in contributing to the renal effects of PPV. ADH acts to permit diffusion of water out of renal-collecting tubules into the interstitium, resulting in hyperosmolar urine excretion. In the absence of ADH, the collecting ducts are impermeable to water and a dilute urine is produced. An increased ADH concentration would alter renal function in a manner consistent with the clinical findings of water retention and hyponatremia observed in patients described by several investigators. Baratz and Ingraham (12) measured a large increase in ADH associated with oliguria in dogs receiving PPV. Hemmer et al. (13) demonstrated a significant rise in ADH in patients receiving PPV, which subsequently declined as PPV was withdrawn. Other studies demonstrating similar elevations in ADH were not accompanied by expected changes in urine osmolarity and free water clearance. This would argue against a primary role of ADH in the pathogenesis of oliguria in subjects receiving PPV. Finally, a 1987 study by Payen et al. (14) failed to demonstrate any rise in plasma levels of ADH in patients receiving PPV. Because ADH also is a potent vasoconstrictor, some experts have suggested that elevations in ADH are in response to a decline in cardiac output and that they may assist in restoring compromised hemodynamics, rather than primarily affecting renal function. At present, the contribution of ADH to the decline in renal function remains unclear.

Renin-Angiotensin-Aldosterone

The renin-angiotensin-aldosterone hormonal pathway has been shown to contribute to the decline in renal function associated with PPV. Renin, an enzyme produced by renal juxtaglomerular cells, is released in response to renal blood flow changes, renal sympathetic stimulation, and the fluid composition in the distal tubule. It has no known physiologic actions, but it acts on its substrate angiotensinogen to release angiotensin I. Angiotensin I is rapidly converted to angiotensin II, a potent systemic and renal vasoconstrictor. Angiotensin II is also a major factor stimulating the release of aldosterone. Elevations in aldosterone act on the kidney to decrease urinary sodium excretion.

Positive-pressure ventilation has been cited as a potential stimulant for the renin-angiotensin-aldosterone cascade. PPV in dogs produced an increase in renin concentration and an expected decrease in urine volume (15). Additionally, an increase in plasma renin concentration was also demonstrated in dogs with a single denervated kidney (15). This would suggest that renal innervation is not necessary for the release of renin. Annat et al. (6) studied seven patients receiving PPV and demonstrated a simultaneous rise in plasma renin activity and aldosterone levels in addition to a decline in urine output. They attributed these findings, however, as most likely mediated by changes in renal perfusion or renal sympathetic stimulation rather than directly by PPV. Although studies are inconclusive, the renin-angiotensin-aldosterone cascade appears to play a significant role in PPV-induced changes in renal function.

Atrial Natriuretic Factor

Another hormone is involved in the antidiuresis associated with PPV. Atrial natriuretic factor is synthesized and stored by the cardiac atria and released in response to increases in atrial distension. Atrial natriuretic factor possesses potent natriuretic and diuretic properties, as well as an inhibitory effect on renin and aldosterone secretion. Conditions that increase atrial distension (e.g., congestive heart failure and volume loading) increase plasma levels of atrial natriuretic factor and promote diuresis. Conversely, conditions that decrease atrial distension would be expected to decrease the release of atrial natriuretic factor and provoke antidiuresis. PPV with PEEP has been demonstrated to decrease atrial distension by two mechanisms: direct compression by the lungs and reductions in venous return to the heart. Leithner et al. (16) studied seven patients and six healthy volunteers exposed to PPV with PEEP. Significant declines in atrial natriuretic factor were observed in response to increases in PEEP support, which returned toward baseline as PEEP support was withdrawn. Andrivet et al. (17) demonstrated that the application of PPV with PEEP reduced atrial transmural pressure (stretch), lowered plasma atrial natriuretic factor levels, and was associated with a decrease in urine output and urine sodium excretion. Additionally, they demonstrated that restoration of venous return and central blood volume without fluid loading raised atrial natriuretic factor levels and returned urine output and sodium excretion to baseline levels. Although these studies are preliminary, they strongly suggest that atrial natriuretic factor plays a significant role in PPV-induced renal changes.

Investigators studying the renal effects of PPV have used a wide variety of experimental designs. An important difference among these studies was the mode of PPV employed and its effect on intrathoracic pressure. Subjects receiving PPV with high levels of PEEP would be expected to have greater increases in intrathoracic pressure than those ventilated without PEEP. Likewise, those subjects with normal lung compliance receiving PPV would be expected to demonstrate greater increases in intrathoracic pressure than those subjects with noncompliant lungs. It is clear that an individual change in renal function in response to PPV is proportional to the degree of change in intrathoracic pressure. The greater the increase in intrathoracic pressure, the greater the decline in renal function.

Several mechanisms have been cited as contributing to the adverse renal effects associated with PPV. Direct effects secondary to a decrease in cardiac output, renal blood flow redistribution, and changes in renal venous pressure play an important role in these adverse effects.

Despite the demonstrated role of both direct and indirect effects of PPV on renal function, it is virtually impossible to predict the exact mechanism responsible in each patient. As the interaction among respiratory, cardiovascular, endocrine, and renal systems is further clarified, successful techniques for preserving renal function during PPV may be developed.

POSITIVE-PRESSURE VENTILATION: HEPATIC AND GASTROINTESTINAL FUNCTION

Severe impairment in hepatic and gastrointestinal function is frequently observed in critically ill patients. PPV has been demonstrated to play a role in contributing to those adverse conditions. The mechanisms whereby PPV affects hepatic and gastrointestinal functions are unclear, but they appear to be multifactorial:

Decreased cardiac output
Increased hepatic vascular resistance
    Elevated venous pressure
    Elevated intraabdominal pressure
    Diaphragmatic compression
Elevated bile duct pressure

Hepatic Function

The normal adult liver has a dual blood flow and oxygen supply. Approximately two thirds of hepatic blood flow and one half of the oxygen supply are provided by the portal vein; the remainder is derived from the hepatic artery. Factors that inhibit hepatic perfusion via either of these routes would be expected to affect hepatic function adversely.

Decreased Cardiac Output

It is widely accepted that cardiac output is significantly reduced in patients receiving PPV. The decline in cardiac output associated with PPV has been implicated as contributing to hepatic dysfunction. Several animal studies have demonstrated alteration in hepatic perfusion due to PPV. Manny et al. (18) recorded an approximate 50% decline in hepatic arterial blood flow in dogs receiving PPV associated with a similar decline in cardiac output.

Bredenberg and Paskanik (19) demonstrated that PPV simultaneously reduced cardiac output and portal venous blood flow. Correction of cardiac output by volume expansion returned portal blood flow to baseline levels. Matuschak et al. (20) demonstrated that global hepatic blood flow reductions during PPV were proportional to the reductions in cardiac output. The reduction in hepatic blood flow is preventable by returning cardiac output to baseline levels by volume expansion.

Bonnet et al. (21) studied eight critically ill patients receiving PPV. These patients had no evidence of hepatic dysfunction at the study onset. Cardiac output was measured by thermodilution via a pulmonary artery catheter. Total hepatic blood flow was determined by measuring the clearance of indocyanine green dye, previously demonstrated to be an accurate measurement of hepatic flow. PPV without PEEP was not associated with a fall in hepatic blood flow. A significant fall, however, in hepatic blood flow was demonstrated with increasing levels of PEEP. The peak decrease in hepatic blood flow reached 32% of control at 20 cmH_2O of PEEP and a positive linear regression between PEEP and hepatic blood flow was found. A linear correlation was found between cardiac output and hepatic blood flow so that hepatic blood flow remained a constant 15% fraction of cardiac output. The authors concluded the PEEP-induced decline in cardiac output was primarily responsible for the simultaneously measured decline in hepatic blood flow.

Increased Hepatic Vascular Resistance

An increase in hepatic vascular resistance has been cited as another mechanism responsible for PPV-induced hepatic dysfunction. An increase in hepatic vascular resistance, either arterial or portal, would be expected to result in a decrease in hepatic blood flow and possible ischemia. Factors demonstrated to contribute to an increase in hepatic vascular resistance include elevations in hepatic venous pressure and mechanical compression of the liver, either directly or indirectly through increases in intraabdominal pressure.

An elevation in hepatic venous pressure would be expected to induce an increase in hepatic vascular resistance and result in a decrease in hepatic arterial perfusion pressure. PPV may increase hepatic venous pressure by increasing inferior vena caval pressure as a result of increased intrathoracic pressure. This so-called "venous back pressure" has been demonstrated in laboratory animals (18).

Mechanical compression of the liver has been postulated to reduce portal venous flow. Descent of the diaphragm during PPV (especially with large tidal volumes) may directly compress the hepatic parenchyma (22). In addition, the descending diaphragm could produce a dramatic rise in intraabdominal pressure (22). Ultimately, the combination of these forces would resist portal venous flow. Johnson and Hedley-Whyte (23) demonstrated a significant decline in portal venous flow, as well as a simultaneous increase in portal pressure in dogs subjected to PPV. Portal blood flow and pressure both returned to normal with PPV cessation. These authors claimed that the elevation in pressure as flow decreased indicates that the reduction in flow was not solely a reflection of reduced mesenteric blood flow due to a decline in cardiac output. Furthermore, they suggest that compression of the liver, either directly by the descending diaphragm or by an increase in intraabdominal pressure, was responsible for an increase in portal resistance accompanied by an increase in portal pressure and a reduction in portal flow. Their study failed, however, to demonstrate either an increase in intraabdominal pressure or evidence of diaphragmatic hepatic compression. Additionally, Sussman et al. (24) demonstrated no correlation between the level of PEEP and direct measurement of intraabdominal pressure in a study of 15 surgical patients. However, the study was limited to PEEP levels of 0–15 cmH$_2$O (24). Thus, the contribution of mechanical compression of the liver to the observed hepatic dysfunction in subjects on PPV remains speculative.

Increased Bile Duct Pressure

An increased resistance to the flow of bile through the common bile duct has been shown to influence liver function. Common bile duct resistance increased by 21% in dogs receiving PPV and returned to normal when PPV was removed (23). The suggested mechanism is that vascular engorgement of the duct was responsible for the increased resistance. Whether this increased resistance would be sufficient to impair hepatic performance is unclear.

A decrease in hepatic blood flow and function secondary to the effects of PPV could have important consequences in critically ill patients. Medications that are cleared by the liver may accumulate and result in unanticipated adverse effects. The literature strongly suggests that the decline in cardiac output that occurs in subjects receiving PPV is responsible for the possible hepatic dysfunction.

Gastrointestinal Function

Gastrointestinal changes frequently occur in critically ill patients receiving PPV. The incidence of gastrointestinal bleeding is >40% in patients receiving mechanical ventilation for more than 3 days (5). Unlike many other vascular beds, the gastric arterial system probably does not have autoregulatory capabilities. Gastric blood flow, therefore, is highly dependent on arterial pressure. In addition, an increase in gastric venous pressure would be expected to decrease flow further. PPV has been demonstrated to be possibly responsible for a reduction in arterial pressure and an increase in venous pressure. This combination could result in ischemia of the highly susceptible gastrointestinal mucosa and lead to ulceration and bleeding (5,25).

In patients with decreased lung compliance, PPV use could lead to gastrointestinal distension and, potentially, to barotrauma. The etiologic mechanism appears to be secondary to high airway pressure, causing an inspiratory gas leak around the artificial airway (26). In addition, case reports have described tension pneumoperitoneum in patients receiving PPV as a result of transdiaphragmatic passage of gases postoperatively. These patients had surgical disruption of both the diaphragm and the tracheobronchial tree. PPV generated sufficient pressure to disrupt surgical closure and allow for passage of inspired gases to migrate into the peritoneum (27).

CONCLUSION

In conclusion, airway pressure therapy is associated with alterations in renal, hepatic, and gastrointestinal function. Many of the adverse effects appear to directly result from increased intrathoracic pressure and a reduction in cardiac output, although several other reasonable explanations demonstrate the multifactorial nature of the issue.

References

1. Drury D, Henry J, Goodman J. The effects of continuous pressure breathing on kidney function. J Clin Invest 26:945–995, 1947.
2. Hall S, Johnson E, Hedley-Whyte J. Renal hemodynamics and function with continuous positive-pressure ventilation in dogs. Anesthesiology 41:452–461, 1984.
3. Gammanpila S, Bevan D, Bhudu R. Effect of positive and negative expiratory pressure on renal function. Br J Anaesth 49:199–205, 1977.
4. Sladen A, Laver M, Pontoppidan H. Pulmonary complications and water retention in prolonged mechanical ventilation. N Engl J Med 279:448–453, 1968.
5. Geiger K, Georgieff M, Lutz H. Side effects of positive pressure ventilation on hepatic function and splanchnic circulation. Int J Clin Monit Comput 12:103–106, 1986.
6. Annat G, Viale JP, Bui Xuan B, et al. Effect of PEEP ventilation on renal function, plasma

renin, aldosterone, neurophysins and urinary ADH, and prostaglandins. Anesthesiology 58: 136–141, 1983.

 7. Priebe H, Heimann J, Hedley–Whyte J. Mechanisms of renal dysfunction during PEEP ventilation. J Appl Physiol 50:643–649, 1981.

 8. Venus B, Mathru M, Smith R, et al. Renal function during application of PEEP in swine: effects of hydration. Anesthesiology 62:765–769, 1985.

 9. Katz M, Shear L. Effect of renal nerves on renal hemodynamics. Nephron 14:246–256, 1976.

10. Berne R. Hemodynamics and sodium excretion of denervated kidney in anesthetized and unanesthetized dog. Am J Physiol 171:148–158, 1952.

11. Fewell J, Bond G. Role of sinoaortic baroreceptors in initiating the renal response to continuous positive pressure ventilation in the dog. Anesthesiology 52:408–413, 1980.

12. Baratz R, Ingraham R. Renal hemodynamics and antidiuretic hormone release associated with volume regulation. Am J Physiol 198:565–570, 1960.

13. Hemmer M, Viquerat C, Suter P, et al. Urinary antidiuretic hormone excretion during mechanical ventilation and weaning in man. Anesthesiology 52:395–400, 1980.

14. Payen D, Farge D, Beloucif S, et al. No involvement of ADH in acute antidiuresis during PEEP ventilation in humans. Anesthesiology 66:17–23, 1987.

15. Berry A. Respiratory support and renal function. Anesthesiology 55:655–667, 1981.

16. Leithner C, Frass M, Pacher R, et al. Mechanical ventilation with PEEP decreases release of alpha-atrial natriuretic peptide. Crit Care Med 15:484–488, 1987.

17. Andrivet P, Adnot S, Brun-Buisson C, et al. Involvement of ANF in the acute antidiuresis during PEEP ventilation. J Appl Physiol 65:1967–1974, 1988.

18. Manny J, Justice R, Hechtman H. Abnormalities in organ blood flow and its distribution during PEEP. Surgery 85:425–432, 1979.

19. Bredenberg C, Paskanik A. Relation of portal hemodynamics to cardiac output during mechanical ventilation with PEEP. Ann Surg 198:218–222, 1983.

20. Matuschak G, Pinsky M, Rogers R. Effects of PEEP on hepatic blood flow and performance. J Appl Physiol 62:1377–1383, 1987.

21. Bonnet F, Richard C, Glaser P, et al. Changes in hepatic flow induced by continuous positive pressure ventilation in critically ill patients. Crit Care Med 10:703–705, 1982.

22. Johnson E. Splanchnic hemodynamic response to passive hyperventilation. J Appl Physiol 38: 156–162, 1975.

23. Johnson E, Hedley-Whyte J. Continuous positive-pressure ventilation and choledochoduodenal flow resistance. J Appl Physiol 39:937–942, 1985.

24. Sussman A, Boyd C, Williams J, et al. Effect of positive end-expiratory pressure on intraabdominal pressure. South Med J 84:697–700, 1991.

25. Johnson E, Hedley-Whyte J. Continuous positive-pressure ventilation and portal flow in dogs with pulmonary edema. J Appl Physiol 33:385–389, 1982.

26. Barker SJ, Karagianes T. Gastric barotrauma: a case report and theoretical considerations. Anesth Analg 64:1026–1027, 1985.

27. Schwartz R, Pham S, Bierman M, et al. Tension pneumoperitoneum after heart-lung transplantation. Ann Thorac Surg 57:478–481, 1994.

Suggested Readings

Baratz R, Philbin D, Patterson R. Plasma antidiuretic hormone and urinary output during continuous positive-pressure breathing in dogs. Anesthesiology 34:510–513, 1971.

Berry A, Geer R, Marshall C, et al. The effect of long-term controlled mechanical ventilation with PEEP on renal function in dogs. Anesthesiology 61:406–415, 1984.

Fewell J, Bond G. Renal denervation eliminates the renal response to continuous positive pressure ventilation. Proc Soc Exp Biol Med 161:574–579, 1979.

Gett P, Jones E, Shepherd G. Pulmonary oedema associated with sodium retention during ventilator treatment. Br J Anaesth 43:460–470, 1971.

Kumar A, Pontoppidan H, Baratz R, et al. Inappropriate response to increased plasma ADH during mechanical ventilation in acute respiratory failure. Anesthesiology 40: 215–221, 1974.

Sha M, Saito Y, Yokoyama K, et al. Effects of continuous positive-pressure ventilation on hepatic blood flow and intrahepatic oxygen delivery in dogs. Crit Care Med 15: 1040–1043, 1987.

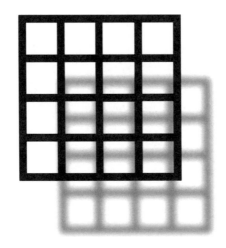

Section II
Ventilatory Modes

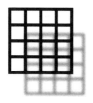

7
Control Mode Ventilation and Assist/Control Ventilation

Theodore W. Marcy • John J. Marini

Mechanical ventilation is used by physicians to support critically ill patients with refractory hypoxemia, depressed ventilatory drive, respiratory muscle fatigue signs, excessive cardiac or ventilatory workload, or life-threatening disturbances in acid-base balance. Under these conditions, the goals of mechanical ventilation are to (*a*) improve arterial blood oxygenation by applying high levels of inspired oxygen (F_IO_2), by improving ventilation/perfusion mismatching, or by recruiting previously nonventilated alveoli; (*b*) decrease or eliminate the energy consumed by the respiratory muscles by having the ventilator provide some or all of the power required to breathe; and (*c*) control the rate of alveolar ventilation of the patient who is either unable to meet the ventilatory demand or, conversely, who has excessive or inadequate central respiratory drive.

To accomplish these mechanical ventilation goals, the physician must be certain that the ventilator parameters of F_IO_2, tidal volume (V_T), respiratory rate, positive end-expiratory pressure (PEEP), and ventilation modes are set so that the ventilator maintains appropriate lung volumes and delivers an appropriate F_IO_2 and minute ventilation. This chapter presents the generally accepted guidelines for selecting the initial ventilator settings (Table 7.1). It then describes in detail the mode of ventilation most frequently used when patients are first placed on mechanical ventilation—the assist/control (A/CMV) mode in both of its current iterations: flow controlled, volume-cycled ventilation; and pressure controlled, time-cycled ventilation. Finally, we present case examples of two patients in whom these guidelines are applied to resolve problems that may occur during mechanical ventilation.

INITIAL VENTILATOR SETTINGS

Fractional Inspired Oxygen Concentration

Oxygen is crucial in the production of high energy stores of adenosine triphosphate (ATP) through oxidative phosphorylation. Severely hypoxemic patients sup-

Table 7.1. Initial Ventilator Settings

Mode of ventilation	Assist/Control
Tidal volume	10–12 ml/kg
Respiratory rate	10–12/minute or a rate that provides 80% of minute ventilation
Fraction of inspired oxygen	0.6 (60%)

plement ATP formation via anaerobic metabolism, but this pathway is vastly less efficient than oxidative phosphorylation and it generates lactic acid. The goal of oxygen therapy is to increase oxygen delivery (O_2 Del) to the tissues so that oxidative phosphorylation and other oxygen-dependent metabolic processes can continue.

Cardiac output (CO), hemoglobin (Hgb) concentration, and hemoglobin oxygen saturation are the primary determinants of tissue O_2 Del.

$$O_2 \text{ Del} = CO \times \text{Arterial Oxygen Content}$$

$$(O_2 \text{ Del} \approx CO \text{ (ml/min)} \times (\text{Hgb Concentration (g/dl)} \times O_2 \text{ Saturation} \times 1.3)$$

Increasing the F_IO_2 alters only one of these primary determinants (i.e., hemoglobin O_2 saturation). Once the arterial oxygen tension (PaO_2) is increased sufficiently to fully saturate hemoglobin, only small additional amounts of O_2 dissolve in the plasma with additional increases in PaO_2. The sigmoidal shape of the oxygen saturation curve predicts that there will be little change in hemoglobin saturation with small changes in PaO_2 at saturations >90% (corresponding approximately to a PaO_2 of 55–65 mmHg). Therefore, in normal practice, the F_IO_2 or other interventions initiated to improve PaO_2 should be adjusted to maintain the hemoglobin saturation in this range. However, the safe lower limit of PaO_2 may be lower for certain individuals if their hemoglobin concentration is normal, if they can generate a higher (compensating) cardiac output to maintain O_2 delivery, and if their tissues extract O_2 efficiently from blood.

There are risks associated with administering high F_IO_2 levels. First, potent cellular toxins—most notably free oxygen radicals—are created at high partial pressures of oxygen. If the concentration of free oxygen radicals overwhelms the lung's antioxidant defenses, cellular injury, with subsequent inflammation, edema, and pulmonary fibrosis, will ensue. The F_IO_2 level and the therapy duration associated with significant oxygen toxicity in the critically ill patient are not well defined. However, because both time and concentration are important, it is prudent to maintain the F_IO_2 at 65% or lower in patients who require oxygen supplementation for extended periods (1).

Another risk of breathing very high concentrations of inspired oxygen is that poorly ventilated alveoli may collapse as oxygen is rapidly absorbed from the alveolus into capillary blood. At an F_IO_2 well below 100%, these alveoli maintain their volume because of the splinting effect of nitrogen, which exists in virtual equilibrium with nitrogen dissolved in the blood and interstitial fluids. However, at very high concentrations of F_IO_2, nitrogen is washed out of the lung and oxygen becomes the predominant gas. The gradient between high alveolar and low pulmonary arterial PO_2 leads to rapid absorption of this gas and instability of the alveolus unless adequate alveolar ventilation is provided. This process, termed *absorption atelectasis,* can intensify a shunt, thereby increasing hypoxemia significantly. Moreover, it may evolve in less than an hour at an F_IO_2 of 100% (2).

A third problem in high inspired oxygen concentration use often occurs in spontaneously breathing patients with chronic hypercapnia. High concentrations of inspired O_2 can worsen CO_2 retention and respiratory acidosis. This phenomenon has been attributed to the blunting of the hypoxic drive in patients who do not have an appropriate response to hypercapnia. However, when the minute ventilation is actually measured in these patients while administrating a high F_IO_2, the small decrease in minute ventilation observed does not explain entirely the observed rise in arterial carbon dioxide ($PaCO_2$) (3,4). It has been suggested that, in such patients, oxygen therapy may increase dead-space ventilation and contribute to the increased hypercapnia by reducing the efficiency of CO_2 excretion.

The appropriate F_IO_2 to deliver depends on the etiology of the hypoxemia. In general, the pathophysiology of hypoxemia in the acutely ill patient usually involves one or more of the following mechanisms: hypoventilation, ventilation/ perfusion ($\dot{V}A/\dot{Q}$) mismatching, or shunt (venous admixture). In the presence of lung pathology, an imbalance of oxygen consumption to oxygen delivery may cause mixed venous blood to desaturate abnormally, adding to the hypoxemia as the profoundly desaturated venous blood exacerbates venous admixture. Patients who are hypoxemic secondary to hypoventilation or $\dot{V}A/\dot{Q}$ mismatching usually respond impressively to relatively small increments of $F_IO_2 > 21\%$. Some examples of clinical conditions in which these are the predominant mechanisms of hypoxia are uncomplicated overdose of sedative drugs, chronic bronchitis, asthma, and emphysema.

By contrast, patients who are hypoxemic from intrapulmonary or intracardiac shunting are refractory to inspired oxygen and require a high F_IO_2. Pulmonary edema, pneumonia, and atelectasis are common clinical conditions in which shunting is the primary mechanism responsible for hypoxemia. If the shunt fraction exceeds 40%, it is not possible to obtain an adequate PaO_2, even on an F_IO_2 of 100%. In this situation, nonventilated alveoli must be recruited to reduce the shunt fraction. Increasing the mean alveolar pressure with PEEP or inverse-ratio ventilation (discussed in Chapters 9, Intermittent Mandatory Ventilation, and 13, Differential Lung Ventilation) may open collapsed alveoli or shift fluid out of alveoli that are flooded from pulmonary edema into the interstitial spaces. Disproportionate alveolar collapse and regional shunting in dorsal and basilar regions may be aided by prone positioning. It has also been shown that if cardiac output falls in response to higher lung pressures, shunt flow and venous admixture also decline (5).

Often, the disease responsible for the patient's hypoxemia is not well defined nor is the oxygenation status known. In these situations, the patient can be placed on an F_1O_2 of 100% for a short period until measurements of PaO_2 are made. The F_1O_2 then can be adjusted to achieve a hemoglobin saturation rate of 90%.

Tidal Volume and Respiratory Rate

Positive-pressure ventilators inflate the lung by producing a pressure difference across the lungs and chest wall. The total inflation pressure during positive-pressure ventilation is composed of three primary elements (Fig. 7.1): (*a*) the pressure driving gas to the alveolar level against airway resistance (airway pressure minus alveolar pressure: Paw − Palv; (*b*) the pressure distending the lung against elastic forces (alveolar pressure minus pleural pressure: Palv − Ppl; and (*c*) the pressure

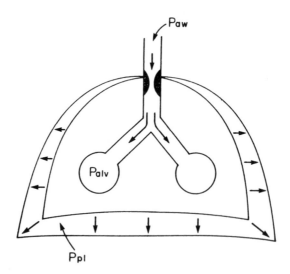

Figure 7.1. The pressures relevant to inflating the chest and lung during passive positive-pressure ventilation are illustrated in this figure. The pressure gradient driving gas to the alveolar level against resistive forces is the airway pressure (Paw) minus the alveolar pressure (Palv). The pressure gradient expanding the lung against elastic forces is Palv minus pleural pressure (Ppl). The pressure gradient expanding the chest wall against elastic forces is pleural pressure minus atmospheric pressure. The transpulmonary pressure is airway pressure minus atmospheric pressure.

across the chest wall. In a passively inflated patient, the latter gradient is pleural pressure minus atmospheric pressure (Ppl − Patm). In a spontaneously breathing patient, the pressure relevant to the chest wall is generated by the respiratory muscles and is inaccessible to a measuring instrument.

Many of the first mechanical ventilators were pure pressure generators in that they delivered gas to the airway opening until a fixed pressure target was achieved. This type of ventilatory pattern is called *pressure-cycled ventilation* (Fig. 7.2). The rate of air flowing into the chest decreases as the alveolar pressure rises with increasing alveolar volume. Flow ceases entirely when alveolar pressure equals the applied airway pressure. The rate at which this equilibrium occurs is determined by the mechanical properties of the chest: the airway resistance and the joint compliance of the lung and chest wall.

The patient is not guaranteed a constant V_T or specific flow pattern when a set level of pressure is applied to the airway. Instead, the delivered V_T is a function of the mechanical properties of the chest, the time allotted for inspiration, and the alveolar pressure at the beginning of inspiration. As compliance decreases, less volume enters the lung for any applied airway pressure. When airway resistance increases, inspiratory air flow may decrease to the point that alveolar and airway pressures do not equilibrate at the end of the available inspiratory time; consequently, the alveoli do not reach their full equilibrium volume. If there is positive pressure in the alveolus at the beginning of inspiration because of air-trapping or applied PEEP, then higher applied pressure is required to maintain V_T.

There is an obvious disadvantage to not being able to guarantee V_T in a ventilated patient. During pressure-cycled ventilation, V_T can rise or fall if compliance or airway resistance change—a common occurrence in unstable patients with underlying respiratory disease. Therefore, ventilators were developed that are *flow* generators in that they provide specified patterns of gas flow to the airway—whatever pressure is required. Although a constant (square wave) pattern of inspiratory flow has traditionally been selected, it can be sinusoidal or decelerating as well. (The latter is gaining increasing popularity for two reasons: (*a*) ventilation distribution may occur more efficiently in a heterogenous lung, and (*b*) the most rapid inspiratory flow occurs in the first part of inspiration, when the flow demands of the dyspneic patient are greatest.) In any case, in contrast to pressure-cycled ventilation, the flow rate is predictable and predetermined. Inspiratory flow ends when a preset V_T or a preset inspiratory time has been achieved. This type of ventilatory pattern is called *flow controlled, volume-cycled ventilation* (see Fig. 7.2). This is the most common ventilatory algorithm used in adult patients.

The necessary pressure to maintain the flow pattern against opposing resistive and elastic forces is applied to the airway over the inspiratory phase of the respiratory cycle. For a similar V_T and mean flow rate, the peak airway pressures usually will exceed those seen during pressure-cycled ventilation because the same flow rate is maintained even at high alveolar volume (see Fig. 7.2). Under some circum-

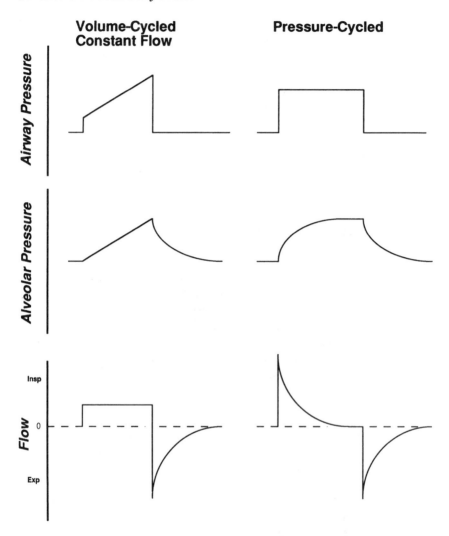

Figure 7.2. Idealized airway pressure, alveolar pressure, and flow tracings during volume-cycled ventilation (with constant flow) and pressure-cycled ventilation.

stances, excessive peak pressures may contribute to lung injury (6), illustrating a possible disadvantage of volume-cycled ventilation in comparison to pressure-cycled ventilation.

The minute ventilation is the product of V_T and respiratory rate. In a spontaneously breathing, healthy adult, the normal minute ventilation is ~6 L/minute—an average V_T of 500 ml multiplied by an average respiratory rate of 12/

minute. The minute ventilation required to maintain acid-base balance in an intubated adult intensive care unit (ICU) patient of average size may range from 6 L to 30 L or more, varying with metabolic demands and the proportion of minute ventilation that constitutes dead space (wasted ventilation).

When a patient is first intubated and placed on mechanical ventilation, the initial settings for V_T and respiratory rate provide only a rough estimate of the patient's required minute ventilation. The desired V_T is chosen not only to satisfy minute ventilation requirements, but also to arrest the progressive atelectasis that can occur in supine patients when they are ventilated monotonously with only a physiologic V_T of 5 ml/kg. Thus, in most patients, the V_T is set at 10–12 ml/kg, up to a maximum of approximately 1 L. Lower V_Ts may be selected in patients with severe airway obstruction where there is a concern about air-trapping (discussed later), in patients with only one lung, or in patients in whom the pressure required to deliver a V_T of 10–12 ml/kg is sufficiently high (>50 cmH$_2$O) to injure the lung (6).

With V_T set at 10–12 ml/kg, an initial respiratory rate of 10–12/minute will provide a minute ventilation more than sufficient to meet the ventilatory requirements of a normal subject. With the guidance of arterial blood gas analysis, adjustments in the respiratory rate are made to alter the delivered minute ventilation to match the patient's metabolic needs and to compensate for dead-space ventilation.

Inspiratory Flow Rate and the Inspiratory: Expiratory (I/E) Ratio

When initiating volume-cycled ventilation, the clinician must select an inspiratory flow rate, measured in L/minute, that determines how quickly the V_T is delivered. The time required to complete inspiration is a function of the average flow rate and V_T; it is called the *inspiratory time* (T_I).

$$T_I = V_T / \text{Flow Rate}$$

The time during which the patient can exhale (the expiratory time or T_E) is determined jointly by the inspiratory flow rate and frequency. For example, in a patient with a respiratory rate of 10 breaths per minute, the total time of each respiratory cycle or breath (T_{tot}) is 6 seconds. If a 1-L V_T is delivered at an average flow rate of 60 L/minute then:

$$T_I = V_T / \text{Average Flow Rate} = 1\text{-L}/60 \text{ L/minute} = 1 \text{ second}$$

$$T_E = T_{tot} - T_I = 5 \text{ seconds}$$

The ratio of the inspiratory time to the expiratory time is called the inspiratory-to-expiratory (I/E) time ratio. In this example, the I/E ratio is 1:5. The inspiratory flow pattern also has an impact on inspiratory time and the I/E ratio. During constant flow, the average flow rate is about equal to the peak inspiratory flow rate set on the ventilator. During decelerating or sinusoidal flow patterns, the inspiratory flow rate set on the ventilator is again equal to the peak inspiratory flow rate, but the average flow rate is lower and the inspiratory time is, therefore, longer for the same settings of peak flow and V_T (Fig. 7.3).

There are several considerations guiding flow rate selection. First, faster flows

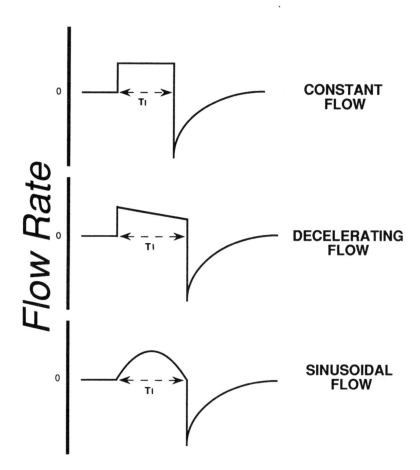

Figure 7.3. Comparison of different inspiratory flow patterns available when using volume-cycled ventilation. Note that the inspiratory time (Tı) is longer with the decelerating and sinusoidal flow patterns than with constant flow, even though the delivered volumes and peak inspiratory flow rates are equal. Under these conditions, expiratory time with decelerating and sinusoidal flow patterns will be shorter than with the constant flow pattern.

require greater central airway pressures to deliver the same V_T. Although airway resistance tends to dissipate high airway pressures proximal to the alveolar level, some pathways may allow alveolar pressure to approach that of the airway opening. Second, the rapid volume changes at higher flow rates may increase shear forces, thereby risking further airway and parenchymal damage. Third, in certain patients, there is a higher inspiratory flow demand because the respiratory center signals that gas be delivered to the lung at a faster rate, particularly if the minute ventilation requirements are high. If the machine flow rate is set lower than the patient's inspiratory flow demand, then the patient will pull or fight against the ventilator, increasing energy consumption and contributing to anxiety. Fourth, as explained previously, because a low inspiratory flow rate shortens the available expiratory time, dangerous air-trapping can occur in patients with air flow obstruction if the flow rate is set too low (7).

Several guidelines can be used when selecting a flow rate. Patients with high ventilatory requirements usually require a peak flow rate in the constant flow mode of at least four times the minute ventilation (e.g., a flow setting of 80 L/minute is appropriate for a patient with a minute ventilation of 20 L/minute). In patients who initiate breaths spontaneously, the flow rate should be adjusted at the bedside to match inspiratory effort. Because flow demands are highest in the beginning of inspiration, a decelerating flow profile often proves helpful. For the same inspiratory V_T and inspiratory time, peak flow should be set ~20–25% higher than in the constant flow mode. Relatively higher flow rates should be used for patients with air flow obstruction.

During pressure-cycled ventilation, the inspiratory flow rate has a decelerating pattern determined as a function of the driving pressure, the airway resistance, and the respiratory system (lungs and chest wall) compliance. The flow rate cannot be adjusted independently from these variables. Instead, the inspiratory time is adjusted by a timing mechanism that cycles the ventilator between inspiration and expiration.

On some pressure-cycled ventilators, the clinician sets a desired I/E ratio, which the timing mechanism then maintains for the set respiratory rate. In most circumstances, the I/E ratio is set at about 33%. Lower I/E ratios provide longer expiratory times. However, under conditions of high airway resistance, a short inspiratory time will result in a lower V_T, because the alveoli do not achieve their full equilibrium volume. If the I/E ratio is too high (>50%, or 1:1) air-trapping may result. I/E ratios greater than 1:1 are generally avoided except under special circumstances where it may be desirable (see Chapter 12, Inverse Ratio Ventilation and the Inspiratory/Expiratory Ratio) (8–10).

Inspiratory Pause

Physicians can maintain a patient's lung inflation at full inspiration by setting an inspiratory pause or plateau. The inspiratory pause control occludes the expiratory port (preventing exhalation) for a set time following the delivery of the V_T. By this method, physicians can vary the I/E ratio during volume-cycled ventilation independently of the flow rate. An inspiratory pause shortens the expiratory phase of the respiratory cycle, increasing the I/E ratio.

There are two circumstances where this feature is useful. First, the physician or therapist can estimate alveolar pressure at end-inflation by setting an inspiratory pause during one respiratory cycle. With flow in the airway stopped, alveolar pressure equilibrates with that measured at the proximal airway by the ventilator's manometer. If total end-expiratory alveolar pressure (Pex) is known (PEEP plus auto-PEEP), static compliance of the respiratory system can then be estimated (Fig. 7.4) (11):

$$\text{Compliance} = V_T / (\text{Palv} - \text{Pex})$$

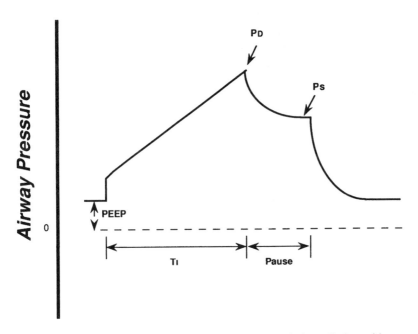

Figure 7.4. An airway pressure tracing during volume-cycled ventilation with a constant inspiratory flow pattern and an inspiratory pause set to stop flow at the end of inspiration. The peak airway pressure (*P*D) occurs at the end of the inspiratory time (*T*I) when inspiratory flow stops. With a pause added, alveolar pressure will equilibrate with that measured at the proximal airway and will be equal to the plateau pressure (*P*S). Static compliance of the respiratory system can be estimated by dividing the delivered tidal volume (*V*T) by the quantity of estimated alveolar pressure (PALV) minus the end-expiratory pressure (PEX: PEEP or auto-PEEP).

Differences in a plateau pressure for sequential breaths of a fixed tidal volume and PEEP separated by an artificially prolonged expiratory time quantifies auto-PEEP. A second use of the end-inspiratory pause in volume-cycled ventilation is to implement inverse-ratio ventilation (IRV) (8). This option, which can only be exercised in well-sedated, passive patients, may have some advantages over the alternative of pressure-cycled ventilation with a long I/E ratio, including a guaranteed V_T, and ready access in patients already on volume-cycled ventilators.

Mode of Ventilation

The choice of V_T and respiratory rate are straightforward in a paralyzed patient or in a patient otherwise unable to ventilate spontaneously: the respiratory rate and V_T are set to provide the appropriate minute ventilation. The situation is more complex when the patient can initiate a breath. Under these conditions, the physician must determine how the ventilator responds and interacts with the patient's own ventilatory efforts. The selected algorithm for this interaction of the patient with the ventilator is called the *mode of ventilation.*

The different modes available to physicians can be illustrated by the pressure and flow wave forms they apply to a patient's airway in response to the patient's efforts and in response to apnea (Fig. 7.5). That response can be characterized by whether the ventilator ignores patient efforts (controlled mechanical ventilation—CMV); whether it allows the patient to breathe passively through the ventilator circuit continuously or alternating with machine assistance (continuous positive airway pressure—CPAP and intermittent mandatory ventilation—IMV); or whether the ventilator delivers the same pressure to the airway in response to the patient's inspiratory efforts (assist/control ventilation—A/CMV and pressure support ventilation).

The appropriate mode to choose depends on the patient's circumstances. When the patient is first intubated, or during periods of instability, A/CMV ventilation is customarily used because it provides maximal ventilatory assistance and guarantees a lower limit of delivered ventilation. When the patient is being evaluated for removal of machine support, or when machine support is being gradually withdrawn, pressure support ventilation, IMV, CPAP, or combinations of these modes are employed. These latter modes are discussed in subsequent chapters.

Alarms

Alarms on ventilators warn about potentially dangerous problems: disconnection of the patient from the ventilator, apneic episodes, and dangerously high airway pressures. Patients with respiratory failure, particularly if they are sedated or paralyzed, are extremely vulnerable to failure of the ventilator to deliver the set tidal volume, to circuit disruption, or to inadvertent disconnection of the

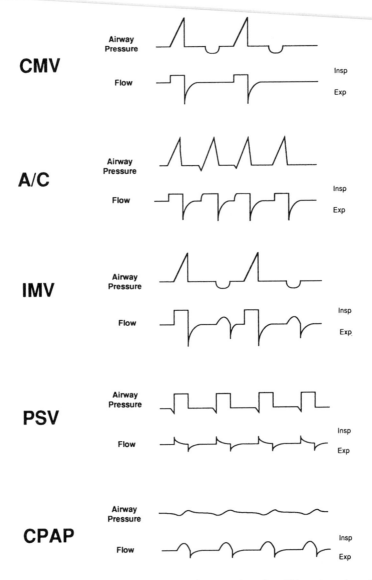

Figure 7.5. Schematic airway pressure and flow tracings for different modes of mechanical ventilation. Note that during controlled mechanical ventilation (*CMV*) no airflow occurs when the patient attempts to breathe spontaneously (when the airway pressure is negative in relation to atmosphere). By contrast, during assist/control ventilation (*A/C*) when the patient attempts to breathe spontaneously (negative airway pressure deflections), the flow rate is adjusted by the machine to equal that during a control breath. During intermittent mandatory ventilation (*IMV*) and continuous positive airway pressure breathing (*CPAP*) the patient determines the inspiratory flow rate on spontaneous breaths. During pressure support ventilation (*PSV*), each spontaneous inspiratory effort is supported by applied positive airway pressure.

ventilator. The low exhaled volume and low pressure alarms detect inadequate volume or pressure delivery to the airway and alert personnel in the ICU to the possibility of machine failure, circuit disruption, ventilator disconnection, or even large bronchopleural fistulas. If patients are breathing spontaneously through the ventilator circuit (CPAP, pressure support ventilation, or IMV), the ventilator can be set to alarm automatically or to provide backup positive-pressure breaths if it does not detect spontaneous breaths within a specified period.

The high pressure alarm prevents the ventilator from delivering excessive pressure to the airway during volume-cycled ventilation. If the airway pressure exceeds the high pressure limit, then the ventilator depressurizes the airway, shunting the remaining tidal volume into the opened expiratory port. While protecting the airway against high pressures, this alarm system reduces delivered V_T. Often, the high pressure limit is reached during coughing efforts or during the dyssynchronous efforts of an agitated patient. Repeated alarming of the high pressure limit should prompt a careful reassessment of the patient, searching for endotracheal tube kinking, mucus plugging, bronchospasm, intubation of the right main bronchus, or a tension pneumothorax.

CONTROL AND ASSIST/CONTROL VENTILATION

CMV and A/CMV ventilation are full support modes in that a ventilator in either of these modes performs most or all of the work necessary to maintain an adequate minute ventilation. Full support modes are advantageous in the acutely ill patient who requires a guaranteed and often high minute ventilation. These modes also reduce the oxygen and energy consumed by respiratory muscles. For these reasons, full support modes tend to be preferable in the following circumstances: (*a*) when patients are first intubated, prior to a full evaluation; (*b*) in patients who require a high minute ventilation; (*c*) in patients who have an unstable respiratory drive; (*d*) in patients who have respiratory muscle fatigue with need for maximal rest of these muscles; and (*e*) in patients with a poor cardiac output in whom it is advantageous to reduce oxygen consumption by the respiratory muscles. Although both pressure-preset and volume-cycled ventilators can be used in CMV and A/CMV modes, in adults, these two modes are most frequently used with volume-cycled ventilation.

Historically, CMV was the first mode developed for mechanical ventilators. In this mode, the ventilator delivers gas to the airway at a fixed rate despite the patient's respiratory efforts. CMV is mechanically the simplest and, therefore, the most mechanically reliable mode of ventilation. However, CMV has several major problems. First, it is usually dysphoric to the patient who attempts to ventilate spontaneously. The patient can neither trigger a positive-pressure breath nor inspire air through the ventilator circuit. To prevent dysphoria and agitation, the patient's respiratory efforts must be suppressed by either intentional overventilation or sedation, supplemented if necessary with paralytic medications. These approaches add certain risks: alkalosis, apnea during ventilator disconnection, and adverse pharmacologic effects on the patient's underlying medical problems. Second, this mode is unresponsive to the changing minute ventilation requirements of the patient. The physician must maintain constant vigilance so that appropriate adjustments are made in the delivered minute ventilation to avoid acid-base disturbances. Finally, total mechanical support of ventilation inhibits contraction of the respiratory muscles, which are then prone to atrophy.

A/CMV ventilation is an adaptation of CMV that allows the patient to initiate a volume-cycled or pressure-cycled breath at a rate greater than the set, or backup, respiratory rate. The patient can adjust the rate of positive-pressure breaths to meet the ventilatory requirement, provided adequate central respiratory drive and respiratory muscle strength are available to trigger the ventilator at an appropriate rate.

The backup rate on A/CMV ventilation is a safety feature: if the patient's respiratory rate falls below it, the ventilator will automatically cycle at the backup rate. Critically ill patients will not trigger the ventilator appropriately if they have an unstable respiratory drive, or if they are unable to contract respiratory muscles forcefully secondary to neuromuscular disease or fatigue. Conditions can change quickly in the ICU. A patient who is spontaneously triggering the ventilator at one time may be incapable of doing so a brief time later because of a changing medical status or the administration of a sedative. A good strategy is to set the backup rate to provide about 80% of the baseline minute ventilation.

Respiratory muscles still consume energy during A/CMV ventilation if the patient is breathing faster than the backup rate. Although each patient-initiated breath on A/CMV ventilation is machine supported, the inspiratory muscles must first generate a negative pressure to trigger the ventilator. Even when the ventilator begins applying positive pressure to the airway, these inspiratory muscles continue to contract, contributing significantly to the work of breathing (12,13).

Spontaneous efforts during A/CMV ventilation can prevent or delay respiratory muscle atrophy. However, in a dyspneic patient with unstable angina or a low cardiac output, this extra oxygen consumed by the respiratory muscles may represent an unnecessary burden for the overtaxed cardiovascular system. For this type of patient, it may be desirable to set the backup rate above the patient's respiratory rate, thereby achieving control and eliminating respiratory muscle work. There are other circumstances when the backup rate should be set above the respiratory rate of the patient: if the patient's respiratory drive is unstable; if the pH or $PaCO_2$ must be tightly controlled; or in patients with a flail chest in whom vigorous inspiratory efforts may interfere with healing. Alternatively, the patient's contribution to the work of breathing can be reduced or eliminated by sedation that is sufficient to suppress respiratory drive, thereby preventing triggering of the ventilator above the backup rate. This strategy is often used for patients with high levels of respiratory drive and in those with significant respiratory alkalosis.

To actuate an assisted breath, the patient must generate negative pressure in the airway sufficient to be sensed by the ventilator. Trigger sensitivity can be adjusted, but a setting that is too sensitive can cause positive-pressure breaths to be activated by extraneous movements of the patient or transient fluctuations in circuit pressure. Sensitivity set too low requires increased patient effort and energy expenditure (12) or results in the patient being "locked out"—unable to trigger the ventilator—creating the same problems that occur in CMV.

There are several potential disadvantages of A/CMV ventilation. First, as the respiratory rate increases with A/CMV ventilation, the mean intrathoracic pressure rises. Venous return to the heart may be impaired by high mean intrathoracic pressures and cardiac output may fall because of the subsequent decrease in preload to the left ventricle. Alternative ventilation modes, such as IMV, which permit unsupported (negative pressure) breaths, have comparatively less effect on cardiac output because the unsupported breaths will reduce mean intrathoracic pressure. Although the rising intrapleural pressure tends to impede venous return, it simultaneously decreases the afterload to the left ventricle that it helps to generate the intracavitary systemic arterial pressure. Both effects may prove beneficial to a patient with volume overload of a failing left ventricle; institution of mechanical ventilatory support may prove a crucial point of therapy in this setting, both because it favorably influences the left ventricular loading conditions and because it reduces systemic oxygen demands.

Pressure Preset (Pressure Targeted) Ventilation

Modern high capacity ventilators provide pressure preset or pressure targeted ventilatory modes (e.g., pressure control or pressure support) as options for full or partial ventilatory assistance. Once the breath is initiated, these modes apply and maintain a targeted amount of pressure at the airway opening until a specified time (pressure control or flow) pressure support cycling criterion is met. Maximal pressure is regulated, but tidal volume is a complex function of applied pressure and its rate of approach to target pressure, available inspiratory time, and the impedance to breathing (compliance, inspiratory and expiratory resistance, and auto-PEEP). High flow capacity, pressure targeted ventilation compensates well for small air leaks and, therefore, it is quite appropriate for use with leaking or uncuffed endotracheal (ET) tubes, as in neonatal or pediatric patients. Because of its virtually "unlimited" ability to deliver flow and its decelerating flow profile, pressure targeted ventilation is also an appropriate choice for spontaneously breathing patients with high inspiratory flow demands that usually peak early in the ventilatory cycle. Decelerating flow profiles also tend to improve the distribution of ventilation in a lung with heterogeneous mechanical properties (widely varying time constants). Apart from their application in limiting the lung's exposure to high airway pressure and barotrauma, pressure targeted modes may also prove helpful in adult patients in whom the airway cannot be completely sealed (e.g., bronchopleural fistula).

Differences Between Pressure and Volume Targeted Ventilation

The fundamental difference between pressure and volume targeted ventilation is implicit in their names; pressure targeted modes guarantee pressure at the expense of letting tidal volume vary; volume targeted modes guarantee flow—and consequently the column provided to the circuit in the allowed inspiratory time (tidal volume)—at the expense of letting airway pressure vary.

Flow and tidal volumes are important variables to monitor in pressure targeting; pressure is of parallel importance in volume targeting. Gas stored in compressible circuit elements does not contribute to effective alveolar ventilation. In adult patients, such losses (2–4 ml/cmH$_2$O of peak pressure) usually constitute a modest fraction of the tidal volume. In infants, however, compressible losses may comprise such a high fraction of the V$_T$ that *effective* ventilation varies markedly with peak cycling pressure. Thus, during volume-cycled ventilation, moment-by-moment changes in chest impedance caused by bronchospasm, secretions, and muscular activity can force both peak airway pressure and compressible circuit volume to rise and effective tidal volume to fall. Finally, because airway pressure is controlled, pressure targeted modes are somewhat less likely to cause barotrauma, a major life-threatening problem in this age group.

Volume targeted modes provide a preset volume unless a specified pressure limit is exceeded. Major advantages to volume targeting are the capacity to deliver unvarying tidal volumes (except in the presence of a gas leak), flexibility of flow and volume adjustments, and power to ventilate difficult patients. All ventilators currently used for continuous support in adults offer volume cycling as a primary option. Unlike pressure controlled ventilators, volume cycled modes cannot ventilate effectively and consistently unless the airway is well sealed. Moreover, flow controlled modes do not respond to variable flow demands, and excessive alveolar pressure may be required to deliver the desired tidal volume.

Another potential disadvantage of the A/CMV ventilation mode as conventionally applied, is its potential to result in more lung injury related to barotrauma than that seen with pressure-controlled ventilation delivered at lower V$_T$s or with modes that assign part of the minute ventilation burden to the patient (IMV, pressure support ventilation). Barotrauma is a frequent and serious complication of mechanical ventilation that can manifest as a pneumothorax, pneumomediastinum, subcutaneous emphysema, or tension air cysts. The incidence of barotrauma increases with higher peak airway pressures, PEEP, and with certain pulmonary diseases, specifically, necrotizing pneumonia and gastric aspiration (15,16).

Experimental studies suggest that excessive alveolar distension and high alveolar pressures predispose to barotrauma (15). A/CMV ventilation at high respiratory rates and fixed V_Ts will increase mean alveolar pressure and may increase alveolar distension. At least one retrospective study has demonstrated that patients on IMV ventilation had a lower incidence of barotrauma than patients on A/CMV ventilation (17). A prospective study of the incidence of barotrauma during the two modes of ventilation has not been reported and it is not possible to recommend a specific mode of ventilation for patients at risk for barotrauma. Instead, it may be more appropriate to reduce the cycling pressures by decreasing the V_T or inspiratory flow rate, to reduce secretion retention and to decrease the patient's respiratory rate and agitation with the use of sedation.

The third potential problem with A/CMV ventilation is that patients who have an abnormally increased central respiratory drive (e.g., who have sepsis, aspirin overdose, cirrhosis, or agitation) may become significantly alkalemic during fully supported A/CMV ventilation. IMV is often instituted in these situations because patient-initiated breaths above the backup rate are not supported. However, several studies suggest that there is a lower set point for $PaCO_2$ in these patients, and they will increase their minute ventilation to maintain the lower $PaCO_2$ whatever the mode of ventilation selected, provided they have sufficient strength (18–20). If this is true, then the patient with a higher central respiratory drive may consume more energy when on IMV as opposed to A/CMV. If severe respiratory alkalosis persists, despite the use of IMV and treatment of the underlying etiology, sedation may be necessary.

EXAMPLES OF SPECIAL CIRCUMSTANCES

Auto-PEEP in a Patient with Airway Obstruction

A 60-year-old man with a history of chronic bronchitis and emphysema was brought to the emergency room lethargic with labored respirations. The initial arterial blood gas showed a pH of 7.03, a $PaCO_2$ of 125 mmHg, and a PaO_2 of 100 mmHg on supplemental oxygen. The patient was intubated and vigorously ventilated with a manual resuscitation bag. Within several minutes, he became hypotensive and bilateral chest tubes were placed because of the clinical suspicion of tension pneumothoraxes by the emergency room staff. However, no air leak was confirmed, and a subsequent chest radiograph showed no pneumothorax. Whenever ventilation was suspended to allow airway suctioning, the patient's blood pressure improved. After this observation, the ventilatory rate was reduced and the patient's blood pressure stabilized, allowing transfer to the ICU. What are the considerations in the initial ventilator orders?

This patient had elevated expiratory airway resistance that slowed the expiratory flow rate. With vigorous positive pressure breathing, the patient did not have sufficient expiratory time for the alveoli to empty to their resting volume. At higher end-expiratory volumes, elastic forces generate a positive pressure in the alveolus. Eventually, a new equilibrium is reached in which this end-expiratory alveolar pressure (auto-PEEP or intrinsic PEEP) increases expiratory gas flow to the point that the inhaled volume equals the exhaled volume (7,21).

Unfortunately, auto-PEEP has several adverse effects: it decreases cardiac output because the higher intrathoracic pressures reduce venous return; it can artifactually increase pressures measured by central venous or pulmonary artery catheters; and it increases the energy the patient must expend to trigger the ventilator. Patients who have auto-PEEP must first generate a negative intrathoracic pressure that equals the auto-PEEP value before they can generate the negative central airway pressure needed to trigger the ventilator (22). Often, the trigger sensitivity of the ventilator in this situation can be improved by adding low levels of applied PEEP (22). Unless specifically measured by occluding the ventilator expiratory port at the end of the expiratory cycle (Fig. 7.6), this phenomenon may not be recognized (7,23). Auto-PEEP during A/CMV is best assessed in the passive patient by following the end-inspiration plateau pressure.

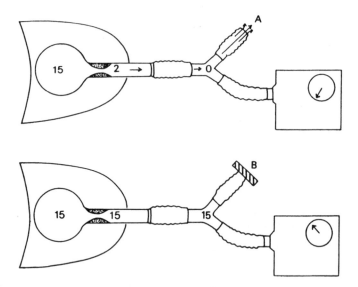

Figure 7.6. The auto-PEEP effect and its measurement. In the presence of severe air flow obstruction and a high minute ventilation, alveolar pressure remains elevated throughout the expiratory cycle as flow is driven by the recoil pressure of the hyperexpanded chest. In this example, although alveolar pressure at end-expiration is 15 cmH$_2$O, the central airway pressure downstream is negligible (**A**). Transiently stopping flow at end-expiration allows equilibration of pressure throughout the circuit and detection of this occult alveolar pressure by the ventilator's manometer (**B**). (From O'Quin R, Marini JJ. Pulmonary artery occlusion pressure: clinical physiology, measurement, and interpretation. Am Rev Respir Dis 128:319–326, 1983.)

Although medical therapies are directed at reducing airway resistance, the goal of ventilatory strategy is to limit end-expiratory alveolar volume and pressure. First, V_T is decreased to 8–10 ml/kg to decrease the volume of gas that must be exhaled on each breath. Next, the respiratory rate is decreased to 8–10/minute to reduce the minute ventilation and increase the expiratory time. Third, a higher inspiratory flow rate is set to increase the expiratory time for each cycle. A decelerating wave form of inspiratory flow may help evenly distribute the tidal volume. Once the patient is allowed to trigger the ventilator, the cautious addition of PEEP (generally <10 cmH_2O) may narrow the differences between alveolar and central airway pressures at end-exhalation, auto-PEEP, making the ventilator easier to trigger.

Tachypnea and Agitation in a Patient With ARDS

A 25-year-old man was admitted with pneumococcal pneumonia and sepsis. His course was complicated within 24 hours of admission by the development of refractory hypoxemia, bilateral infiltrates, and decreased lung compliance without evidence of volume overload or elevated left ventricular filling pressures. He was intubated and placed on A/CMV ventilation at a backup rate of 12/minute, a V_T of 800 ml, an inspiratory flow rate of 40 L/minute, an FiO_2 of 90%, and a PEEP of 5 cmH_2O. On these ventilator settings, he was noted to be diaphoretic and agitated with a respiratory rate of 25/minute, a heart rate of 130/minute, a minute ventilation of 18 L/minute, and arterial blood gas analysis of pH 7.32, $PaCO_2$ of 48 mmHg, and PaO_2 of 60 mmHg. What would be the approach to his agitation, respiratory acidosis, and refractory hypoxemia?

This patient's respiratory problem fits all the diagnostic criteria for ARDS, a syndrome characterized by diffuse injury to the alveolar-capillary membrane and subsequent alveolar edema, with the development of severe hypoxemia and increased physiologic dead space from shunting and $\dot{V}A/\dot{Q}$ mismatching. There are a number of clinical conditions that predispose to this syndrome, including bacterial sepsis, as was present in this patient. Currently, the approach to patients with this syndrome is to treat the underlying illness and provide ventilatory support until the lung heals adequately from the injury.

The patient's problems with agitation, respiratory acidosis, and hypoxemia may be due, in part, to the ventilator settings. Although agitation can be caused by pain or psychosis, in this patient, a large component of agitation could be from dyspnea related to poor matching of the ventilator settings to the patient's ventilatory needs. First, the patient is triggering the ventilator at a rate of 25/minute, and expending significant respiratory muscle effort far in excess of the backup rate setting (12,13). Even at this high respiratory rate, the patient has a respiratory acidosis related to a high CO_2 production and to a high physiologic dead space. Second, the inspiratory flow rate of 4 L/minute is lower than his predicted inspiratory flow demand (minute ventilation $\times$ 4 = 72 L/minute) and will contribute to the patient's work of breathing and agitation (13).

When the inspiratory flow rate was increased to 70 L/minute additional sedation and an increased backup rate of 28/minute succeeded in controlling ventilation. The patient's agitation resolved and his heart rate decreased to 90/minute. With these changes in the ventilator settings, the patient's oxygenation also improved. With less agitation and respiratory muscle effort, his oxygen consumption decreased, increasing his mixed venous saturation. (For any given shunt fraction, higher mixed venous saturation will increase the PaO_2) (5). In addition, relaxation of the expiratory muscles may allow PEEP to recruit collapsed or flooded alveoli more effectively, thereby decreasing the shunt fraction (24).

References

1. Gilbe CE, Salt JC, Branthwaite MA. Pulmonary function after prolonged mechanical ventilation with high concentrations of oxygen. Thorax 35:907, 1980.
2. Nunn JF. Applied Respiratory Physiology, 3rd ed. Boston, Butterworths, 1987, pp 442–443.
3. Aubier M, Murciano D, Milic-Emili J, et al. Effects of O_2 administration on ventilation and blood gases in acute respiratory failure of patients with chronic obstructive lung disease. Am Rev Respir Dis 122:747–754, 1980.
4. Milic-Emili J. Recent advances in clinical assessment of control of breathing. Lung 160:1–17, 1982.
5. Dantzker DR. Gas exchange in the adult respiratory distress syndrome. Clin Chest Med 3:57, 1982.
6. Kolobow T, Moretti MP, Fumagalli R, et al. Severe impairment in lung function induced by high peak airway pressure during mechanical ventilation: an experimental study. Am Rev Respir Dis 135:312–315, 1987.
7. Pepe PE, Marini JJ. Occult positive end-expiratory pressure in mechanically ventilated patients with airflow obstruction: the auto-PEEP effect. Am Rev Respir Dis 126:166–170, 1982.
8. Cole AGH, Weller SF, Sykes MK. Inverse ratio ventilation compared with PEEP in adult respiratory failure. Intensive Care Med 10:227–232, 1984.
9. Gurevitch MJ, Van Dyke J, Young ES, et al. Improved oxygenation and lower peak airway pressure in severe adult respiratory distress syndrome: treatment with inverse ratio ventilation. Chest 89:211–213, 1986.
10. Tharratt RS, Allen RP, Albertson TE. Pressure controlled inverse ratio ventilation in severe adult respiratory failure. Chest 94:755–762, 1988.
11. Truwit JD, Marini JJ. Evaluation of thoracic mechanics in the ventilated patient. Part 1: primary measurements. J Crit Care 3:133–150, 1988.
12. Marini JJ, Capps JS, Culver BH. The inspiratory work of breathing during assisted mechanical ventilation. Chest 87:612–618, 1985.
13. Marini JJ, Rodriquez RM, Lamb V. The inspiratory workload of patient-initiated mechanical ventilation. Am Rev Respir Dis 134:902–909, 1986.
14. Mathru M, Rao TLK, El-Etr AA, et al. Hemodynamic responses to changes in ventilatory patterns in patients with normal and poor left ventricular reserve. Crit Care Med 10:423, 1982.
15. Haake R, Schlichtig R, Ulstad DR, Henschen RR. Barotrauma: pathophysiology, risk factors, and prevention. Chest 91:608–613, 1987.
16. Maunder RJ, Pierson DJ, Hudson LD. Subcutaneous and mediastinal emphysema: pathophysiology, diagnosis, and management. Arch Intern Med 144:1447–1453, 1984.
17. Mathru M, Venus B. Ventilator-induced barotrauma in controlled mechanical ventilation versus intermittent mandatory ventilation. Crit Care Med 11:359–361, 1983.
18. Culpepper JA, Rinaldo JE, Rogers RM. Effect of mechanical ventilator mode on tendency towards respiratory alkalosis. Am Rev Respir Dis 132:1075–1077, 1985.
19. Hudson LD, Hurlow RS, Craig KC, et al. Does intermittent mandatory ventilation correct respiratory acidosis in patients receiving assisted mechanical ventilation? Am Rev Respir Dis 132:1701–1704, 1985.
20. Hooper RG, Browning M. Acid-base changes and ventilator mode during maintenance ventilation. Crit Care Med 13:44, 1985.
21. Marini JJ. Mechanical ventilation. In: Simmons (ed). Current pulmonology. Chicago, Year Book Medical Publishers, Inc., 1988.

22. Smith TC, Marini JJ. Impact of PEEP on lung mechanics and work of breathing in severe airflow obstruction. J Appl Physiol 65:1488–1499, 1988.
23. Rossi A, Gottfried SB, Zocchi L, et al. Measurement of static compliance of the total respiratory system in patients with acute respiratory failure during mechanical ventilation: the effect of intrinsic positive end-expiratory pressure. Am Rev Respir Dis 131:672, 1985.
24. Coggeshall JW, Marini JJ, Newman JH. Improved oxygenation after muscle relaxation in adult respiratory distress syndrome. Arch Intern Med 145:1718–1720, 1985.

8
Breathing Circuits for Spontaneous Ventilation and the Work of Breathing
Robert A. Smith

Mechanical ventilation has not been observed to significantly blunt or reverse pathophysiology associated with human acute respiratory insufficiency. Mechanical ventilatory support, however, may promote further damage to injured lung and injure remaining healthy lung. When patients with acute lung injury are capable of adequate spontaneous breathing, they are often treated with continuous positive airway pressure (CPAP). CPAP is also used to improve left ventricular performance in patients with congestive heart failure and reduce inspiratory work of breathing in patients with chronic obstructive pulmonary disease (see Chapter 10, Positive End-Expiratory Pressure (PEEP) and Continuous Airway Pressure (CPAP)). CPAP should be applied with a circuit that provides adequate gas flow with minimal inspiratory effort and incorporates an expiratory valve that generates predictable pressure at end-exhalation, independent of gas flow rate. Apparatus-imposed work of breathing varies widely among devices used for the application of CPAP. Clinicians who prescribe CPAP must be cognizant of the capabilities and limitations of available devices. Assessment of respiratory muscle work and use of equipment that imposes minimal resistance are important considerations in the management of patients receiving CPAP therapy.

WORK OF BREATHING

Respiratory muscles contract during spontaneous inspiration, thereby enlarging the thorax, further decreasing intrapleural pressure (Ppl). As the volume of gas that occupies the alveoli increases, the intra-alveolar pressure decreases below airway pressure and air flows into the lungs. The pressure gradient between the airway pressure and visceral pleura surface pressure, which is approximately equal to Ppl, is called the transpulmonary pressure (P_L). Transpulmonary pressure is not uniform because Ppl is not uniform. Regional Ppl is determined primarily by body position relative to the gravity vector (~0.2 cmH_2O/cm of vertical distance down the lungs) and regional lung volume. In general, Ppl becomes less subatmospheric and P_L decreases as lung regions become more gravity dependent. Nonuniform P_L notwithstanding, distensibility of the respiratory system during spontaneous inspiration is often quantified by calculating dynamic respiratory system compliance, which is determined with the following equation:

$$C_{RS} = \Delta V_L / \Delta P_L$$

where ΔV_L = change in lung volume or tidal volume (V_T) and ΔP_L = change in transpulmonary pressure (see Chapter 10). Dynamic respiratory system compliance represents primarily the elastic forces (those that develop in the tissues attendant with a change in volume), resistive forces (resistance offered by the airways to the flow of gas and by the deformation of nonelastic tissue), and inertial forces (associated with the mass of the gases and tissues) acting to oppose the respiratory muscles during spontaneous inspiration. Inertial forces are presumed inconsequential and are not usually considered when determining work of breathing. Because the transthoracic pressure gradient (atmospheric minus intrapleural) is not acting to distend the thorax during spontaneous inspiration, thoracic compliance cannot be directly determined.

Mechanical work is quantified physically as the product of force and displacement. In a pneumatic system, work of breathing (W) may be determined with the following relationship:

$$W = \int PdV$$

where P = the cumulative product of the trans-structural pressure gradient (e.g., transpulmonary pressure) and dV = the volume of gas moved at each instant. Mechanical work of breathing is measured in joules (J) and the rate at which respiratory muscles perform work (power) is quantified in watts (1 watt = 1 J/second). Work and power are often represented clinically as J/L and J/minute; and, in normal young adults, they average 0.5 J/L and 4.0 J/minute, respectively.

Mechanical work of breathing includes the work required to change lung volume and thoracic volume. Mechanical work done moving the thorax cannot be assessed during spontaneous breathing because there is no method available to quantify the mechanical work done by the muscles of breathing on themselves. However, mechanical work performed on the lungs may be computed electronically by integrating the product of the transpulmonary pressure and attendant change in lung volume ($\int PdV$). Work of breathing may also be determined graphically by measuring the area under the curve produced by plotting the change in intrapleural pressure against the change in lung volume.

Clinically, esophageal pressure (Pes) is used indirectly to estimate changes in intrapleural pressure and to determine transpulmonary pressure. Simultaneous determinations of Pes and Ppl correlate well when Pes is carefully and correctly measured. Esophageal pressure is measured with a pneumatic pressure transducer

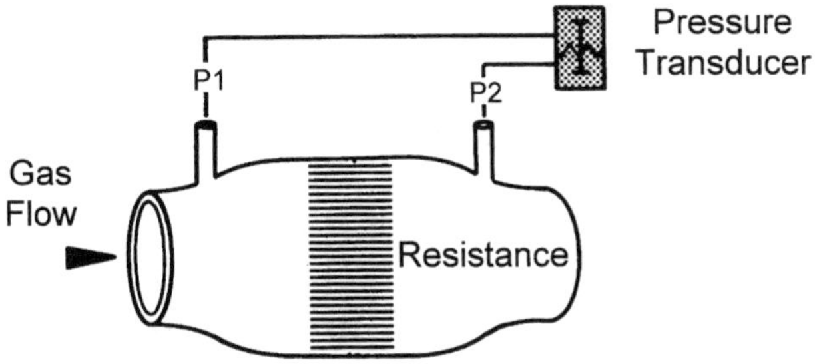

Figure 8.1. Schematic illustration of a pneumotachograph incorporating a hydraulic resistance head and differential pressure transducer. See text for details.

linked with a polyethylene balloon attached to a polyurethane radiopaque catheter. The balloon is inflated with 0.5 to 0.8 ml of air, inserted oro- or nasopharyngeally, passed into the esophagus while observing the pressure, and advanced until the balloon resides in the stomach. Supra-atmospheric pressure during spontaneous inspiration indicates that the balloon is beyond the cardiac sphincter. Then the catheter is slowly withdrawn retrograde until the Pes at end-expiration becomes subatmospheric and 10 cm (or length of the balloon) further to ensure the entire balloon is in the esophagus. Adequate positioning of the esophageal balloon is confirmed by occluding the airway opening at end-expiration with a pressure measuring device (Pao) and observing the recorded Ppl and Pes during two or three of the patient's inspiratory efforts. A ΔPes/ΔPao ratio ≥ 0.80 indicates position of the esophageal balloon is adequate to reflect accurately the changes in intrapleural pressure. The ΔPes/ΔPao ratio should be assessed when the patient's body position is altered. For example, in the supine position, the heart may compress the esophagus and increase baseline Pes. Therefore, in the supine position Pes should not be expected to reflect absolute Ppl, but the changes in Pes are likely representative of the changes in Ppl.

Graphic estimation of the work of breathing was introduced by Rohrer in 1925 and expanded by Campbell in 1958 to employ esophageal pressure. Airway opening gas flow and pressure are measured with a pneumotachograph (Fig. 8.1). The pneumotachograph incorporates a hydraulic resistor and a differential pressure transducer. The function of the pneumotachograph is based on the pneumatic equivalent of Ohm's law, where

$$\text{Gas flow } (\dot{V}) = \frac{\text{Pressure differential (P1} - \text{P2)}}{\text{Fixed resistance of the pneumotachograph (e.g., 0.5 cmH}_2\text{O/L·s)}}$$

Gas volume is computed as the time integral of gas flow ($\int \dot{V}dt$) and corrected to body temperature and pressure saturated (BTPS). The total work of breathing is determined by integrating the area subtended by change in Pes versus change in lung volume during inspiration and expiration (Fig. 8.2). Inspiratory and expiratory resistive work is distinguished by constructing a line between points of no gas flow (end-expiration and end-inspiration). This line (AC) reflects the esophageal pressure developed opposing the elastic forces of the respiratory system (Pel) as lung volume changes (slope of line AB represents the static respiratory system compliance); the area to the right represents inspiratory resistive work (ABCA); and the area to the left (ACEA) represents expiratory resistive work. The total work performed by the inspiratory respiratory muscles to increase the gas volume of the lungs from the relaxation volume is represented by the area ABCDEA. Elastic work done by the inspiratory respiratory muscles to increase the gas volume of the lungs from the relaxation volume is represented by the area ACDEA. When expiration is passive (i.e., area ACDEA is greater than area ACEA), the resistive work is accomplished by the energy (potential energy) stored in elastic tissues during inspiration. Work of breathing is increased by an increase in the resistive or the elastic forces opposing the respiratory muscles during inspiration (Fig. 8.3).

When patients have an artificial airway, change in lung volume should be assessed using the change in intratracheal pressure (tracheal tubes are commercially

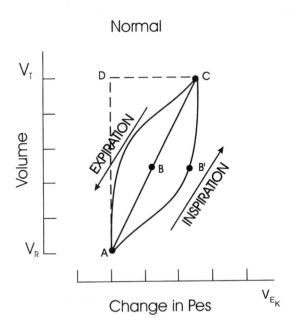

Figure 8.2. Schematic rendition of the change in lung volume plotted against the change in esophageal pressure during inspiration and expiration with a normal respiratory system compliance. See text for explanation.

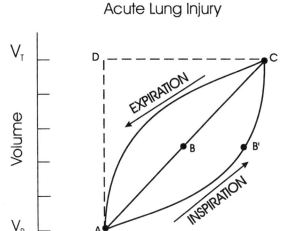

Figure 8.3. Schematic rendition of the change in lung volume plotted against the change in esophageal pressure during inspiration and expiration with a respiratory system compliance characteristic of acute lung injury. See text for explanation.

available that incorporate a lumen imbedded in the wall that exits near the distal end of the tube). The tracheal tube acts like a resistor connected in series between the breathing circuit and conducting airways of the respiratory system. The pressure gradient required to effect gas flow through a tracheal tube is primarily determined by the internal diameter and length and averages 3 to 6 cmH$_2$O/L/second in tubes used in adults. During mechanical ventilation, measuring pressure at the airway opening overestimates alveolar pressure during inspiration and underestimates alveolar pressure during expiration. During spontaneous breathing, airway pressure underestimates the reduction in alveolar pressure during inspiration and underestimates alveolar pressure during expiration. Indeed, in patients with acute lung injury, most of the resistive work is associated with tracheal tube resistance (and other apparatus-imposed load) rather than anatomic airways resistance.

In summary, the primary determinants of the amount of respiratory muscle work done on the lungs during spontaneous breathing include lung distensibility, breathing depth (tidal volume), anatomy airway gas flow resistance, inspiratory gas flow rate, and apparatus-imposed resistance (e.g., artificial airway components of the breathing circuit). Monitoring work of breathing and the contributing elements may facilitate efficacious application of positive airway pressure while minimizing apparatus-imposed loading of the respiratory muscles in spontaneously breathing patients.

BREATHING CIRCUITS

Access to atmospheric air is virtually boundless during normal spontaneous breathing; thus, airway pressure is nearly constant and the work of breathing is minimal. Normally we breathe with a CPAP (atmospheric pressure) equal to 760 mmHg at sea level. When an artificial airway is inserted into the trachea and connected to a breathing circuit, the patient's work of breathing is increased. If the flow of gas available from the breathing circuit is less than the patient's inspiratory flow rate, even transiently, airway pressure will decrease and work of breathing will increase. Apparatus-imposed inspiratory load frequently is not recognized by clinicians directing the patient's therapy, yet may be significant and represent the difference between therapeutic success and failure. Proper equipment and settings are essential for efficient and successful positive airway pressure breathing.

Gas flow in a circuit that permits spontaneous breathing may be provided continuously or with a demand valve designed to generate gas flow in response to patient effort. The potential gas flow with either method must exceed the patient's peak inspiratory flow. Therefore, a continuous gas flow system often must include a reservoir. A typical circuit used for the application of positive airway pressure with a continuous gas flow and reservoir is represented schematically in Figure 8.4. The reservoir bag provides an additional source of gas to the bias flow during inspiration. Ideally, the size and elastic properties of the reservoir bag should be such that constant pressure is exerted, despite alteration in volume. The continuous gas flow rate should be adjusted to sustain reservoir bag inflation during the inspiratory phase of the respiratory cycle. When the volume of the reservoir bag is large (e.g., 10 L) relative to the patient's VT and is constructed of thin, highly compliant rubber, gas flow rate need only be slightly greater than the patient's minute volume. Thus the variation in flow across the pressure relief valve is decreased and airway pressure fluctuation minimized during tidal breathing. Optimal pressure stability can be achieved by placing the gas reservoir near the tracheal tube connection of the breathing circuit (i.e., distal to the humidification mechanism). However, condensate may accumulate and the reservoir should incorporate a water vent. An inspiratory airway pressure reduction or an expiratory airway pressure increase >4 cmH$_2$O represents an unacceptable degree of resistance and the increased work of breathing may not be tolerated. Breathing circuit pressure changes during the inspiratory and expiratory phases of the respiratory cycle can be evaluated with a pressure manometer interfaced at the airway opening. An idealized rendition of airway pressure and esophageal pressure during CPAP are illustrated in Figure 8.5. Note that the change in esophageal pressure is similar

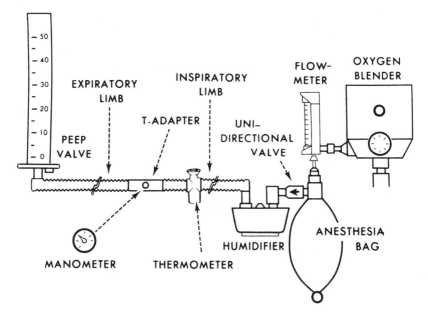

Figure 8.4. Schematic representation of a breathing circuit in which positive pressure is maintained throughout the respiratory cycle.

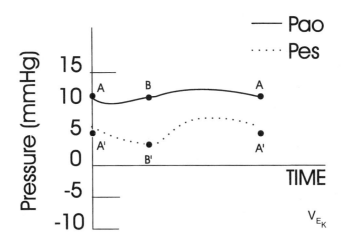

Figure 8.5. Schematic rendition of the airway opening pressure (Pao) and esophageal pressure (Pes) during inspiration (path A and A' to B and B', respectively) and expiration (path B and B' to A and A', respectively) with CPAP.

to that illustrated in Figure 8.6, when fluctuations in airway pressure are minimized during normal breathing at atmospheric pressure.

Continuous positive airway pressure can be administered with a circuit providing gas at a high flow rate (Fig. 8.7), thus obviating the need for a gas reservoir. Source gas, usually oxygen, is metered to a constriction (jet), and as the gas is accelerated, a subatmospheric pressure is created (Bernoulli factor) and gas is entrained into the tube (Venturi factor). The delivered gas is a mixture of jet gas (usually 100% oxygen) and entrained gas (room air); typically it provides 30% to 40% oxygen. Because ambient air entrainment increases the relative humidity of compressed oxygen, added humidification may be unnecessary. However, a compressed air-powered nebulizer can be coupled with the entrainment port to moisten inspired gas further.

Continuous positive airway pressure also can be applied with a circuit in which gas is provided on demand by a regulator. Ideally, demand regulators generate gas flow at a constant pressure. Gas flow is initiated in response to a decrement in airway pressure resulting from the patient's inspiratory effort. The opening pressure (trigger sensitivity) of the gas regulator is usually selected by the clinician. Response time of a pressure-triggered gas flow generator to an inspiratory effort may be significantly reduced when pressure is detected at the distal end of the tracheal tube. The resistive and response latency characteristics of demand gas flow regulators vary widely.

Another potential source of increased work of breathing during positive pressure breathing therapy is the humidification device, particularly when the gas flow

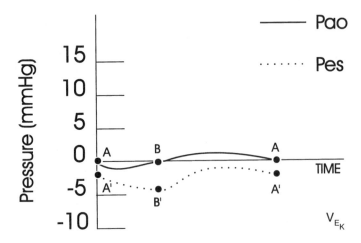

Figure 8.6. Schematic rendition of the airway opening pressure (Pao) and esophageal pressure (Pes) during inspiration (path A and A' to B and B', respectively) and expiration (path B and B' to A and A', respectively) at atmospheric pressure.

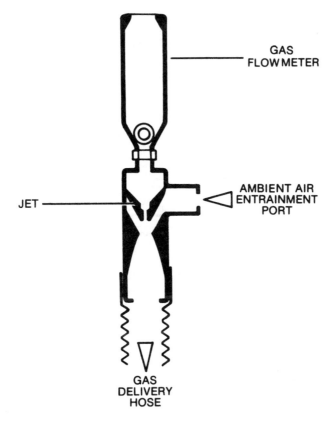

Figure 8.7. Schematic illustration of gas injector. See text for details.

is diverted through a submerged mechanism. If the patient's inspiratory flow demand exceeds circuit flow, the patient must inspire reservoir gas through the humidifier. Most humidifiers have extremely high-flow resistance and significantly increase the work of breathing. Although passover-type humidifiers (passive humidification) tend to offer less resistance to flow, gas is not adequately moistened at high-flow rates. Wick-type humidifiers capable of humidifying gas at flow rates up to 60 L/minute are ideal.

A wide variety of pressure valves are commercially available. By design, they are either gravity-dependent or gravity-independent. Gravity-dependent valves typically incorporate a weighted ball or hydrostatic mechanism. An example of a hydrostatic pressure valve is illustrated in Figure 8.8. To function properly, these valves must be aligned parallel to the gravity vector. Gravity-independent pressure valves use pneumatic, magnetic, electromagnetic, or spring-tension mechanisms that function independently of spatial orientation. An example of a gravity-inde-

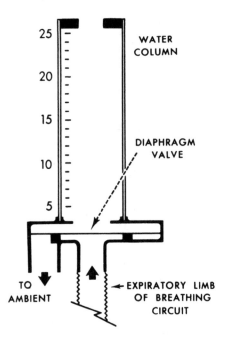

Figure 8.8. A schematic design of a hydrostatic PEEP valve. Gas flow from the expiratory limb of a breathing circuit is directed against the diaphragm weighted by a column of water. The force opposing gas flow is determined by the weight of the column of water and diaphragm.

pendent pressure valve is illustrated in Figure 8.9. Pressure is determined by the tension developed by two curved springs applied to a disc valve. A curved, rather than linear orientation is used to avoid the inherent length-tension fluctuations characteristic of springs. Therefore, applied force on the disc valve remains nearly constant whether opened or closed. Otherwise, flow resistance is unacceptably high.

An ideal pressure valve would produce a predictable pressure independent of gas flow rate. Although most pressure valves are designed to function at a given threshold pressure, their response to gas flow rate is highly variable. Pressure generated by structural resistance to gas flow is not easily controlled and may be detrimental to the patient because of the increased work of breathing. Emphasis has been placed on the inspiratory load contributed by the gas delivery mechanism. However, expiratory valve flow resistance also can influence the inspiratory work of breathing. This situation is unique to CPAP systems using bias gas flow because a portion of the expiratory pressure is derived from resistance to gas flow traversing the expiratory circuit. The pressure contributed by expiratory circuit resistance

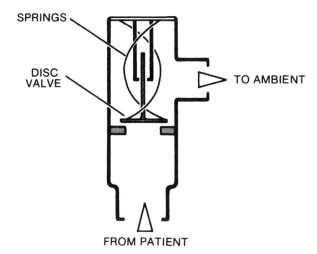

SPRINGS

DISC
VALVE

TO AMBIENT

FROM PATIENT

Figure 8.9. A schematic illustration of a spring-tension PEEP valve. Gas flow from the expiratory limb of a breathing circuit is directed against a disc valve. The force opposing gas flow is determined by the spring-tension and weight of the disc. When positioned the valve is upright.

primarily is due to the expiratory pressure valve. CPAP circuits, incorporating valves that produce pressure derived from gas flow resistance, will result in exaggerated reductions in airway pressure during spontaneous inspiration. During spontaneous inspiration, flow is diverted from the expiratory pressure device to the lungs, which reduces the corresponding circuit pressure. The more flow resistance, the greater the decrement in airway pressure during inspiration and the greater the increment in airway pressure during exhalation, hence, the greater the work of breathing. A decline in the airway pressure during inspiration might be interpreted as a sign of insufficient continuous gas flow. Paradoxically, the apparent remedy will compound the problem: When the gas flow rate is increased, the CPAP level will climb, thus the "selected" valve pressure must be reduced to reestablish the original CPAP. An even larger portion of the CPAP is composed of pressure derived from flow resistance offered by the valve, causing a larger decrement in pressure during inspiration. The effect of the flow-resistive characteristics of the pressure valve on the inspiratory work of breathing can be minimized by using a low-flow, large-volume, highly compliant reservoir CPAP circuit.

SUMMARY

As dynamic respiratory system compliance decreases during acute lung injury, the intrapleural pressure change increases because the stiff lung requires a greater decrease in intrapleural pressure to accomplish tidal breathing and a progressive increase in the work of breathing results. After the application of positive airway pressure to restore functional residual capacity, a reduction in the work of breathing may be observed, but only if inspiratory reduction in airway pressure is small. During CPAP, potential gas flow must be available at a rate equaling or exceeding the patient's inspiratory flow rate. Therefore, airway pressure fluctuates minimally throughout the respiratory cycle. The goal of positive pressure breathing therapy should be to minimize the patient's work of breathing.

Suggested Readings

Baydur A, Cha EJ, Sassoon C. Validation of esophageal balloon technique at different lung volumes and postures. J Appl Physiol 62:315–321, 1987.

Beydon L, Chasse M, Harf A, et al. Inspiratory work of breathing during spontaneous ventilation using demand valves and continuous flow systems. Am Rev Respir Dis 138: 300–304, 1988.

Campbell EJM, Agostoni E, Davis JN (eds). The respiratory muscles: mechanics and neural control. Philadelphia, WB Saunders, 1970.

Cox D, Niblett DJ. Studies on continuous positive airway pressure breathing systems. Br J Anaesth 56:905–911, 1984.

Douglas ME, Downs JB. Cardiopulmonary effects of PEEP and CPAP (Special Correspondence). Anesth Analg 57:346–350, 1978.

Katz JA, Marks JD. Inspiratory work with and without continuous positive airway pressure in patients with acute respiratory failure. Anesthesiology 63:598–607, 1985.

Marini JJ, Culver BH, Kirk W. Flow resistance of exhalation valves and positive end-expiratory pressure devices used in mechanical ventilation. Am Rev Respir Dis 131: 850–854, 1985.

Moran JL, Homan S, O'Fathartaigh M, et al. Inspiratory work imposed by continuous positive airway pressure (CPAP) machines: the effect of CPAP level and endotracheal size. Intensive Care Med 18:148–154, 1992.

Milic-Emili J. Work of breathing. In: Crystal RG, West JB (eds). The Lung: scientific foundations. New York, Raven Press, 1991, pp 1065–1075.

Nunn JF. Nunn's applied respiratory physiology, 4th ed. Oxford, Buterworth-Heinemann Ltd, 1993, pp 117–128.

Rodarte JR, Rehder K. Dynamics of respiration. In: Machlem PT, Mead J (eds). Handbook of physiology, Section 3: The respiratory system, Vol. III. Mechanics of breathing, Part 1. Bethesda, MD: American Physiological Society, 1986, pp 131–144.

Rohrer F. Physiologie der atembewegung. Handbuch der Normalen und Pathologischen Physiologie 2:70–127, 1925. In: West JB (ed). Translations in respiratory physiology. Stroudsburg, PA, Dowden, Hutchinson & Ross, Inc., 1975, pp 161–167.

Sturgeon CL, Douglas ME, Downs JB, et al. PEEP and CPAP: cardiopulmonary effects during spontaneous ventilation. Anesth Analg 56:633–641, 1977.

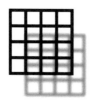

9
Intermittent Mandatory Ventilation
Robert R. Kirby

In the first edition of this text (1) I wrote that intermittent mandatory ventilation (IMV) and synchronized intermittent mandatory ventilation (SIMV) "largely supplanted other forms of ventilatory support." This statement was based on my personal experience and the results of a survey of more than 1000 U.S. hospitals concerning the most frequently used techniques of mechanical ventilatory support and weaning (2). I noted also that despite the apparent popularity of IMV/SIMV at the grass roots level, considerable controversy still surrounded the scant scientific basis existing for their use and the outcome thereof.

Although the chapter in which these considerations appeared was published in 1992, it was written in 1990. This current revision was born in April 1995. Thus, 5 years have passed, and a look to see what, if anything, has changed is in order.

HISTORICAL CONSIDERATIONS

Neonatal

Although *interpretation* of historical *facts* frequently varies, the facts themselves remain reasonably constant. The impetus for the development of IMV/SIMV grew out of a general dissatisfaction with the results of conventional mechanical ventilation techniques used in neonates with hyaline membrane disease. In the 1960s, when large-scale support evolved for the treatment of this problem, only assisted (patient-triggered) mechanical ventilation and controlled mechanical ventilation (CMV) techniques were available.

The common failing of both assisted and CMV techniques was matching the patient's needs (low tidal volume [V_T] and rapid respiratory rates) to what the ventilator was capable of delivering. Sensing mechanisms for assisted ventilation frequently were not sufficiently responsive to the small airway pressure fluctuations generated by the struggling infant's efforts to breathe. As a result, the ventilator often failed to cycle on, and the infant became progressively hypoxemic and hypercapnic. With the substitution of the control mode, unless it was set exactly right (difficult under the best of circumstances), the infant attempted to breathe but received no fresh gas flow between the preset cycles. Again, hypoxemia and hypercapnia usually occurred.

For many years, anesthesiologists had used Ayre's T-piece and several modifications thereof to provide ventilatory support for infants and small children in the operating room. In its simplest form (Fig. 9.1), the device provided a continuous flow of gas through the T-piece, from which the infant could breathe spontaneously. Periodic occlusion of one end of the T-piece by the anesthesiologist's thumb diverted gas, under pressure, into the infant's lungs. Thus, a combination of spontaneous and manual inflations was provided in the desired ratio. Later modifications included various arrangements of valves and reservoir bags that allowed more precise control.

Existing mechanical ventilators could not provide a continuous gas flow that allowed infants to breathe spontaneously. Thus, every breath had to be delivered by the ventilator; spontaneous attempts to breathe—"fighting the ventilator"—were controlled by deliberate hyperventilation, neuromuscular paralysis, sedation, or a combination of these. In 1971, a prototype ventilator was developed that provided a continual gas flow and incorporated a timing mechanism, which closed the exhalation valve in a manner similar to the placement of the anesthesiologist's

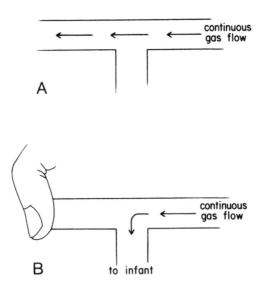

Figure 9.1. Modification of the Ayre's T-piece is the basis of intermittent mandatory ventilation in most neonatal ventilators. **A,** Continuous gas flow allows spontaneous breathing. **B,** Occlusion of the end of the T-tube diverts the flow into the infant's lungs. A positive-pressure inflation results, the volume of which is controlled by the gas flow rate and duration of occlusion.

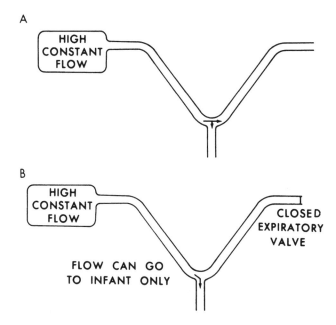

Figure 9.2. Schematic configuration of neonatal intermittent mandatory ventilator. Compare with Figure 9.1. **A,** High continuous gas flow for spontaneous breathing. **B,** Pneumatic or electronic control mechanism periodically closes the exhalation valve diverting gas flow into the infant's lungs. In principle, the method of ventilation is identical to thumb occlusion of the Ayre's T-piece.

thumb over the end of the Ayre's T-piece (3) (Fig. 9.2). Combined mechanical and spontaneous breathing could then be provided for long periods, and continuous positive airway pressure (CPAP) was incorporated with specially designed valve assemblies, changes in the continual gas flow, or both. This method of ventilation was termed IMV (Fig. 9.3).

From 1975 to the present, most ventilators designed for neonatal and infant applications incorporated IMV as the primary ventilatory mode. It was simple, relatively foolproof, easy to convert to more aggressive support (e.g., CMV) or to lower level applications (CPAP), and was supplemented easily by positive end-expiratory pressure (PEEP).

Adult

The success of IMV in neonatal care led investigators to study its use in adults. Again, experience in the operating room provided much of the background information necessary. Anesthesia circuits were equipped with a reservoir bag. A spontaneously breathing patient obtained gas from two sources. The first was a fresh

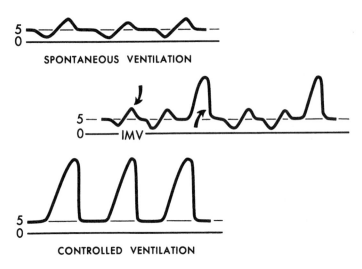

Figure 9.3. Airway pressure tracings during spontaneous ventilation, intermittent mandatory ventilation (IMV), and controlled ventilation. Note that IMV has characteristics of both spontaneous and controlled ventilation. Because both fewer mechanical breaths generally are delivered with IMV than with controlled ventilation and airway and pleural pressures are reduced with the spontaneous breaths, lower intrapleural pressures result, and venous return, cardiac output, and blood pressure tend to be higher (see, also, Fig. 9.7).

gas flow from the anesthesia machine gas manifold. The peak inspiratory flow required, however, often was in excess of 30 L/minute. The flow deficit was made up from gas in a 3- to 5-L reservoir bag. The reservoir bag also served a second function. If the patient's respiratory efforts were not sufficient to maintain satisfactory ventilation, the anesthesiologist could augment gas flow by squeezing the bag synchronously with the second, third, or fourth breath, or some multiple of these. Thus, any desired combination of spontaneous and manually assisted breathing was available, allowing precise control of minute ventilation, $PaCO_2$, and pHa.

The apparent advantages of such assisted ventilation in the operating room could not be carried over to the postanesthesia care areas or intensive care unit (ICU) because existent adult ventilators had no means to supply the requisite continuous gas flow for spontaneous breathing. An adult, with a V_T of several hundred milliliters and inspiratory flow rates >20–30 L/minute, needed considerably higher circuit flows that were wasteful and expensive. The solution to this problem initially was provided by the development of an open-ended system (4), followed shortly thereafter by a closed reservoir system (5) (Fig. 9.4). Subsequently,

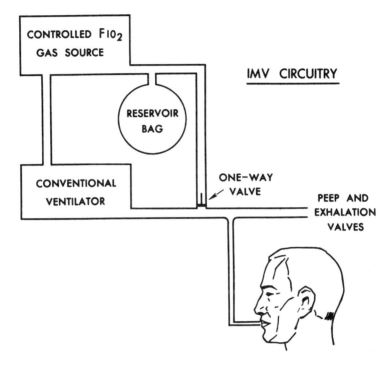

Figure 9.4. Adult closed reservoir bag system to provide intermittent mandatory ventilation (IMV). Spontaneous breaths are obtained from the reservoir bag between mechanical cycles. This system is used with some Emerson IMV ventilators. Gas flow is continuous.

a variety of demand regulators largely replaced the reservoir bag (Fig. 9.5). Because they responded only to the patient's inspiratory effort, gas flow was intermittent and more economic.

Synchronization of the ventilator-delivered V_T (the mandated breath) with the patient's spontaneous inspiratory effort soon followed. SIMV differed from IMV in that the mandated breath could not be delivered until the next spontaneous inspiratory effort occurred (Fig. 9.6), thereby preventing the possibility of the ventilator *stacking* a mechanical V_T on top of a spontaneous one.

Within a decade, SIMV largely replaced IMV in adult ventilation, although the latter technique remained pre-eminent for neonatal applications. From the mid-1980s on, the primary modification to traditional IMV/SIMV (and indeed to all ventilator modes) was the introduction of microprocessor technology that allowed more precise applications and expanded capabilities (6).

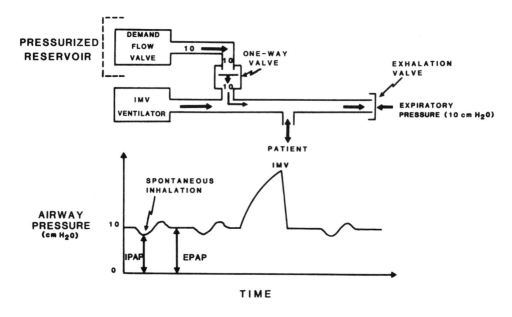

(CPAP = IPAP + EPAP)

Figure 9.5. A demand flow valve provides the means for spontaneous breathing in most new intermittent mandatory ventilation (IMV) ventilator systems. Flow is provided only during inspiration rather than continuously with the reservoir bag system depicted in Figure 9.4. *IPAP,* inspiratory positive airway pressure; *EPAP,* expiratory positive airway pressure.

CLINICAL APPLICATIONS

Reputed advantages and disadvantages of IMV/SIMV are summarized in Tables 9.1 and 9.2 (6). Some effects that seemed very important years ago appear less so today.

Reputed Advantages

AVOIDANCE OF RESPIRATORY ALKALOSIS

IMV/SIMV decrease the incidence and severity of respiratory alkalosis with *statistically* significant decreases in pH and increases in $PaCO_2$ compared with assisted or controlled ventilation. Whether the differences are clinically relevant and what the mechanism producing such differences may be are debatable.

Proponents of IMV/SIMV claim that the reduction in alkalosis results from

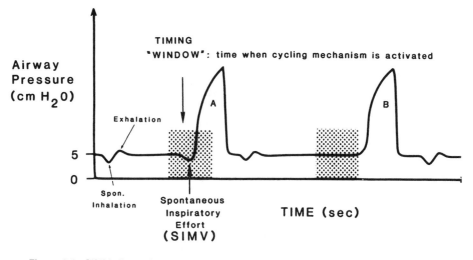

Figure 9.6. SIMV allows the mechanical breath to be delivered only in response to the patient's spontaneous inspiratory effort. **A,** Spontaneous effort triggers the ventilator-delivered breath. **B,** No spontaneous effort occurred. The ventilator then delivers a breath automatically as a safety backup measure.

the patient's ability to set both the rate and V_T of spontaneous breathing to meet his or her physiologic requirements (4). The ventilator is used only to augment insufficient ventilation, bringing it to a normal level in terms of CO_2 elimination. Hence, normal pHa and $PaCO_2$ are predictable.

Opponents argue that the only reason that pH and $PaCO_2$ are better with IMV/SIMV is that CO_2 production is increased as a result of increased respiratory muscle activity associated with the spontaneous breathing component (7) and not from improved ventilation/perfusion ($\dot{V}_A/\dot{Q}$) relationships suggested by previous investigations. Groeger et al. (8), however, reported no overall difference in CO_2

Table 9.1 Reputed Advantages of IMV[a]

Avoidance of respiratory alkalosis
Decreased requirement for sedation/muscle relaxation
Lower mean airway pressure
Better matching of ventilation and perfusion
Expedited weaning
Prevention of respiratory muscle atrophy/discoordination
Reduced likelihood of cardiac decompensation

[a] *Modified from Weisman IM, Rinaldo JE, Rogers RM, et al. State of the art: intermittent mandatory ventilation. Am Rev Respir Dis 127:641, 1983.*

Table 9.2 Reputed Disadvantages of IMV[a]

Increased risk of CO_2 retention
Increased work of breathing
Respiratory muscle fatigue
Prolongation of weaning
Increased likelihood of cardiac decompensation

[a] Modified from Weisman IM, Rinaldo JE, Rogers RM, et al. State of the art: intermittent mandatory ventilation. Am Rev Respir Dis 127:641, 1983.

production, energy expenditure, or oxygen consumption (reflective of work of breathing) between SIMV and assist/control ventilation.

With respect to the clinical relevance of a reduction in respiratory alkalosis, one must judge each case individually. For some patients, the difference may be slight or even nonexistent. For others, it will be much greater and of correspondingly increased importance. Respiratory alkalosis has well-documented adverse effects, including a reduction of cardiac output, decreased cerebral blood flow, altered metabolic function, reduction of Ca^{2+}, and a transient rightward shift of the oxyhemoglobin dissociation curve. IMV/SIMV probably do maintain more nearly normal $PaCO_2$ and pHa, but the impact of this homeostasis seems to be minimal in most cases.

DECREASED REQUIREMENT FOR SEDATION/MUSCLE RELAXATION

Because the goals of IMV/SIMV, real or apparent, can be achieved only through a maximization of spontaneous breathing, muscle relaxant drugs are not used. Sedatives and narcotics are employed to achieve endpoints for which they were originally intended—sleep, relief of anxiety, and pain—not spontaneous ventilation suppression.

LOWER MEAN AIRWAY PRESSURE

Because spontaneous breathing reduces airway pressure, whereas mechanical ventilation increases it, a technique that combines the two will result in a lower mean airway pressure than one in which only mechanically delivered positive-pressure breaths are used (Figs. 9.3 and 9.7). Two advantages perhaps accrue to a reduction of airway pressure. First, with fewer high peak inflation pressure, large V_T mechanical breaths, the risk of pulmonary barotrauma is reduced (9) significantly. Second, the lower mean airway and, hence, intrapleural pressure represent less of an impediment to venous return and cardiac output.

The relative importance of this well-described effect must be tempered by the

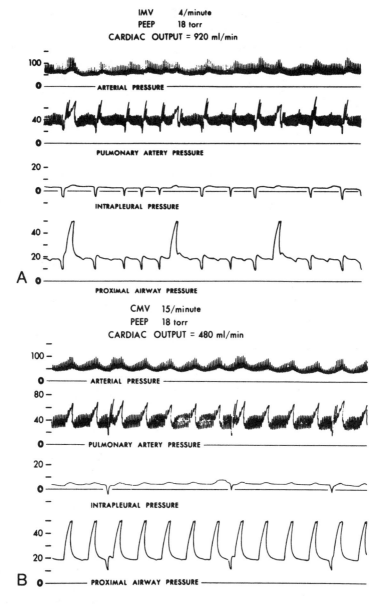

Figure 9.7. Lower mean airway pressure and fewer mechanical breaths with intermittent mandatory ventilation (**A**) result in higher blood pressure and cardiac output than with controlled ventilation (**B**). This relationship holds even with the high level of positive end-expiratory pressure (18 mmHg or 25 cmH$_2$O) (see also Fig. 9.3).

fact that our knowledge of ventilator-induced cardiopulmonary changes is far more complex (and confusing) than it was when IMV and SIMV were developed. Pressure transmission obviously is affected by lung and chest wall alterations. Normal lungs transmit more of a change in airway pressure to the heart and great vessels than do those with significantly reduced compliance (increased stiffness) or higher airways resistance. Significant reductions in airway and pleural pressures increase left ventricular afterload, decrease pulmonary interlobar vascular resistance, and increase alveolar septal vascular resistance. Additionally, leftward displacement of the interventricular septum may occur, thereby reducing left ventricular compliance.

All of these changes can be modified (positively or negatively) by the degree of intravascular volume excess or deficit and by the state of myocardial contractility. Thus, our ability to predict the effect of any variable, such as IMV/SIMV, on a given patient's circulatory status is marginal at best. Pinsky provides an excellent review of this subject matter (10).

As a general rule, higher levels of PEEP/CPAP can be employed safely with IMV/SIMV in patients with particularly severe cases of respiratory failure than can be used effectively with assist or control ventilation (11). For reasons that are unclear, we do not seem to see these cases with nearly the frequency we did in the 1970s (or maybe we are not as aggressive as we once were). However, when they occur, the lower mean airway pressures associated with IMV/SIMV lend themselves to higher PEEP/CPAP.

BETTER MATCHING OF VENTILATION/PERFUSION

Most patients are supine when they are mechanically ventilated. In normal subjects, a reduction of functional residual capacity (FRC) averaging 500 ml occurs when they move from upright to supine. When they breathe spontaneously, however, most ventilation occurs in the dependent (posterior) lung areas, where most pulmonary perfusion is directed. Less ventilation and perfusion are present in the nondependent (anterior) regions (12). Accordingly, overall $\dot{V}_A/\dot{Q}$ matching tends to be retained, even in the face of a reduced FRC.

If the diaphragm is rendered flaccid by muscle relaxant drugs or it does not contract because spontaneous breathing is eliminated for any reason, $\dot{V}_A/\dot{Q}$ relationships are altered dramatically. Now most of the ventilation is directed to the nondependent regions (12) (less impedance from the abdominal viscera exists here), while most of the perfusion remains dependent. Hence, an increase of dead space results anteriorly ($\dot{V}_A > \dot{Q}$), while an increase of shunting occurs posteriorly ($\dot{V}_A < \dot{Q}$).

Because of the decrease in mechanical breaths and increase in spontaneous effort, IMV/SIMV tends to reduce these ventilator-induced $\dot{V}_A/\dot{Q}$ relationships, bringing them toward normal as an increasing proportion of total ventilation is assumed spontaneously. Obviously, ventilation is best served by moving patients to a variety of positions (even prone). However, many ICU patients have injuries or illness that preclude such changes. Hence, any technique that minimizes the obligatory ($\dot{V}_A/\dot{Q}$) abnormalities that the supine position and mechanical ventilation impose must be viewed as advantageous.

EXPEDITED WEANING

Of all the reported advantages of IMV/SIMV, weaning is perhaps most controversial and hardest to establish (4,13). For every paper that has been published showing that weaning is expedited with IMV/SIMV, another is published saying it is not. Weaning is *not* a major problem for most mechanically ventilated patients. When the reason for ventilatory support no longer exists, discontinuation is easy in most instances. Because most published studies used patients for whom weaning was not problematic, one technique is as likely to prove efficacious as another.

Weaning criteria most often employed as an alternative to IMV/SIMV, lack precision and are not well defined (Table 9.3). Applicability of the criteria listed in Table 9.3 deserves attention. Note the variability in the "acceptable" values. As an example, the vital capacity that is accepted in one institution may be 10 ml/kg, whereas in another it is 20 ml/kg—a 100% difference. A patient in the first hospital who can generate the requisite 10 ml/kg (along with other designated tests) would be weaned and extubated, whereas the same patient in the second hospital would have "failed" and would be continued for an additional period of intubation and ventilation. Although the patient is the same, the arbitrary selection

Table 9.3 Criteria for Weaning from Mechanical Ventilation[a]

	Normal	Acceptable
PaO_2 (mmHg)	>80 (room air) >500 ($F_IO_2 = 1.0$)	70–100 ($F_IO_2 = 0.5$–0.6)
P(A-a)O_2 (mmHg) ($F_IO_2 = 1.0$)	<100	<300–450
$PaCO_2$ (mmHg)	35–45	30–55 (in absence of previous hypercapnia)
Vital capacity (mg/kg)	70	10–20
Peak negative pressure (cmH_2O)	−50 to −100	−20 to −30
V_D/V_T	0.3	<0.55 to 0.6
Minute ventilation (L/minute)	4–5	<10; doubled on command

[a] *Abbreviations used in this table: PaO_2, arterial oxygen tension; $P_{A-a}O_2$, arterial alveolar oxygen tension; $PaCO_2$, carbon dioxide tension; V_D/V_T, dead space/tidal volume ratio; F_IO_2, fraction of inspired oxygen.*

of specific criteria determine the eventual treatment. Far preferable, in my view, is to reduce the rate of ventilator cycling using IMV/SIMV and to observe whether spontaneous breathing over a period of time can be maintained satisfactorily.

In the final analysis, a good clinician will be prepared to vary the weaning approach based on the individual patient's requirements. Some modifications in ventilatory technology, discussed later, have expanded and improved our ability to use IMV/SIMV, potentially lessening the weaning difficulties alluded to in the past.

PREVENTION OF RESPIRATORY MUSCLE ATROPHY/DISCOORDINATION

Prolonged skeletal muscle disuse leads to atrophy and perhaps to discoordination of diaphragmatic and accessory muscle contraction. IMV/SIMV have been suggested to minimize this problem because continuous *exercise* occurs with whatever level of spontaneous breathing the patient is able to maintain. Forcing a patient to breathe beyond his or her capabilities, however, leads to fatigue and to the development of discoordination and paradoxic thoracoabdominal respiratory muscle contraction. Under these circumstances, it is preferable to place the respiratory muscles at rest and to provide full ventilatory support. In this regard, graded pressure support ventilation (PSV) in conjunction with direct measurement of the total patient and ventilator work of breathing allows selection of appropriate workloads that will not be fatiguing, on the one hand, nor lead to muscle atrophy on the other (14–17). Precise ventilator support titration of IMV/SIMV and PSV is possible.

REDUCED LIKELIHOOD OF CARDIAC DECOMPENSATION

The primary effects of IMV/SIMV on cardiovascular function have been mentioned. In general, these involve intrapleural pressure reduction, venous return augmentation, as well as cardiac output and systemic blood pressure maintenance (8). However, as discussed, the complexity of ventilator and cardiopulmonary interactions (10) defies any attempt to predict the precise effect likely in a given patient.

Reputed Disadvantages

The reputed disadvantages of IMV/SIMV have received a great deal of attention, both by critics of the techniques and by their proponents who seek to improve their clinical use. They include the following considerations (see Table 9.2) (6).

INCREASED RISK OF CARBON DIOXIDE RETENTION

IMV/SIMV depend on the patient's maintenance of spontaneous ventilation. At low ventilator rates, any decrease of this component can result in significant

CO_2 retention and respiratory acidemia. The technique should be reserved, therefore, for patients with stable central nervous system respiratory control mechanisms. Additionally, patients should not be unduly sedated or depressed with narcotics or anesthetic agents; muscle relaxants are absolutely contraindicated. Inappropriate use of IMV/SIMV in patients who are not suitable candidates for such therapy is responsible for adverse effects rather than the techniques themselves. Careful patient assessment should be no less than with any other form of ventilatory support.

INCREASED WORK OF BREATHING

Increased work of breathing can and does occur with IMV/SIMV. Inadequate circuit design with high inspiratory resistance, an endotracheal tube with too small a diameter (14), and highly flow-resistant PEEP/CPAP valves may preclude satisfactory clinical application. Many older ventilators and even some new ones have intrinsic design flaws in their patient circuits that add significantly to the work of breathing (18,19). The combination of this "external" imposed workload and that resulting from the patient's intrinsic disease process may lead to weaning failure and prolonged ventilator therapy (19–22).

RESPIRATORY MUSCLE FATIGUE

Although respiratory muscle conditioning may benefit from the judicious use of IMV/SIMV, overly zealous application can produce muscle fatigue (16,18,20,21,23). Forcing a patient to breathe spontaneously when he or she is incapable of such effort, or does so only with an inordinate increase of metabolic stress, is counterproductive. Frequent assessment and clinical judgment are essential in preventing this problem. Low resistance ventilator circuits, PSV, and measurement of work of breathing should largely obviate this problem in most individuals (14–22).

PROLONGATION OF WEANING

Weisman et al. state: "IMV, with its gradual reduction of mechanical ventilatory rate, allows desultory physicians to unnecessarily delay the weaning process" (6). In other words, if a ventilator rate reduction from 6 per minute to 4 per minute is successful, but the attending physician then delays the order for a further decrease until 4 hours later, slower weaning may well result. Other problems are related to obligatory delays incidental to obtaining the results of laboratory tests. Thus, a physician or respiratory therapist might have to wait up to an hour for the results of a blood gas analysis before deciding whether to proceed with weaning. However, pulse oximetry and capnography largely circumvent these problems;

when combined with careful patient observation, they *can* make this criticism a thing of the past.

INCREASED LIKELIHOOD OF CARDIAC DECOMPENSATION

The decreased likelihood of cardiac decompensation has been discussed earlier under the purported advantages of IMV/SIMV. This apparent discrepancy has been discussed in detail and will not be considered further. Again, the complex interactions between ventilator and patient make oversimplification risky (10).

CONCLUSIONS

In standing the "test of time" with respect to demonstrated efficacy in ventilatory support, the popularity of IMV/SIMV is well deserved. However, neither IMV nor SIMV is a panacea for all that befalls a patient with respiratory failure. They must be used and monitored just as carefully as any other technique; the clinician should be knowledgeable regarding both their theory and application. In particular, limitations of equipment design and the problems such limitations impose in patient care must be well understood. Ease of care should not lull one into a false sense of security. Continued vigilance and a recognition of the unique characteristics of each patient with respiratory failure should prevent most of the problems that have been described. Careful equipment selection and the addition of other techniques, such as PSV and permissive hypercapnia, reportedly associated with a significant reduction of mortality in adult respiratory distress syndrome (23), may result in improved outcome and reduced morbidity.

References

1. Kirby RR. Intermittent mandatory ventilation. In Perel A, Stock MC (eds). Handbook of mechanical ventilatory support, 1st ed. Baltimore, Williams & Wilkins, 1992, pp 101–116.
2. Venus B, Smith R, Mathru M. National survey of methods and criteria used for weaning from mechanical ventilation. Crit Care Med 15:530, 1987.
3. Kirby RR, Robison EJ, Schulz J, et al. A new pediatric volume ventilator. Anesth Analg 50:533, 1971.
4. Downs JB, Klein EF, Desautels D, et al. Intermittent mandatory ventilation: a new approach to weaning patients from mechanical ventilation. Chest 64:331, 1973.
5. Desautels DA, Bartlett JL. Methods of administering intermittent mandatory ventilation (IMV). Respir Care 19:187, 1974.
6. Weisman IM, Rinaldo JE, Rogers RM, et al. State of the art: intermittent mandatory ventilation. Am Rev Respir Dis 127:641, 1983.
7. Hudson LD, Hurlow RS, Craig KC, et al. Does intermittent mandatory ventilation correct respiratory alkalosis in patients receiving assisted mechanical ventilation? Am Rev Respir Dis 132:1075, 1985.

8. Groeger JS, Levinson MR, Carlon GC. Assist control vs synchronized intermittent mandatory ventilation during acute respiratory failure. Crit Care Med 17:612, 1989.
9. Kirby RR. Barotrauma. In: Webb WR, Besson A (eds). Thoracic surgery: surgical management of chest injuries. St. Louis, Mosby Year Book, 1994, pp 64–71.
10. Pinsky MR. Cardiovascular effects of ventilatory support and withdrawal. Anesth Analg 79:567, 1994.
11. Kirby RR, Downs JB, Civetta JM, et al. High level positive end-expiratory pressure (PEEP) in acute respiratory failure. Chest 67:156, 1975.
12. Froese AB, Bryan AC. Effects of anesthesia and paralysis on diaphragmatic mechanisms in man. Anesthesiology 41:242, 1974.
13. Sahn SA, Lakshmenarayan S, Petty TL. Weaning from mechanical ventilation. JAMA 235:2208, 1976.
14. Brochard L, Rua F, Lorino H. Inspiratory pressure support compensate for the additional work of breathing caused by the endotracheal tube. Anesthesiology 75:739, 1991.
15. Banner MJ, Kirby RR, MacIntyre NR. Patient and ventilator work of breathing and ventilatory muscle loads at different levels of pressure support ventilation. Chest 100:531, 1991.
16. Banner MJ, Blanch PB, Kirby RR. Imposed work of breathing and methods of triggering a demand-flow continuous positive airway pressure system. Crit Care Med 21:183, 1993.
17. Banner MJ. Respiratory muscle function and the work of breathing. Crit Care Med 2:1, 1995.
18. Gibney RTN, Wilson RS, Pontoppidan H. Comparison of work of breathing on high gas flow and demand valve continuous positive airway pressure systems. Chest 82:692, 1982.
19. Civetta JM. Nosocomial respiratory failure or iatrogenic ventilator dependency. Crit Care Med 21:171, 1993.
20. Banner MJ, Jaeger MJ, Kirby RR. Components of work of breathing and implications for monitoring ventilator-dependent patients. Crit Care Med 22:515, 1994.
21. Sassoon CS, Giron AE, Ely EA. Inspiratory work of breathing on flow-by and demand-flow continuous positive airway pressure. Crit Care Med 17:1108, 1989.
22. Banner MJ, Kirby RR, Gabrielli A, et al. Partially and totally unloading the respiratory muscles based on real time measurements of work of breathing: a clinical approach. Chest 106:1835, 1994.
23. Hickling KG, Walsh J, Henderson S, et al. Low mortality rate in adult respiratory distress syndrome using low-volume, pressure-limited ventilation with permissive hypercapnia: a prospective study. Crit Care Med 22:1568, 1994.

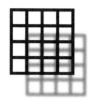

10
Positive End-Expiratory Pressure (PEEP) and Continuous Positive Airway Pressure (CPAP)

Robert A. Smith

End-expiratory pressure may be applied during continuous mechanical ventilation (positive end-expiratory pressure, PEEP) or spontaneous breathing with or without partial ventilatory support (continuous positive airway pressure, CPAP). PEEP and CPAP typically are used to reduce or prevent expiratory atelectasis in patients with acute lung injury. PEEP and CPAP also are administered to increase intrathoracic pressure and reduce left ventricular afterload in patients with congestive heart failure. PEEP and CPAP have been observed to reduce inspiratory load in patients with chronic obstructive disease who experience incomplete exhalation (air trapping). The effects of PEEP and CPAP on lung mechanics may be similar, but they have potentially a different effect on the distribution of ventilation and perfusion ratios and cardiovascular function. The physiologic effects of end-expiratory pressure are predicated on application method, lung and heart condition, and intravascular volume status. This chapter reviews the technical and physiologic aspects associated with PEEP and CPAP therapy.

TECHNICAL CONSIDERATIONS

Flow during expiration may be interrupted by a pressure relief valve if a selected level of end-expiratory pressure has been attained, terminating expiration before it has been completed and thus increasing intrapulmonary gas volume. Various valves are used to produce end-expiratory pressure, including hydrostatic-tension valves, spring-tension valves, pneumatic valves, permanent magnet or electromagnetic valves, or weighted-ball valves. Figure 10.1 illustrates a schematic representation of an electromagnetic exhalation valve (see Chapter 8, Breathing Circuits for Spontaneous Ventilation and the Work of Breathing). The exhalation valve incorporates a metallic disc imbedded into a silicone rubber membrane that is enclosed in a plastic housing. The valve is closed with a linear drive electronic motor. During inspiration, electric current is passed through the coil, creating an

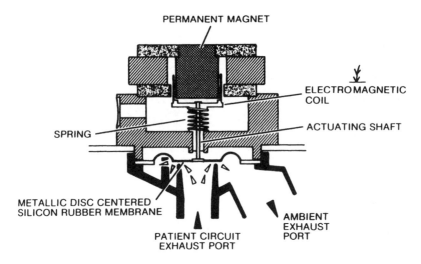

Figure 10.1. Schematic illustration of an electromagnetic exhalation/ positive end-expiratory pressure valve.

electromagnetic field with the same polarity as the permanent magnet. Thus, the silicone membrane is seated by the downward motion of the actuating shaft, which also compresses a spring. Normal exhalation occurs when the current switches off, eliminating the electromagnetic field. When end-expiratory pressure is selected, the electromagnetic mechanism seats the valve at the appropriate circuit pressure. The weight of the coil and actuating shaft are offset by the spring tension; thus, valve resistance is minimized and the exhalation valve is allowed to open.

Ideally, an end-expiratory pressure mechanism should permit unrestricted expiration (i.e., offer no resistance to gas flow rate up to 100 L/minute) until the pressure in the breathing circuit reaches the level of PEEP selected. Because expira-

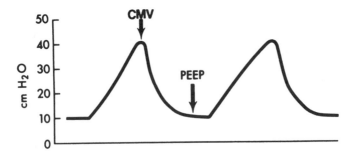

Figure 10.2. Schematic rendition of airway pressure during continuous mechanical ventilation (CMV) and positive end-expiratory pressure (PEEP).

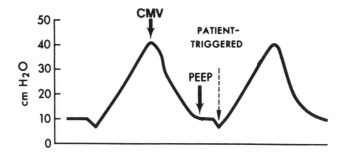

Figure 10.3. Schematic rendition of the airway pressure during patient-triggered continuous mechanical ventilation (CMV) and positive end-expiratory pressure (PEEP).

tory resistance increases mean intrapleural pressure, the increase in intrapleural pressure associated with a given level of end-expiratory pressure also depends on the function of the valve. Because many harmful effects of end-expiratory pressure are associated with mean intrapleural pressure, only valves offering minimal resistance to gas flow should be used.

End-expiratory pressure can be administered in conjunction with control mode ventilation (CMV + PEEP), which may be either controlled (Fig. 10.2) or initiated by the patient (assist mode ventilation + PEEP) (Fig. 10.3). End-expiratory pressure may be applied during spontaneous ventilation (e.g., CPAP) (Fig. 10.4).

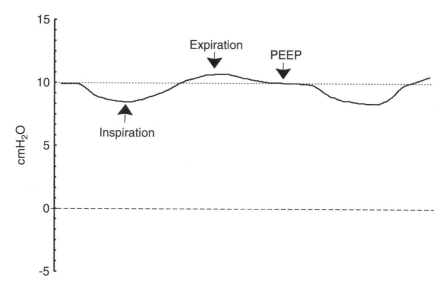

Figure 10.4. Schematic representation of the airway pressure during continuous positive airway pressure (CPAP).

CPAP can be administered with or without partial ventilatory support (e.g., intermittent mandatory ventilation [IMV], airway pressure release ventilation, or biphasic CPAP). CPAP may be delivered to patients via an artificial airway or a face mask.

PHYSIOLOGIC CONSIDERATIONS

Both PEEP and CPAP have long been observed to reduce venous admixture or physiologic shunt (Qsp/Qt) in patients with acute lung injury. Reduction in Qsp/Qt at a given inspired oxygen concentration may be facilitated by a (*a*) reduction in blood flow to non- or under-ventilated lung regions, (*b*) increase in ventilation to under-ventilated lung regions, or (*c*) recruitment and ventilation of previously nonventilated alveoli. The principal difference between PEEP and CPAP occurs during inspiration. During CMV + PEEP, the pressure gradient responsible for inspiratory gas flow is generated by a mechanical ventilator and intrapleural pressure increases. Whereas during CPAP, the pressure gradient required for inspiration is generated by the respiratory muscles and intrapleural pressure decreases.

Respiratory Gas Exchange

Arterial blood gas tensions represent the mean partial pressure of carbon dioxide (PCO_2) and oxygen (PO_2) in perfused gas-exchanging alveoli. End-capillary PCO_2 and PO_2 depend on alveolar gas composition and the degree to which venous blood equilibrates with alveolar gas. Alveolar gas composition is determined by the interaction of the inspired oxygen concentration, the relationship between alveolar ventilation ($\dot{V}_A$) and perfusion ($\dot{Q}$), and the gas tensions in venous blood. Unventilated perfused alveoli (right to left intrapulmonary venous blood shunting), are unable to modify the gas tensions of venous blood. In lung regions with very low $\dot{V}_A/\dot{Q}$ (e.g., <0.1), end-capillary gas tensions are only slightly altered from those in venous blood. The fraction of total cardiac output ($\dot{Q}t$) perfusing unventilated and under- ventilated alveoli ($\dot{Q}va$) is defined as the venous admixture ($\dot{Q}sp/\dot{Q}t$) ratio. When $0.1 < \dot{V}_A/\dot{Q} \leq 10$, end-capillary gas tension reflects alveolar gas composition. Normally, mean $\dot{V}_A/\dot{Q}$ is 0.8 (e.g., $\dot{V}_A = 4.0$ L/minute and $\dot{Q} = 5$ L/minute) and $\dot{Q}sp/\dot{Q}t \cdot 100$ is about 3% to 5% of $\dot{Q}$ (accounted for mostly by anatomic right- to-left shunting). Acute lung injury often is characterized by a decrease in FRC (because lung compliance declines without much alteration in chest wall compliance) causing an increase in $\dot{Q}sp/\dot{Q}t$, usually dominated by shunting (see Chapter 18, Extracorporeal Techniques to Support Ventilation).

Respiratory System Mechanics

Because the majority of gas exchange occurs during expiration, effective improvement in $\dot{Q}sp/\dot{Q}t$ must occur primarily during expiration. During passive expiration, the gas flow is approximately laminar and proportional to the pressure gradient between the alveoli (Palv) and airway pressure (Paw). The Palv to Paw gradient is related to the volume of the lungs (ΔV_L) in excess of functional residual capacity (FRC) of the coupled lungs and chest wall (*infra vide*), assuming near constant elastic recoil forces. As a result, there is a relationship between the rate of lung emptying and the ΔV_L in excess of FRC (i.e., "inspired" tidal volume) and it is commonly expressed with an exponential model using a wash-out function of the form:

$$V_E = \Delta V_L \cdot e^{(-t/C_{RS} \cdot Raw)}$$

where V_E = expired volume ("expired" tidal volume), e = base of natural logarithm, t = time, C_{RS} = compliance of the respiratory system during expiration calculated as the dividend of ΔV_L and associated change in the Paw and intrapleural pressure gradient (transpulmonary pressure gradient), and Raw = airways resistance determined as the dividend of associated transpulmonary pressure gradient and the flow rate of V_E (Fig. 10.5). According to the exponential model,

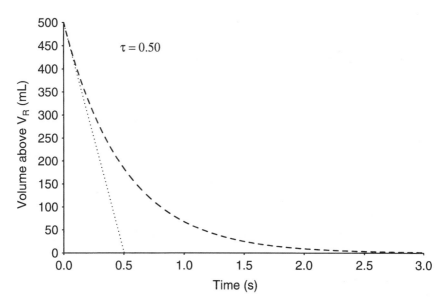

Figure 10.5. Schematic representation of the change of lung volume during passive exhalation with a time constant (τ) of 0.5 second. See text for details.

when V_E reaches steady state, $-t/C_{RS} \cdot Raw = 0$, the time must be infinite. Although the exponential model provides a reasonable representation of reality, from a practical standpoint, expiration does "cease" in a finite time. A convenient unit of time measurement may be obtained by letting the exponent of $e = -1$ and solve for t:

$$t = C_{RS} \cdot Raw.$$

The product of respiratory system compliance and Raw is defined as the time constant (τ) of the exponential function. For example, if respiratory system compliance $= 0.1$ L/cmH$_2$O and Raw $= 6$ cmH$_2$O/L $\cdot$ second, then $\tau = 0.6$ second. Thus, expiration would be completed in 0.6 second if the initial rate of lung emptying was sustained. However, during passive expiration, the initial rate of emptying is not sustained; it progressively decreases according to the wash-out function. Approximately 63%, 86%, 95%, 98%, or 99% of V_E is washed-out in one, two, three, four, or five time constants, respectively. Thus, knowing τ facilitates estimation of adequate expiratory time. For example when $\tau = 0.6$ second, an expiratory time of 2.4 seconds would permit 98% emptying of V_E ("expired" tidal volume).

The thorax and lungs are mechanically coupled (via parietal and visceral pleural surface contact, respectively) elastic structures with different resting states. However, with intact pleura, the thorax and lungs are mechanically interdependent. At the end of a normal exhalation, when the respiratory muscles are relaxed, the tendency of the lungs to recoil inward and that of the thorax to recoil outward is balanced (i.e., the recoil forces are equal and opposite). The mean intrapleural pressure is ~5 cmH$_2$O less than atmospheric pressure, and the lungs are at their FRC. When the balance is upset (e.g., acute lung injury) where the recoil forces of the lungs are increased, the FRC decreases.

Alveolar collapse (atelectasis) and alveolar size reduction caused by hydrostatic compression (pulmonary edema) and reduced surface tension (damage to surfactant) are primarily responsible for the increase in the recoil forces of the lungs (quantified as a reduction in respiratory system compliance), the reduction in FRC, and increase in Raw (due to the reduction in radial traction of peripheral airways attendant with FRC). The reduction in respiratory system compliance is dominant, thus the expiratory time constant is reduced. The rapid rate of lung recoil to an abnormally low FRC is detected by pulmonary baroreceptors and the respiratory control center mediates a tachypnea and glottic narrowing during expiration. Baroreceptor-induced tachypnea is a compensatory mechanism to increase resident lung volume; it often precedes manifestation of gas exchange abnormalities (e.g., arterial hypoxemia). Glottic narrowing is another physiologic compensation to "brake" gas flow, thus increasing the expiratory time constant and resident lung volume in patients without an artificial airway (e.g., expiratory grunting). However, this process does not effectively prevent, but merely delays development of expiratory atelectasis. Indeed, alveoli that are recruited and derecruited during tidal ventilation may eventually become unrecruitable because the surfactant lining is damaged by the rhythmic reopening and collapsing. Moreover, rhythmic alveoli expansion and collapse causes shear forces often associated with parenchymal damage (e.g., barotrauma).

Mechanical ventilation usually is not effective in improving oxygenation because $\dot{Q}sp/\dot{Q}t$ is only affected during inspiration. When inspiration terminates and expiration begins, alveolar collapse recurs. During inspiration, recruitable alveoli are inflated when sufficient distending pressure (recruitment pressure) is applied (Fig. 10.6). Once opened, alveolar patency can be sustained by applying end-expiratory pressure equal to the derecruitment pressure (Fig. 10.7). Derecruitment is prevented with less pressure than was required for recruitment. This phenomenon is called "hysteresis" and is characteristic of elastic structures where recoil forces are less than expansion forces. When successful, end-expiratory pressure acts as a counterforce at a given lung volume, preventing alveolar collapse. Prevention of alveolar collapse tends to increase respiratory system compliance (i.e., decreases lung recoil forces), decrease recoil rate (i.e., increases expiratory time constant), reduce baroreceptor-mediated tachypnea, and improve arterial oxygenation at a given level of inspired oxygen concentration (i.e., oxygenation tends to be proportional to the gas-exchanging surface area of the lungs). When the elastic recoil forces of the lungs are reduced, the efficiency of spontaneous breathing usually improves, thus reducing or obviating the requirement for me-

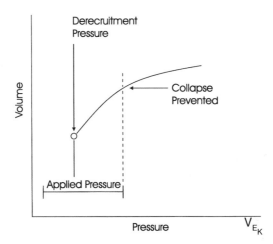

Figure 10.6. Schematic illustration of alveolar recruitment during inspiration and derecruitment during expiration. See text for details.

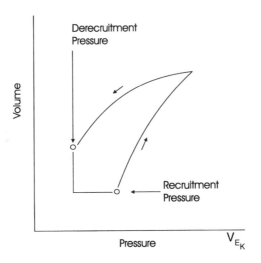

Figure 10.7. Schematic illustration of alveolar recruitment during inspiration and prevention of derecruitment by the application of positive end-expiratory pressure (PEEP). See text for details.

chanical ventilation. Moreover, prevention of rhythmic alveolar reopening and collapse may preserve surfactant function and decrease the shear forces responsible for lung parenchymal damage.

Relaxation volume is increased by an amount equal to the product of end-expiratory pressure and respiratory system compliance. Because alveoli in patients with acute lung injury tend to be either healthy and recruitable or diseased and not recruitable, the effect of end-expiratory pressure on FRC is variable. End-expiratory pressure tends to cause relative hyperinflation and a decrease in respiratory system compliance of healthy alveoli. End-expiratory pressure applied equal to alveolar derecruitment pressure will prevent expiratory collapse and improve respiratory system compliance in recruited alveoli. Thus, end-expiratory pressure has conflicting effects on regional alveolar volume and respiratory system compliance. Appropriate therapy includes assessment of the competing effects of end-expiratory pressure.

Relaxation volume of the respiratory system may be similar with a given level of end-expiratory pressure regardless of whether patients receive PEEP or CPAP, but ventilation distribution is different. In supine, spontaneously breathing patients, inspired gas is preferentially distributed to lung regions that are relatively gravity dependent. Because blood tends to be directed to gravity-dependent alveoli, ventilation and perfusion tend to be well matched during spontaneous breathing. In contrast, during CMV, inspired gas is preferentially distributed to non-dependent lung regions where alveoli are under- or nonperfused. Thus, physiologic dead space tends to be greater during PEEP versus a comparable level of CPAP.

Because end-expiratory pressure increases FRC, many clinicians believed end-expiratory pressure was contraindicated in patients with chronic obstructive pulmonary disease (COPD) characterized by abnormally increased FRC and a prolonged expiratory time constant resulting from abnormally increased respiratory system compliance (emphysema) and Raw (bronchitis). COPD patients often experience incomplete expiration (i.e., failure to achieve VR because expiration is interrupted by the subsequent inspiration). Failure to reach FRC was initially called "air trapping." Because air-trapping causes a positive elastic recoil pressure at the end of expiration, the terms occult-PEEP, inadvertent PEEP, and dynamic hyperinflation have evolved as descriptive terms. Air trapping in a spontaneously breathing patient requires that the inspiratory muscles generate sufficient force to overcome the opposing positive recoil pressure to create a gradient between the alveoli and airway opening to initiate airflow. Air trapping, therefore, increases the inspiratory load for respiratory muscles in spontaneously breathing patients or patients undergoing assisted CMV. Application of PEEP (during assisted mechanical ventilation) or CPAP counterbalances and reduces the inspiratory load imposed by air trapping, thus reducing the work of breathing and perhaps improving ventilation efficiency.

CARDIOVASCULAR EFFECTS

The respiratory system affects cardiovascular function primarily by variation in venous blood return. When cardiac function is normal, venous return is the predominant determinant of cardiac output. The rate at which systemic venous blood returns to thoracic veins depends on the transthoracic vascular pressure gradient (i.e., extrathoracic pressure minus intrathoracic pressure). The transthoracic pressure gradient is determined largely by intrapleural pressure, which is normally subatmospheric. Intrapleural pressure is created by two opposing forces: lung recoil (visceral pleura) and chest wall retraction (parietal pleura). Any change in either of these forces will alter intrapleural pressure and the transthoracic vascular pressure gradient. As the volume of the thorax increases during spontaneous inhalation, intrapleural pressure decreases from an average of 5 cmH_2O to 10 cmH_2O below atmospheric pressure. The vena caval, pulmonary arterial, and aortic pressures decrease immediately because the vessels dilate when the extramural pressure decreases. Both the cardiac output and the systemic arterial pressure decrease because of the momentary increase in pulmonary vascular capacitance. As the transthoracic vascular pressure gradient increases, so do venous return and right ventricular stroke volume. At end-inspiration, the pulmonary arterial and aortic pressures as well as the cardiac output taper as venous blood flow increases and fills the expanded pulmonary vascular capacitance. During spontaneous exhal-

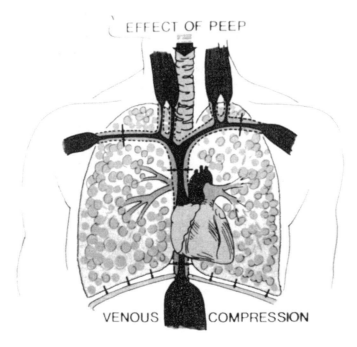

Figure 10.8. Artist's rendition of the effect of positive end-expiratory pressure (PEEP)-induced increase of intrathoracic pressure on thoracic vascular structures. See text for explanation.

ation, intrapleural pressure and pulmonary artery blood flow return to baseline; the cardiac output and systemic arterial pressure increase as pulmonary vascular capacitance diminishes. Thus, cardiac output and systemic arterial pressure fluctuate with breathing patterns, reflecting phasic alterations in blood flow into and out of the thorax.

This process is reversed during mechanical ventilation because intrapleural pressure increases when mechanical inspiration is initiated. Intrapleural pressure also increases after the application of end-expiratory pressure, thereby decreasing transthoracic vascular pressure gradient, venous inflow, right ventricular stroke volume, left ventricular stroke volume, and cardiac output (Fig. 10.8). The fractional transmission of end-expiratory pressure to the pleura depends on the mechanical properties of the lung and chest wall. End-expiratory pressure will increase intrapleural pressure by an amount determined by the following relationship:

$$\Delta Ppl = EEP - \Delta FRC/C_{RS}$$

where ΔPpl = change in intrapleural pressure; EEP = end-expiratory pressure;

and C_{RS} = respiratory system compliance. The increase in intrapleural pressure and pericardial pressure affect the hemodynamic response to end-expiratory pressure. If the pericardium does not limit diastolic filling (e.g., right and/or left ventricular overdistension, and/or compression of cardiac fossa by overdistension of the lung), intrapleural pressure can be used to estimate pericardial pressure.

When end-expiratory pressure is employed with spontaneous ventilation (CPAP), it affects cardiovascular functions differently than when it is provided with mechanical ventilation (CMV + PEEP). Expiratory intrapleural pressure varies little with different respiratory patterns, as long as end-expiratory pressure is similar. Therefore, at a given level of end-expiratory pressure, the most important determinant of mean airway pressure, intrapleural pressure, and transthoracic vascular pressure gradient is the inspiratory airway pressure pattern. During inspiration with mechanical ventilation, transthoracic vascular pressure gradient diminishes, venous return is lowered, and cardiac output decreases. This is not the case during spontaneous breathing. During spontaneous exhalation, intrapleural pressure and venous return are similar to those observed during mechanical ventilation with the same end-expiratory pressure level. However, during inhalation, intrapleural pressure decreases, increasing venous influx to the right side of the heart. The magnitude of venous inflow during spontaneous inspiration depends on the change in transthoracic vascular pressure gradient. Thus, harmful effects of end-expiratory pressure on venous return and cardiac output are minimized by maintaining spontaneous ventilation.

End-expiratory pressure may reduce or increase pulmonary vascular resistance. Principal respiratory factors that affect pulmonary vascular resistance, pulmonary perfusion, and blood flow distribution are airway pressure, lung volume, and hypoxic pulmonary vasoconstriction. When FRC is normal, pulmonary vascular resistance is minimal. Changes in lung volume above or below normal FRC increase pulmonary vascular resistance. Therefore, FRC should be normalized whenever possible. End-expiratory pressure titrated to restore FRC should improve the cross-sectional area of the pulmonary vascular bed. End-expiratory pressure also recruits perfused, but nonventilated lung units, thus improving PaO_2 and relieving hypoxic pulmonary vasoconstriction. Pulmonary blood flow also is affected by the ventilatory mode. During CMV, pulmonary blood flow is increased during expiration and reduced during inspiration. However, during spontaneous breathing with end-expiratory pressure blood flow decreases during expiration. Thus, ventilation and perfusion distribution may vary within a breathing cycle depending on the mode of ventilation (i.e., CMV + PEEP or CPAP) and attendant change in intrathoracic pressure.

Patients with congestive heart failure may benefit from the hemodynamic consequences of end-expiratory pressure. Left ventricular failure causes an increase in left atrial and pulmonary venous pressure. As pulmonary venous pressure continues to rise, the transvascular fluid flux increases and eventually the interstitial space is maximally expanded, the lymphatic clearance mechanism is overwhelmed, alveoli become flooded, and respiratory system compliance, FRC, and expiratory time constant decrease. Spontaneously breathing patients in congestive heart failure are typically tachypneic and have intercostal and/or epigastric retractions during inspiratory efforts caused by unusual reductions in intrapleural pressure. Alterations in intrapleural pressure may significantly alter left ventricular function. Reductions in pleural pressure may impede left ventricular ejection by increasing the transmural wall pressure gradient for ejection (i.e., left ventricular end-diastolic pressure minus epicardial surface pressure or intrapleural pressure). Increase in pleural pressure may facilitate left ventricular ejection by decreasing the transmural left ventricular end-diastolic pressure gradient for ejection. When the pericardium or cardiac fossa do not limit the dimension of the left ventricle, transmural left ventricular end-diastolic pressure is equal to the left ventricular end-diastolic pressure relative to atmospheric pressure minus epicardial surface pressure relative to atmospheric pressure, which is approximated by the intrapleural pressure relative to atmospheric pressure. In congestive heart failure, in which left ventricular contractility is reduced and relatively unresponsive to changes in preload, decreasing left ventricular afterload improves cardiac output. Because increased pleural pressure reduces left ventricular afterload, end-expiratory pressure may improve cardiac performance and lung function in patients suffering from congestive heart failure.

When distending pressure is increased by end-expiratory pressure, the change in alveolar volume is not consistent. Lung units with relatively high respiratory system compliance become hyperinflated and compress juxtaposed pulmonary capillaries. Increased pulmonary vascular resistance reduces local blood flow and may divert it to under-ventilated regions, thereby increasing $\dot{Q}sp/\dot{Q}t$. Hyperinflation causes overventilation and underperfusion (i.e., dead space ventilation), usually defined as $\dot{V}_A/\dot{Q} > 100$. Clinical indications of hyperinflation include: increased arterial to end-tidal CO_2 gradient, increased $PaCO_2$, increased inflation pressure during mechanical ventilation, increased pulmonary vascular resistance, and radiographic evidence of hyperinflation.

Fluid retention and diminished urinary output are commonly observed in patients receiving end-expiratory pressure, particularly in conjunction with mechanical ventilation. Mechanical ventilation and PEEP reportedly increase antidiuretic hormone, decrease mean renal artery perfusion pressure, redistribute perfusion from the cortex, reduce urine flow, reduce creatinine clearance, and diminish fractional sodium excretion. The observed effects of PEEP on glomerular filtration rate, total kidney perfusion, and the renin-angiotensin mechanism are conflicting. Low-dose dopamine infusion and intravascular hydration have been shown to improve renal function during mechanical ventilation and PEEP. CPAP is less detrimental to renal function than mechanical ventilation with comparable PEEP.

Because end-expiratory pressure reduces the transthoracic vascular pressure gradient, venous return from the brain is impeded. Venous congestion may cause increased intracranial pressure and may reduce cerebral perfusion pressure. Spontaneous ventilation and/or elevation of the head 10 to 15 degrees may increase the transthoracic vascular pressure gradient and intracranial pressure and improve cerebral perfusion. However, data regarding the effect of end-expiratory pressure on intracranial pressure are contradictory.

EXTRAVASCULAR LUNG WATER

End-expiratory pressure was originally thought to reduce extravascular lung water because abrupt discontinuation of PEEP or CPAP was often followed by violent ejection of frothy, sanguineous fluid from the tracheal tube. However, no evidence indicates that extravascular lung water is reduced by end-expiratory pressure. End-expiratory pressure may facilitate the redistribution of fluid from alveoli into the interstitium, thus improving gas exchange but not pulmonary edema.

PULMONARY BAROTRAUMA

In 1970, Mead et al. observed "at a transpulmonary pressure of 30 cmH_2O, the pressure tending to expand an atelectatic region surrounded by a fully expanded lung would be approximately 140 cmH_2O." Alveolar rupture associated with positive pressure therapy may lead to pulmonary interstitial emphysema, subcutaneous emphysema, pneumothorax, pneumomediastinum, and pneumoperitoneum. Hyperinflation may result in alveolar rupture with dissection of air through the perivascular and peribronchiolar interstitial tissue to the hilum. Air may continue to distribute throughout the fascial planes of the soft tissues (e.g., subcutaneous emphysema or pneumoperitoneum) or rupture visceral pleura (e.g., pneumomediastinum or pneumothorax). The incidence of barotrauma complicating mechanical ventilation with PEEP ranges from 10% to 20% in most investigations. Barotrauma occurs less frequently in critically ill patients who are ventilated with IMV than with comparable continuous mechanical ventilation (controlled or patient-initiated) with comparable levels of end-expiratory pressure, and is probably more closely related to high peak inspiratory pressure and severity of parenchymal disease than to the level of end-expiratory pressure.

Although subcutaneous and mediastinal gas is harmless, either should alert clinicians to the possibility of pneumothorax. Although pulmonary interstitial emphysema can lead to pneumothorax, no consistent relationship exists between the two. No causal association between pulmonary barotrauma and the use or level of end-expiratory pressure has been established. However, mechanical ventilation with PEEP may perpetuate air leak (bronchopleural fistula) once pneumothorax has occurred.

PHYSIOLOGIC PEEP/CPAP

In patients recovering from acute lung injury, data suggest that 2 to 5 cm H_2O of PEEP or CPAP provide lung function and gas exchange similar to that encountered after tracheal extubation. Extubation from atmospheric pressure is accompanied by a significant increase in VR and gas exchange, suggesting that glottic function may be an important determinant of expiratory lung volume when VR is reduced, especially when associated with a low-compliance breathing pattern characterized by limited vital capacity, reduced tidal volume, and increased respiratory rate.

TITRATING PEEP/CPAP THERAPY

Because derecruitment pressure is not uniform throughout the lung, end-expiratory pressure is usually titrated to some desirable end-point (e.g., reduced respiratory rate, increased pulmonary compliance, reduced $\dot{Q}sp/\dot{Q}t$, or increased PaO_2/F_IO_2 ratio). Controversy surrounds the end-point for PEEP therapy. A conservative approach is to titrate the PEEP to achieve an adequate PaO_2 (usually >60 to 65 torr or SaO_2 >90%) with a "nontoxic" F_IO_2 (i.e., <0.5 at sea level) without causing a significant reduction in cardiac output. If cardiac output declines, PEEP/CPAP is reduced despite F_IO_2. Another approach is to titrate PEEP to achieve optimal respiratory system compliance (i.e., "best PEEP"). A more aggressive regimen involves the titration of PEEP/CPAP until the $\dot{Q}sp/\dot{Q}t$ is ≤15% (i.e., "optimal PEEP"). If the cardiac output deteriorates before achieving optimal PEEP, the patient undergoes intravascular volume expansion in an effort to restore hemodynamics. The end-point for intravascular volume expansion is usually judged by restoration of cardiac output or a transmural pulmonary artery occlusion pressure or left atrial pressure of 18 to 20 mmHg with normal systemic vascular resistance and a competent mitral valve. If intravascular volume expansion fails to restore cardiac output, then inotropic agents are used (e.g., dopamine or dobutamine).

Respiratory system mechanics and gas exchange are evaluated as PEEP/CPAP is titrated. Once optimal CPAP is obtained with patients who are managed with IMV, mechanical support can often be reduced, as long as arterial pH remains >7.35. Simultaneously, the inspired oxygen concentration is reduced to a level that will preserve PaO_2 at an adequate level. Pulmonary gas exchange and mechanics should be evaluated frequently. When considered adequate, CPAP can be reduced without allowing detrimental alterations to occur.

Despite optimal CPAP, some patients are unable to sustain adequate ventilation and partial ventilatory support may be provided with IMV, airway pressure release ventilation, or bilevel CPAP. When partial ventilatory support and CPAP are employed, weaning from mechanical ventilation may commence soon after the initiation of therapy. Patients managed with CMV and PEEP often require large amounts of intravenous fluids to stabilize cardiovascular function because mean airway pressure is significantly higher. When weaning from mechanical support is attempted, such intravascular fluid loading may increase pulmonary capillary hydrostatic pressure and cause deterioration in pulmonary function because of increased extravascular lung water. If spontaneous breathing is allowed to persist in the early phase of therapy and if mechanical ventilatory support is discontinued as soon as possible, intravascular volume expansion is often unnecessary and oxygen and CPAP may be withdrawn more rapidly. If patients are weaned rapidly from mechanical ventilation, exposure to elevated airway pressure and barotrauma may be reduced.

Suggested Readings

Downs JB, Douglas ME, Sanfelippo PM, et al. Ventilatory pattern intrapleural pressure, and cardiac output. Anesth Analg 56:88–96, 1977.

Gattinoni L, Pelosi P, Crotti S, et al. Effects of positive end-expiratory pressure on regional distribution of tidal volume and recruitment in adult respiratory distress syndrome. Am J Respir Crit Care 151:1807–1814, 1995.

Kirby RR, Downs JB, Civetta JM, et al. High level positive end expiratory pressure (PEEP) in acute respiratory insufficiency. Chest 67:156–163, 1975.

Kirby RR, Perry JC, Calderwood HW, et al. Cardiorespiratory effects of high positive end-expiratory pressure. Anesthesiology 43:533–539, 1975.

Marquez JM, Douglas ME, Downs JB, et al. Renal function and cardiovascular responses during positive airway pressure. Anesthesiology 50:393–398, 1979.

Mead J, Takishima T, Leith D. Stress distribution in lung: a model of pulmonary elasticity. J Appl Physiol 28:596–608, 1970.

Qvist J, Pontoppidan H, Wilson RS, et al. Hemodynamic responses to mechanical ventilation with PEEP: the effect of hypervolemia. Anesthesiology 42:45–55, 1975.

Rosi A, Santos C, Roca J, et al. Effects of PEEP on $\dot{V}_A/\dot{Q}$ mismatching in ventilated patients with chronic airflow obstruction. Am J Respir Crit Care Med 149:1077–1084, 1994.

Rosi A, Polese G, Brandi G, et al. Intrinsic positive end-expiratory pressure (PEEPi). Intensive Care Med 21:522–536, 1995.

Sjöstrand UH, Lichtwarck-Aschoff M, Nielsen JB, et al. Different ventilatory approaches to keep the lungs open. Intensive Care Med 21:310–318, 1995.

Smith RA. Physiologic PEEP. Respir Care 33:620–629, 1988.

Smith TC, Marini JJ. Impact of PEEP on lung mechanics and work of breathing in severe airflow obstruction. J Appl Physiol 65:1488–1499, 1988.

Sturgeon CL Jr, Douglas ME, Downs JB, et al. PEEP and CPAP: Cardiopulmonary effects during spontaneous ventilation. Anesth Analg 56:633–641.

Suter PM, Fairley HB, Isenberg MD. Optimum end-expiratory airway pressure in patients with acute pulmonary failure. N Engl J Med 292:284–289, 1975.

Venus B, Cohen LE, Smith RA. Hemodynamics and intrathoracic pressure transmission during controlled mechanical ventilation and positive end-expiratory pressure in normal and low compliant lungs. Crit Care Med 16:686–690, 1988.

Wolf G, Eberhard L, Guttman J, et al. Polymorphous ventilation: a new ventilation concept for distributed time constants. In: Rüegheimer E (ed). New aspects of respiratory failure. Berlin, Springer-Verlag, 1992, pp 235–252.

11
Pressure Support Ventilation

Neil R. McIntyre

Pressure support (PS) is a form of mechanical ventilatory support that supports a patient's spontaneous inspiratory effort with a clinician-selected amount of positive airway pressure (1). This pressure generally can range up to 50 cmH$_2$O. It is designed to be held constant through servocontrol of delivered flow, and it usually is terminated when a certain minimal inspiratory flow is reached (Fig. 11.1) (2). Using American Association for Respiratory Care (AARC) consensus terminology (3), PS is a patient-triggered, pressure-limited, flow-cycled breath.

Because patients have considerable control over breath delivery characteristics (i.e., flow and timing) with PS, it is considered an "interactive" form of ventilatory support. Other forms of interactive breaths available on modern ventilators are listed in Table 11.1 and, as can be seen, there is considerable overlap in design features among these breaths. For instance, PS has design features similar to demand valve controlled continuous positive airway pressure (CPAP); the only difference being that the inspiratory pressure limit in PS is higher than baseline whereas in CPAP it is equal to baseline. Two other interactive breaths that have many features of the pressure support concept are the pressure assist breath (patient-triggered, pressure-limited with time cycling) and the pressure augmented or volume assured PS breath (patient-triggered, pressure-limited with both flow and a tidal volume [V$_T$] cycle mechanism operative) (3,4).

PHYSIOLOGIC EFFECTS OF PRESSURE SUPPORTED BREATHS

Pressure support of a spontaneous breath has several effects on the respiratory system that are different from unsupported spontaneous or other types of ventilator delivered breaths. These differences involve two broad areas: PS interactions with ventilatory muscle function and PS interactions with patient flow demands (synchrony).

Ventilatory Muscle Function

Pressure support, by providing a constant inspiratory pressure "boost," adds to the patient's own efforts to deliver the V$_T$ (5–7) (Fig. 11.2). The patient's

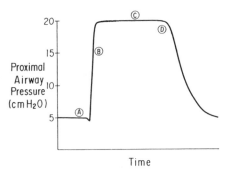

Figure 11.1. Schematic drawing illustrating design features of a pressure supported breath. Plotted is proximal airway pressure over a single inspiratory effort being assisted with 15 cmH_2O pressure support. At point (**A**), a patient's spontaneous inspiratory effort is indicated by a negative pressure deflection. This triggers the demand system to deliver flow to attain the desired pressure support level as rapidly as possible (**B**). Once the pressure support level is attained, ventilator delivered flow is then servo adjusted to patient demand to maintain this pressure plateau (**C**). The inspiratory pressure is terminated when minimal flow criteria is reached (often 25% of peak flow). Airway pressure then returns to baseline (**D**).

response to this boost, however, can be quite varied and appears to depend on the relative load on the ventilatory muscles with respect to muscle strength and endurance capabilities (5,9). A severely overloaded ventilatory muscle system usually is characterized by tachypnea and small tidal breaths (10,11). Adding small amounts of PS to such a patient tends to augment each effort the patient makes to increase the V_T. Overall patient work is reduced by decreasing the needed breath rate. As higher levels of PS are given and the V_T approaches the 4–7 ml/kg

Table 11.1. Interactive Mechanical Breaths

	Trigger	Limit	Cycle
Volume assist	Patient	Flow	Volume
Pressure support	Patient	Pressure	Flow
Pressure assist[a]	Patient	Pressure	Time
Pressure augmented (volume-assured PS)	Patient	Pressure	Flow and volume
IPPB	Patient	Flow	Pressure
CPAP (demand valve system)	Patient	Pressure (held to baseline)	Flow

PS, pressure support; IPPB, intermittent positive pressure breathing; CPAP, continuous positive airway pressure.
[a] Achieved through patient triggering of breaths during pressure "controlled" ventilation.

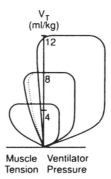

Muscle   Ventilator
Tension   Pressure

Figure 11.2. Schematic diagrams representing the quantity and the characteristics of both the patient's and ventilator's contributions of the work of breathing during various levels of pressure support (PS). Work per tidal breath is depicted as the area inscribed by the pressure-volume relationship during that breath. Patient effort is depicted by leftward directed muscle tension or "intramuscular" pressures, ventilator pressures are depicted by rightward directed airway pressure. The *dashed line* represents a normal pressure-volume relationship. The efforts of various levels of applied PS are represented by the *solid lines.* Patient work quantity is progressively shifted to the ventilator as the level of pressure applied with every breath increases. The pressure-volume work characteristics are also changed with increasing PS to a more normal configuration.

range, the patient's contribution to each breath begins to decrease and the V_T tends to remain constant. Ventilatory muscle work during this range of PS is thus reduced because of tidal breath work being shifted from patient to ventilator. In addition, the pressure-to-volume ratio of the patient's work is shifted to a lower value that is more favorable from an energetics point of view (5,7,12–14). Once enough PS has been given to reduce patient work per breath to very low levels (usually associated with tidal volumes of 7–9 ml/kg), additional PS only serves to passively increase the tidal volume. From these considerations it should be clear that different amounts of PS behave differently in different patients, depending on the state of the patient's ventilatory muscles. For example, 20 cmH$_2$O PS may be just enough to relieve fatigue in a patient with very poor compliance whereas it may overdistend the lung of an overdose patient with normal lungs. PS settings should be adjusted to response (e.g., rate/V_T) rather than to some arbitrary pressure.

Patient-Ventilatory Synchrony

Because PS is an interactive breath, one must consider the three mechanical breath phases (trigger, limit, and cycling) and how their synchrony is achieved with patient effort (15,16).

Trigger synchrony refers to the process of assuring prompt breath initiation on patient demand. A certain amount of dys-synchrony exists on all mechanical ventilators because of the physical separation of the ventilatory muscles and ventilator's sensors and flow controller (see, also, Chapter 8, Breathing Circuits for Spontaneous Ventilation and the Work of Breathing). The ventilator's sensitivity and responsiveness characteristics also can contribute to the dys-synchrony (17–19). Considerable advances have been made in technology to improve triggering function. These include microprocessor controllers, flow-based triggering strategies, and better demand valve designs (17–19). Indeed, the design of a PS breath, which provides a very rapid initial gas flow, can significantly improve trigger response characteristics as compared with flow-limited breaths (18,19). Newer ventilators also have the capability to "fine tune" this response to patient demand using "slope adjustors," or "rise time adjustors" (Fig. 11.3). Despite these advances, triggering loads still can be significant in patients with very active ventilatory devices. An imposed triggering load also can result from intrinsic positive end-expiratory pressure (PEEP) developing in patients with air flow obstruction (21,22). This can sometimes be improved with judicious applications of circuit PEEP (23).

Flow synchrony refers to the ventilator gas delivery process being in accordance with patient efforts. This is important because with any interactive breath, once

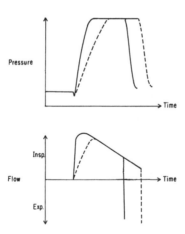

Figure 11.3. The efforts of a pressure slope or inspiratory rise time adjustor on a pressure support (PS) breath. As this is increased, valve responsiveness increases and the rise time to the pressure limit is decreased. Very active patient ventilatory drives may synchronize better with faster rise times; less active patient ventilatory drives may synchronize better with slower rise times. Note that, because maximal flow is affected by this adjustment, flow cycling criteria based on peak flow will affect the inspiratory time.

a patient's effort to breathe has started it continues throughout the breath (24). Flow dys-synchrony is the result of an inadequately delivered inspiratory flow. This is a particular problem with conventional volume-cycled breaths that have a fixed flow pattern, especially in patients being weaned with synchronized intermittent mandatory ventilation (SIMV) (25). An important feature of a pressure-limited breath is a rapid and variable flow that tends to match patient demand better (6). This may be further enhanced by the pressure slope or rise time adjustment as noted (20). In the future, enhanced flow synchrony may come from using either a tracheal (17) or a pleural (6) pressure sensing site to servocontrol inspiratory pressure.

Cycling synchrony refers to matching ventilator breath termination with the end of patient effort. Current systems usually flow-cycle a PS breath at 25%–35% of peak flow. Although this appears reasonable in most patients, both premature and delayed termination can produce cycling dys-synchrony (26). Specifically, early termination may result if the PS level is too low, the initial flow is particularly fast (such that the 25%–35% flow cutoff occurs quite early in the breath), or a patient expiratory reflex develops quickly in response to pressure. Clinician adjustment of the pressure level or the inspiratory rise time may be helpful. Alternatively, setting a fixed inspiratory time (the pressure assist breath; see Table 11.1) or a guaranteed tidal volume (using volume cycling as a backup to flow cycling (see Table 11.1)) (27, 28) can be done to address this issue on some ventilators.

On the other hand, late termination can produce a different type of dys-synchrony. Late termination is usually a result of an excessive PS setting, but it may also occur if the initial flow delivery is too low (thus late occurrence of the cycling criteria). In addition to patient discomfort, an important consequence of delayed termination is inadequate expiratory time and intrinsic PEEP and air-trapping (26). Proper assessment of PS level and inspiratory rise time usually alleviates this problem. Sedatives may be needed as a last resort with abnormal cycling synchrony. Future systems may allow cycling criteria adjustments.

CURRENT APPROACHES TO THE CLINICAL APPLICATION

Three applications of PS currently being used are (*a*) low level PS to overcome patient work associated with an endotracheal tube; (*b*) high level PS to unload ventilatory muscles, especially during weaning; and (*c*) noninvasive applications of PS.

Low level PS uses 2–10 cmH_2O pressure during inspiration to overcome the resistive component of inspiratory work imposed by an endotracheal tube (29, 30). The exact pressure requirement can be calculated by knowing the endotracheal tube diameter and the inspiratory flow characteristics (29). The rationale for this approach is that the air flow resistance associated with an endotracheal tube produces an undesirable workload that may compromise comfort and ventilatory muscle function during spontaneous breaths. Thus, this use of PS may be indicated in any intubated patient taking spontaneous breaths in whom tachypnea, dyspnea, or ventilator-patient asynchrony is felt to be at least partially due to the spontaneous ventilatory muscle work imposed by the endotracheal tube. The hazards of this approach appear minimal, although elevation in mean intrathoracic pressure may compromise cardiovascular function in susceptible individuals.

Higher levels of PS can provide substantial ventilatory support by applying the necessary level of inspiratory pressure for a desired tidal volume and minute ventilation (31). Pressure levels, thus, can range up to 50 cmH$_2$O in patients with large minute ventilation demands and severely impaired ventilatory system mechanics (1). A useful initial setting for PS under these circumstances is one that provides whatever inspiratory pressure is necessary for a V$_T$ of 7–9 ml/kg. This level of PS can reduce patient work to nearly zero and approaches the level of support provided by conventional assist-control volume-cycled ventilation (1,5). Weaning of PS from this point is accomplished by reducing the level of PS, which can generally be guided by the patient's respiratory rate (an indicator of the patient's own sense of load) (11, 31). Elevations in respiratory rate often indicate an excessive ventilatory muscle load and thus represent a requirement for

Table 11.2. Weaning Techniques

	VCV/T-tube	IMV	PSV
Work quantity per minute	All or none	Adjust by number of mandatory breaths	Adjust by level of applied pressure
Work characteristics	Fixed as high P/V by endotracheal tube and disease	Fixed as high P/V by endotracheal tube and disease	P/V reduced by applied pressure
Synchrony	Regular periods of constant load; volume and tidal volume of control breaths are clinician set	Irregular loads; volume and tidal volume of mandatory breaths are clinician set	Regular loads; patient interacts with applied pressure to set volume and tidal volume
Guaranteed MV	All or none guaranteed	Mandatory breath rate guarantees a minimal MV	None guaranteed (unless newer volume-cycled feature present)

VCV, volume-controlled ventilation; IMV, intermittent mandatory ventilation; PSV, pressure support ventilation; MV, mandatory ventilation; P/V, pressure volume ratio.

more ventilatory support in the long-term weaning of a patient. Increases in night support to facilitate sleep may be beneficial.

A common practice in many intensive care units (ICUs) is to combine IMV and moderate to high levels of PS. This approach, in essence, applies two different partial support modes to a patient and it inherently produces a more complex weaning strategy. In a patient with an intact ventilatory drive and with stable or improving lung mechanics (i.e., the patient chosen for partial support and weaning), rarely is there a need for the additional IMV breaths.

The rationale for using a weaning protocol based on PS is to provide patients requiring prolonged ventilatory support with a more comfortable muscle reloading process that may supply a more physiologic type of work than intermittent approaches using spontaneous breaths. Thus, this mode may be particularly useful in those patients who are difficult to make comfortable and who will require a

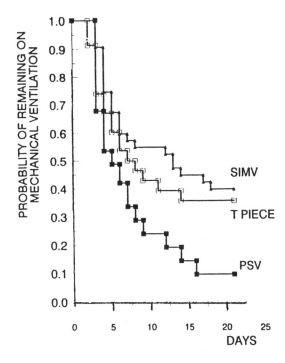

Figure 11.4. Effect of weaning strategy (i.e., T-piece, intermittent mandatory ventilation [IMV] or presure support [PS]) on weaning success in one randomized trial of patients with long-term ventilator dependence. In this trial, PS was associated with a significantly faster weaning time. (Reproduced with permission from Brochard L, Rauss A, Benito S, et al. Comparison of three methods of gradual withdrawal from ventilatory support during weaning from mechanical ventilation. Am J Respir Crit Care Med 1994; 150:896–903.)

prolonged weaning process because of slowly resolving lung disease. The differences between this PS weaning approach and more traditional methods are summarized in Table 11.2. It is important to note that because patients have considerable control over ventilation with PS as a stand-alone mode, only those with a reliable ventilatory drive and stable ventilatory requirements should be selected for stand-alone application. With PS, there is the potential for suboptimal alveolar ventilation in a patient with unstable ventilatory drive or rapidly changing lung impedance. An additional potential hazard to high PS levels is potentially higher mean intrathoracic pressure and consequent cardiovascular compromise.

Two large trials recently have been reported regarding the "best" weaning technique (32,33). Both studies randomly assigned patients to T-piece, IMV, or stand-alone PS protocols. Unfortunately, the relative "aggressiveness" of the three modes was not well-matched in either study, thereby introducing potential biases. Patient populations also were different, particularly in those assigned to the T-piece protocol. Specifically, patients remained mechanically ventilated in one study (32) as compared with the other study (33) prior to entering the weaning protocol. Despite these criticisms of the two studies, one can conclude that more rapidly resolving lung disease seems to benefit from an aggressive weaning protocol (i.e., T-piece) (33), whereas more slowly resolving lung disease seems to benefit from a gradual weaning protocol that is more focused on patient comfort (i.e., PS) (34) (Fig. 11.4).

The third approach to PS is to use it via face mask systems in nonintubated patients who require transient ventilatory support (e.g., overdose, asthma, postoperative chronic obstructive pulmonary disease flare) (see, also, Chapter 15, Noninvasive Ventilation). Effective systems for noninvasive ventilation exist that can deliver up to 20 cmH$_2$O of PS or more (34–35).

CONCLUSIONS

Pressure support is a mode of ventilatory support that offers a means to adjust both the magnitude and the characteristics of patient ventilatory work in a way that is synchronous with patient effort. Clinical data demonstrated that progressive increases in PS transfer work from patient to ventilator, PS provides more synchronous patient-ventilator interactions, and an aggressive PS method of unloading and reloading muscles may have advantages in the slowly recovering patient in need of long-term weaning. Because of these data, the theoretic advantages and the mode's safety in appropriately monitored patients, it is reasonable to consider this mode in any patient needing prolonged partial (i.e., interactive) ventilatory support. At the same time, however, we need further study on the complex process of ventilatory reflexes and muscle reconditioning during mechanical ventilation to understand fully the proper role of PS.

References

1. MacIntyre NR. Respiratory function during pressure support ventilation. Chest 89:677–683, 1986.
2. Kacmarek R. The role of pressure support ventilation in reducing work of breathing. Respir Care 33:99–120, 1988.
3. American Association for Respiratory Care. Consensus statement on essentials of mechanical ventilators 1992. Respir Care 37:1000–1008, 1992.
4. MacIntyre NR. Pressure limited versus volume cycled breath delivery strategies. Crit Care Med 22:4–5, 1994.
5. Brochard L, Harf A, Lorino H, LeMaire F. Inspiratory pressure support prevents diaphragmatic fatigue during weaning from mechanical ventilation. Am Rev Respir Dis 139:513–521, 1989.
6. MacIntyre NR, Nishimura N, Usada Y, et al. The Nagoya Conference on system design and patient ventilator interactions during pressure support ventilation. Chest 97:1463–1466, 1970.
7. Banner MJ, Kirby RR, MacIntyre NR. Patient and ventilator work of breathing and ventilatory muscle loads at different levels of pressure support ventilation. Chest 100:531–533, 1991.
8. MacIntyre NR, Leatherman NE. Ventilatory muscle loads and the frequency-tidal volume pattern during inspiratory pressure assisted (pressure supported) ventilation. Am Rev Respir Dis 141:327–331, 1990.
9. Brochard L, Pluskwa F, LeMaire F. Improved efficacy of spontaneous breathing during inspiratory pressure support. Am Rev Respir Dis 136:411–415, 1987.
10. Rochester DF, Arora NS. Respiratory muscle failure. Med Clin North Am 67(3):573–597, 1983.
11. Young KL, Tobin MJ. A prospective study of indexes predicting the outcome of trials of weaning from mechanical ventilation. N Engl J Med 324:1445–1450, 1991.
12. MacIntyre NR, Leatherman NE. Mechanical loads on the ventilatory muscles: a theoretical analysis. Am Rev Respir Dis 139:968–973, 1989.
13. Campbell EJM, Westlake EK, Cherniack RM. The oxygen consumption and efficiency of the respiratory muscles of young muscle subjects. Clin Sci 18:55–64, 1959.
14. McGregor M, Becklake MR. The relationship of oxygen cost of breathing to inspiratory mechanical work and respiratory force. J Clin Invest 40:971–980, 1961.
15. Marini JJ. Strategies to minimize breathing effort during mechanical ventilation. Crit Care Clin 6:635–661, 1990.
16. MacIntyre NR. Patient ventilator interactions: dys-synchrony and imposed loads. Problems in Respiratory Care 4:150–160, 1991.
17. Banner MJ, Blanch PB, Kirby RR. Imposed work of breathing and methods of triggering a demand flow continuous positive airway pressure system. Crit Care Med 21:183-190, 1993.
18. Sassoon CS, Light RW, Lotia R, Sieck GC, Manhutte CK. Pressure time product during continuous positive airway pressure, pressure support ventilation and T-piece ventilation during weaning from mechanical ventilatory support. Am Rev Resp Dis 143:469–475, 1991.
19. Sassoon CSH. Mechanical ventilation design and function: the trigger variable. Respir Care 37:1056–1069, 1992.
20. Ho LI, MacIntyre NR. Pressure supported breaths; ventilatory effects of breath initiation and breath termination design characteristics. Crit Care Med 17:S26, 1989.
21. Pepe PE, Marini JJ. Occult positive end expiratory pressure in mechanically ventilated patients with airflow obstruction. Am Rev Respir Dis 126:166–170, 1982.
22. Petrof BJ, Legare M, Goldberg P, Milic-Emili J, Gottfried SB. Continuous positive airway pressure reduces work of breathing and dyspnea during weaning from mechanical ventilation in severe COPD. Am Rev Resp Dis 141:20–28, 1990.
23. Gay PG, Rodante JR, Hubmeyer RD. The effects of positive expiratory pressure isovolumic flow

and dynamic hyperinflation in patients receiving mechanical ventilation. Am Rev Resp Dis 139: 621–626, 1989.

24. Flick GR, Bellamy PE, Simmons DH. Diaphage contraction during assisted mechanical ventilation. Chest 1989; 96:130-135.

25. Marini JJ, Smith TC, Lamb VJ. External work output and force generation during synchronized intermittent mandatory ventilation. Am Rev Respir Dis 138:1169–1179, 1988.

26. Vande Graff WB, Gordey K, Dornseif SE, Dries DL, Kleinman BS, et al. Pressure support changes in ventilatory pattern and components of the work of breathing. Chest 100:1082–1088, 1991.

27. MacIntyre NR, Gropper C, Westfall T. Combining pressure-limiting and volume cycling in a patient interactive mechanical breath. Crit Care Med 22:353–357, 1994.

28. Amato MB, Barbas CS, Bonassa J, Saldiva PH, Zin HA, de Carvalho CR. Volume assumed pressure support (VAPSV). A new approach for reducing muscle workload during acute respiratory failure. Chest 102:1225–1234, 1992.

29. Fiastro JF, Habib MP, Quan SF. Pressure support compensation for inspiratory work due to endotracheal tubes and demand CPAP. Chest 93:499–502, 1988.

30. Brochard L, Rue F, Lorino H, Lemaire F, Hart A. Inspiratory pressure support compensates for the additional work of breathing caused by the endotracheal tube. Anesthesiology 75:739–745, 1991.

31. MacIntyre NR. Weaning from mechanical ventilatory support: volume assisting intermittent breaths versus pressure assisting every breath. Respir Care 33:121–125, 1988.

32. Brochard L, Rauss A, Benito S, et al. Comparison of three methods of gradual withdrawal from ventilatory support during weaning from mechanical ventilation. Am J Resp Crit Care Med 150: 896–903, 1994.

33. Esteban A, Frutos F, Tobin M, et al. A comparison of four methods of weaning patients from mechanical ventilation. N Engl J Med 332:545–550, 1995.

34. Meyer TJ, Hill NS. Non-invasive positive pressure ventilation to treat respiratory failure. Ann Intern Med 120:760–770, 1994.

35. Pennock BE, Crenshaw L, Kaplan PD. Non invasive mask ventilation for acute respiratory failure. Chest 105:441–444, 1994.

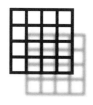

12
Inverse Ratio Ventilation and the Inspiratory/ Expiratory Ratio

Michael Joel Gurevitch

Probably few methods of ventilatory management have been as controversial as pressure-controlled inverse-ratio ventilation (PC-IRV). This modality has been used to ventilate poorly compliant lungs (such as in adult respiratory distress syndrome [ARDS]) and has been intensely scrutinized over the past 10 years since the original report of its potential advantage in 1986.

In a normal respiratory cycle, inspiration is shorter than expiration. The concept of a prolonged inspiratory phase was first investigated in 1971 by Reynolds, who investigated the effect of multiple alterations in mechanical ventilator settings on the pulmonary gas exchange of neonates with hyaline membrane disease. He concluded that the use of a long inspiratory phase resulted in a large increase in partial pressure of oxygen (PO_2) and a decrease in right-to-left shunt. Neonatal and pediatric ventilators were pressure-controlled, time-cycled machines with inspiratory and expiratory times that could be manipulated easily. Methods of increasing the inspiratory time were implemented at many centers for years; however, problems arose because of poor monitoring capabilities with pressure-controlled ventilation. Infants with hyaline membrane disease frequently have significant changes in compliance over short periods allowing the initial appropriate ventilating pressures to result suddenly in larger volumes causing unexpected barotrauma. As a consequence of this phenomenon occurring without early clinical recognition or monitoring, many neonates suffered pneumothoraxes and the concept slowly fell into disfavor among clinicians. In 1976, Fuelihan et al. demonstrated that, in adults with acute respiratory insufficiency, adding an end-inspiratory pause to each mechanical breath resulted in decreased dead space-to-tidal volume ratio (V_D/V_T) and improved ventilatory efficiency. This study, again, demonstrated the efficacy of a slightly prolonged inspiratory time.

As our understanding of physiology and pathophysiology of diseases has increased, we now know that in obstructive airway diseases, such as asthma and emphysema, a short inspiratory phase is necessary. A short inspiratory phase provides the maximal time possible for exhalation to minimize air-trapping; the tendency to increase functional residual capacity (FRC) and partial pressure of carbon dioxide (PCO_2) would be disadvantageous in the core population. On the other hand, patients without air flow obstruction may have diseases that increase lung stiffness (i.e., decreased lung compliance) and promote atelectasis. These patients seem to do better with techniques such as positive end-expiratory pressure (PEEP), which attempts to keep open any segments that might otherwise collapse. In these patients, who begin failing higher levels of traditional PEEP therapy, we consider alternative modes (e.g., pressure-controlled ventilation) and advance to PC-IRV if the clinical situation warrants its use.

TECHNIQUES TO INCREASE INSPIRATORY/ EXPIRATORY RATIO

The most appropriate method to increase the inspiratory time has not been determined. At least three methods are available by which the inspiratory-to-expiratory (I/E) ratio can be prolonged to control completely the patient's ventilation (i.e., no spontaneous ventilatory efforts) as demonstrated in Figure 12.1. Figure 12.1A shows that slowing the flow while maintaining a constant respiratory rate in a volume-controlled breath eventually allows the inspiratory phase to encroach on the expiratory phase. This technique, however, may waste the early portion of inspiration, allowing unstable lung units to continue to empty, despite their being in the inspiratory portion of the cycle (dotted area). In Figure 12.1B, a pause or hold can be added after a preset volume is delivered, thereby increasing the inspiratory time; however, this method results in peak pressures that may overventilate more compliant regions before dropping to a pause or static pressure that may be below the critical pressure necessary to maintain opening of unstable lung units. Figure 12.1C shows the third method of prolonging inspiration using a rapid insufflation with decelerating flow to maintain a preset pressure throughout the inspiratory phase. This method is usually chosen for PC-IRV. Appropriate selection of the I/E ratio and respiratory rate results in a PEEP-like effect, where each new breath begins just before terminal flow being completed from the prior breath. This maneuver effectively traps gas and increases FRC.

Figure 12.2 explains the theory behind this technique. In Figure 12.2A, poorly compliant lung segments completely collapse at end-exhalation; however, with a rapid insufflation and plateau, equilibration occurs throughout all lung units and the next breath occurs just before lung units falling below their closing volume. In essence, this gas trapping has a "PEEP effect" and raises the main airway pressure.

This concept is best understood considering a hypothetical patient who may require 50 cmH$_2$O peak inflation pressure to move a 600-ml V$_T$. If PEEP of 15 cmH$_2$O is added, the peak pressure will rise to 65 cmH$_2$O (50 cmH$_2$O for the V$_T$ on top of a PEEP baseline of 15 cmH$_2$O pressure). With PC-IRV, the 15-cmH$_2$O PEEP-like effect can be achieved in patients who are well ventilated with

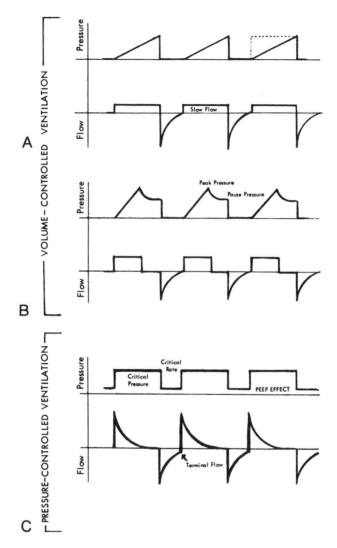

Figure 12.1. Methods used to increase the inspiratory-to-expiratory time (I/E) ratio. **A.** Slowing the flow while at a constant respiratory rate allows the inspiratory phase to encroach onto the expiratory period. This method wastes the early portion of inspiration as many unstable lung units may still be continuing to empty despite being in the inspiratory portion of the cycle (*dotted area*). **B.** Progressive prolongation of an end-inspiratory pause will result in eventual reversal of the I/E ratio. This method results in peak pressures that can overinflate more compliant regions before dropping to a pause (static) pressure that may be below the critical pressure necessary to maintain unstable lung units open. **C.** Rapid insufflation with a decelerating flow maintains a preset pressure throughout inspiration. Appropriate I/E ratio and respiratory rate selection result in a PEEP-like effect. The rate is adjusted while monitoring end-terminal flow, being set to begin each new breath just prior to terminal flow returning to zero.

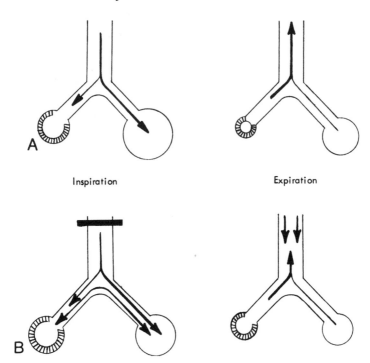

Figure 12.2. Consequences of increasing inspiratory time in lung units with decreased compliance (short time constant). **A.** Short inspiration with longer expiration allows time for unstable lung units to collapse. **B.** Stable, prolonged constant pressure occurs after a rapid insufflation with pressure-controlled ventilation and similarly in volume control with pause. Equilibration occurs between lung units with differing time constants and results in a more even ventilation distribution. If reinflation occurs rapidly after a shortened expiration, a PEEP-like effect occurs, causing further alveoli recruitment and less unstable lung unit collapse.

a peak pressure that may be no >35–40 cmH$_2$O by selecting an appropriate respiratory rate and an I/E ratio that will reinflate the lung before complete emptying. Theoretically, applying a lower constant pressure for a prolonged period may prevent further lung damage while supporting these patients until their underlying lung function improves.

METHOD OF ADMINISTRATION

Once the appropriate patient is selected (i.e., someone failing traditional mechanical ventilation), a ventilator is selected that has PC-IRV capability, (that is an I/E ratio ≥1). Pressure control is available on all newer ventilators, and most can prolong the inspiratory/expiratory ratio. An example of an appropriate patient to consider for this modality is a young patient with severe ARDS, who has been hemodynamically stable (on no pressors), and begins failing traditional ventilatory measures. The PEEP is 15 cmH$_2$O; fraction of inspired oxygen (F$_I$O$_2$) is 0.70; and peak pressures are 65–70 cmH$_2$O, despite full sedation. Radiographic infiltrates are progressing while compliance and arterial oxygen partial pressure (PaO$_2$) are dropping. At this time, IRV application should be considered. Efforts to improve this patient must be started before there is further deterioration. "Onset hypoxemia," which frequently accompanies any modality change, can be noted when starting IRV, and needs to be compensated for should it occur. In addition, it may take up to an hour before any occurring improvement is noted with this modality, making it even more difficult to implement IRV if the patient is already hypoxemic at an F$_I$O$_2$ level of 1.0.

Disposable ventilator circuits are replaced by stiff, noncompliant tubing and then a strip-channel recorder, oscilloscope, or computer module to monitor in-line pressure and flow contours are added. If prior sedation has not been adequate to remove spontaneous respiratory efforts, additional sedation is tried or a neuromuscular blockade added.

The ventilator is switched to its pressure-control mode after 100% oxygen is delivered to allow for an onset hypoxemia with change in mode. The inspiratory time that may have been tried in a normal ratio is slowly advanced from a 1:1 ratio (50% inspiratory time) as is tolerated and then increased to 67% while the pressure-control knob is adjusted to between one half and two thirds of whatever peak cycling pressure had been used in the previous mode. This maneuver should result in a V$_T$ of ~400–600 ml. The respiratory rate is initially and arbitrarily set at 25/minute and then adjusted up or down while watching the terminal flow curve as previously described. A rate is found that causes each new breath to be started just as end-terminal flow approaches baseline (see Fig. 12.1C). The prescribed PEEP level is reduced to no >5–7 cmH$_2$O of pressure and the F$_I$O$_2$ level is returned to its original setting. A complete line of data is then obtained from the ventilator, pulmonary artery catheter, and any noninvasive monitors available (i.e., oximeter or capnograph). A momentary expiratory phase hold measurement is taken to read the "effective PEEP" level and this is also recorded. An arterial blood gas is obtained 15–30 minutes later, after which fine tuning is done by adjusting ventilating pressures, rate, and I/E ratios. Ventilating pressure and rate are adjusted to maintain a desirable arterial carbon dioxide partial pressure (PaCO$_2$), whereas the I/E ratio and rate are adjusted to obtain an "effective PEEP" level for adequate oxygenation. The total inspiratory time can be increased upward with close observation of hemodynamics and O$_2$ delivery to see if a desirable result occurs.

PITFALLS AND COMPLICATIONS

Certain physiologic principles must be understood when using this ventilation mode. Although patients are being ventilated at lower peak airway pressures, these pressures are maintained for a long time and may result in mean airway pressures that are actually higher than what had been noted prior to IRV. The higher mean airway pressure is thought by some to be the reason for improvement in oxygenation. Although correlation between increasing mean airway pressures and PaO_2 exists, mean airway pressure may not be the major determinant of oxygenation. During ventilation at various combinations of inspiratory pressures and I/E ratios, significant changes in blood gas exchange commonly occur, despite a constant mean airway pressure. Interestingly, changes in the respiratory rate do not change mean airway pressure because, in any given minute, the same percentage of time is spent in inspiration at the preset pressure. At I/E ratios of ~2:1, mean airway pressures are usually similar to those attained during conventional ventilation with PEEP, thereby allowing the IRV benefits to be realized without hemodynamic compromise. At ratios approaching 4:1, however, the resultant drop in cardiac output may offset any improvement in PaO_2, thus emphasizing the importance of astute observation when applying IRV to this extreme. If cardiac output falls because of an increased mean airway pressure and decreased venous return, then intravenous fluids should be increased to maintain right ventricular preload much as is done when PEEP levels are increased. Because of this potential hemodynamic compromise, oxygen delivery (O_2 content $\times$ cardiac output) is the important parameter to follow.

Although V_T is not specifically set, it results because of the pressure change in going from an end-expiratory (PEEP) baseline to the preset inspiratory pressure (see Fig. 12.1C). Total PEEP is really a combination of the PEEP dialed into the ventilator plus the PEEP effect, which occurs because of progressively shorter expiratory times. As the I/E ratio or respiratory rate increases, the PEEP baseline rises, causing a smaller pressure differential in going from a new higher baseline to the same preset pressure. The resulting decrease in V_T may cause $PaCO_2$ retention, which can be averted by decreasing the dialed-in ventilator PEEP. At a higher I/E ratio or respiratory rate, the PEEP effect becomes significant even if it is not superimposed on a dialed-in level and, often, the dialed-in PEEP can be set to zero. As an alternative, preset inspiratory pressure can be raised to increase the pressure differential and thereby increase V_T; however, this also increases mean airway pressure, an increase that is usually undesirable.

As expertise is gained, one can frequently look at the expiratory flow tracing to determine whether the patient is a candidate for continued application of the IRV mode. A prolonged expiratory flow suggests increased expiratory resistance or obstruction, and these patients may develop an increasing $PaCO_2$. However, in appropriately selected patients, this mode usually decreases the dead space-to-tidal volume ratio (V_D/V_T) and $PaCO_2$, thereby necessitating a lower minute ventilation than was used in conventional ventilatory modes. In selected patients, there may be improved oxygenation and O_2 delivery at lower peak airway pressures.

CONCLUSIONS AND CONTROVERSY

Prolonged inspiratory time may result in improved alveolar ventilation-to-perfusion matching and decreased V_D/V_T in patients with normal or reduced lung compliance. Although prolonging inspiration to the point of reversing the I/E ratio has limited application, it may be effective in reducing peak airway pressure and improving oxygenation. A PEEP-like effect is created by setting a respiratory rate and an I/E ratio that begin lung insufflation before complete exhalation from the previous breath. A critical inspiratory pressure is maintained throughout the remainder of each ventilatory cycle to provide alveolar stabilization and recruitment. Lower peak airway pressures obtained for a longer period may prevent lung damage caused by excessive shearing forces that develop between inhomogeneous lung units when they are ventilated at high peak and PEEP pressures.

Although many authors have debated the pros and cons of IRV over the last 10 years, recently authors have challenged the desired theoretical benefits that have been described. Ludwigs et al., have studied both volume control-IRV and pressure controlled-IRV using the standard oleic acid-induced lung injury model to understand these ventilatory modes in ARDS. They conclude that neither one seems superior to volume control ventilation with PEEP in terms of oxygenation or effect on lung morphology when extrinsic or intrinsic PEEP and minute ventilation ($\dot{V}_E$) are the same and are carefully controlled.

Shanholtz and Brower raise two interesting potential benefits of IRV that have yet to be evaluated. First, if slower inspiratory flow is provided in a volume-controlled IRV mode, they question whether this use of IRV will reduce volotrauma and improve ARDS outcome by reducing pulmonary parenchymal shear stresses. If proved to be true, volume controlled-IRV might be preferable.

In addition, the scientific studies of ARDS using oleic acid induced injuries are short "snapshot" views as these animals are not studied for any prolonged period. Gradual improvement and potential shunt reduction over hours to days is seen clinically in humans and may be missed in these current animal study designs.

One thing learned from the continued study of ARDS and ventilatory efforts to provide the least lung trauma is that excessive lung distention must be avoided. Clearly, acute lung injury is worsened with overinflation by high airway pressures. Newer approaches seek to reduce this problem by allowing permissive hypercapnea in any mode. To reduce peak airway pressure, many clinicians are advocating pressure control ventilation use with or without the increased inspiratory time to reduce this lung injury. Whether this can be best accomplished with or without the inverse ratio has yet to be shown.

Inverse ratio ventilation should be undertaken only by individuals who are familiar with the equipment being employed and who can provide close observation and monitoring of these critically ill patients.

Suggested Readings

Cole AGH, Weller SF, Sykes MK. Inverse ratio ventilation compared with PEEP in adult respiratory failure. Intensive Care Med 10:227–232, 1984.

Fuelihan SF, Wilson RS, Pontoppidan H. Effect of mechanical ventilation with end-inspiratory pause on blood gas exchange. Anesth Analg 55:122–130, 1976.

Gurevitch MJ. Observations on IRV [letter]. Chest 90:152, 1986.

Gurevitch MJ. Selection of the inspiratory:expiratory ratio. In: Kacmarek Stoller J (ed). Current Respiratory Care. Toronto, BC Decker, 1988, pp 148–152.

Gurevitch MJ, Van Dyke J, Young E, et al. Improved oxygenation and lower peak airway pressure in severe adult respiratory distress syndrome; treatment with inverse ratio ventilation. Chest 89:211–213, 1986.

Lachmann B, Danzmann E, Haendly B, et al. Ventilator settings and gas exchange in respiratory distress syndrome. In: Prakash O (ed). Applied physiology in clinical respiratory care. Boston, Martinus Nijhoff, 1982, p 141.

Ludwigs U, Klingstedt C, Baehrendtz S, et al. A functional and morphologic analysis of pressure controlled inverse ratio ventilation in oleic acid induced lung injury. Chest 106:925–931, 1994.

Ludwigs U, Klingstedt C, Baehrendtz S, et al. Volume-controlled inverse ratio ventilation in oleic acid induced lung injury. Chest 108:804–809, 1995.

Marini JJ. Pressure-targeted, lung-protective ventilator support in acute lung injury. Chest 105 (Suppl. 3):109S–115S, 1994.

Mercat A, Graini L, Teboul JL, et al. Cardiorespiratory effects of pressure-controlled ventilation with and without inverse ratio in the adult respiratory distress syndrome. Chest 104:871–75, 1993.

Reynolds EOR. Effect of alterations in mechanical ventilator settings on pulmonary gas exchange in hyaline membrane disease. Arch Dis Child 46:152–159, 1971.

Shanholtz C, Brower R. Should inverse ratio ventilation be used in adult respiratory distress syndrome? Am J Respir Crit Care Med 149:1354–1358, 1994.

Tharatt RS, Allen RP, Albertson TE. Pressure controlled inverse ratio ventilation in severe adult respiratory failure. Chest 94:755–762, 1988.

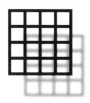

13
Differential Lung Ventilation
Richard D. Branson • James M. Hurst

The eloquent descriptions of ventilatory support in previous chapters usually have relied on a common assumption: the degree of pulmonary dysfunction is equally and homogeneously distributed throughout the lungs. Fortunately, this is most often the case (Fig. 13.1, *top*). Following unilateral lung injury, however, these relationships are altered (Fig. 13.1, *bottom*). The presence of unilateral lung injury also modifies the effects of conventional ventilation and positive end-expiratory pressure (PEEP) on lung mechanics and pulmonary perfusion. Because gas preferentially follows the path of least resistance, a disproportionately large percentage of the tidal volume (V_T) will be delivered to the compliant lung; likewise, it will also have the greatest change in functional residual capacity (FRC) with PEEP application. Hyperinflation of the more compliant lung compresses intraalveolar capillaries, decreasing perfusion in the compliant lung and simultaneously increasing perfusion to the poorly ventilated injured lung (Fig. 13.2, *top*). The cumulative result of these derangements is increased alveolar ventilation-to-perfusion $\dot{V}_A/\dot{Q}$ mismatching, worsening of gas exchange, and, in severe cases, hemodynamic instability and barotrauma.

Early in the treatment of unilateral lung injury, placing the patient in the lateral decubitus position so that the more compliant lung is dependent may improve gas exchange. Lateral positioning uses gravity to increase perfusion to the more normal, dependent lung. This technique may be useful in less severe unilateral lung injury, but has limitations, particularly hindering nursing care. The definitive treatment of unilateral lung injury is the isolation of the lungs with a double-lumen endobronchial tube and differential lung ventilation (DLV) with selective PEEP.

INDICATIONS FOR DIFFERENTIAL LUNG VENTILATION

Clear-cut indications for the initiation of DLV are generally lacking. Usually, a combination of clinical findings and sound clinical intuition are necessary. Initially, the presence of unilateral lung injury is most commonly identified on the

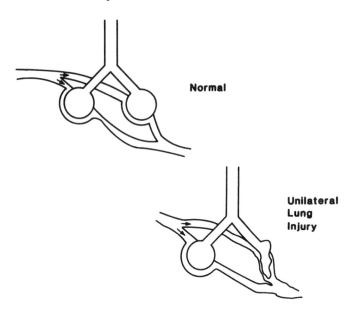

Figure 13.1. *Top:* Normal ventilation/perfusion relationship between the two lungs. *Bottom:* Hypoventilation of the injured lung with little change in perfusion following unilateral lung injury.

chest radiograph. However, radiographic evidence of unilateral lung injury is not of itself an indication for DLV, nor is it a prerequisite. In some cases, radiographic signs of unilateral lung injury may not be apparent until PEEP is applied and hyperexpansion of the normal lung occurs. A fairly firm indication for DLV is the demonstration of a paradoxical response to PEEP along with positive radiographic findings. The paradoxical PEEP effect is manifested by a fall in arterial oxygen partial pressure (PaO_2) and an increase in the intrapulmonary shunt fraction ($\dot{Q}sp/\dot{Q}t$) following increases in PEEP. Placing the patient in the lateral decubitus position (more compliant lung dependent), after demonstration of the paradoxical PEEP response, may offer confirmation of significant unilateral lung injury. If PaO_2 improves and $\dot{Q}sp/\dot{Q}t$ falls with the patient in the lateral position, a trial of DLV is warranted. Siegel et al. suggested analysis of static compliance curves as a method determine if unilateral lung injury exists. If hyperexpansion of the normal lung is present, the compliance curve will have two distinct slopes (Fig. 13.3). This finding is a firm indication for DLV, but its absence does not rule out significant unilateral lung injury. Scrutinizing the nature and cause of the injury may also aid in deciding whether or not to initiate DLV (Table 13.1).

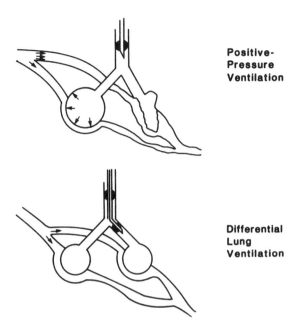

Positive-
Pressure
Ventilation

Differential
Lung
Ventilation

Figure 13.2. *Top:* Positive-pressure ventilation overdistends the compliant lung, shunting blood to the injured, poorly ventilated lung. *Bottom:* Placement of the double-lumen tube and DLV with selective PEEP restores normal $\dot{V}/\dot{Q}$ matching.

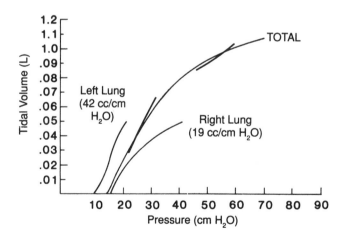

Figure 13.3. Demonstration of two slopes in a static compliance curve as described by Siegel et al. For both lungs at 0.06 L, static compliance is 35 ml/cmH$_2$O; at 0.08 L, it was 32 ml/cmH$_2$O; and at 1.0 L, it was 22 ml/cmH$_2$O. This patient required DLV. Static compliance curves for the individual lungs following the initiation of DLV are shown for comparison. Compliance of the injured lung was 19 ml/cmH$_2$O (0.05 L V$_T$]) and compliance of the normal lung was 42 ml/cmH$_2$O (0.05 L V$_T$).

Table 13.1. List of the Most Common Causes of Unilateral Lung Injury

Unilateral pulmonary contusion
Unilateral aspiration pneumonia
Unilateral lobar pneumonia
Unilateral refractory atelectasis
Unilateral pulmonary edema
Bronchopleural fistula
Pulmonary embolus
Postoperative thoracic surgery (esophagectomy, lung resection)

ENDOBRONCHIAL INTUBATION

Once the decision to initiate DLV has been made, the immediate concern is placement of the double-lumen endobronchial tube. Although double-lumen tubes were introduced in 1949 for bronchospirometry, long-term clinical use has only become practical in the past decade. This limitation was mainly due to the original tube designs. These were commonly made of red rubber (Latex), had low-volume/high-pressure cuffs, and used a carinal hook, which was intended to stabilize the tube. Latex is irritating to tissues; the cuffs tended to inflate asymmetrically (accelerating mucosal damage); and the carinal hook often produced mucosal irritation and puncture. The newest generation features endobronchial tubes made of thermolabile polyvinylchloride; they have radiopaque markers at the tracheal and bronchial openings, use high-volume/low-pressure cuffs, and have an improved cross-section to external diameter ratio (decreased resistance).

Inserting the endobronchial tube is the most difficult technical aspect associated with DLV. Although a skilled clinician may have extensive experience with placement, bronchoscopic guidance is still recommended. Bronchoscopic guidance assures proper placement, reduces procedure time, and improves safety. This is particularly important in that many of these patients are already hypoxic and will not tolerate prolonged intubation attempts. Once proper placement has been radiographically confirmed, the tube should be safely secured (adhesive tape works much better than cloth tape), and the tracheal and bronchial cuffs inflated (we prefer the minimal seal technique). Although bronchial rupture has been reported with use of a double-lumen tube, with proper care it is probably no more common than tracheal rupture associated with single-lumen tubes.

Tube migration, either distally or proximally, is usually associated with change in patient position and can be clinically disastrous. Proximal migration usually manifests itself by a sudden deterioration in patient status, resulting from incomplete isolation of the lungs. This can be detected by monitoring inspired and expired V_Ts. If gas escapes from around the bronchial cuff, expired V_T from the tracheal lumen will be greater than inspired, and expired V_T from the bronchial lumen will be less than delivered. As such, inspired and expired V_Ts should be measured every 2 hours and after every position change (chest x-ray, linen changes, and so forth). Adequate seal of the cuffs should also be checked frequently. Distal migration is a more subtle event and is detected by a rise in peak inspiratory pressure on the bronchial side. Frequently, upper lobe atelectasis accompanies distal migration. This occurs when the bronchial cuff occludes the right upper lobe bronchial orifice. Over time, the right upper lobe collapses from denitrogenation, and the overall decrease in lung volume causes a rise in peak inspiratory pressure for the same delivered V_T. Right upper lobe bronchial occlusion is seen most frequently (due to its proximity to the carina). Recently, National Catheter Corporation (Argyle, NY) modified its double-lumen tube, creating a left- and right-sided tube (Fig. 13.4). The right endobronchial tube has a sigmoidal shaped cuff and Murphy eye, which help to prevent occlusion of the right upper lobe bronchus. Although no recommendations are supported by the literature, we prefer to place the bronchial lumen into the bronchus leading to the uninjured lung.

Other less severe difficulties associated with the endobronchial tube are related to size. These tubes are large (39–41 French) and cause considerable patient discomfort. Topical anesthetic sprays and appropriate use of sedatives may be

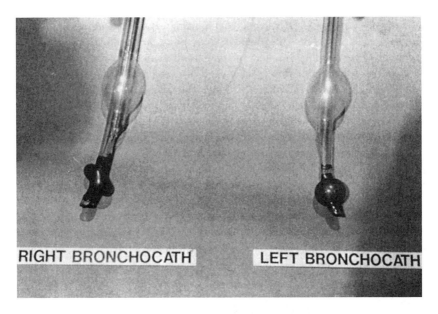

Figure 13.4. Distal third of a left- and right-sided endobronchial tube with tracheal and bronchial cuffs inflated. Note the sigmoidal shape of the bronchial cuff on the right-sided tube. Just below the top side of the cuff is a Murphy eye. Together, these prevent occlusion of the right upper lobe bronchus.

necessary to improve patient tolerance. Despite the overall large outside diameter, individual internal diameters are small. This hinders efforts to suction the tracheobronchial tree. Special suction catheters have been developed to overcome these problems. Specifically, these catheters are longer and more rigid than conventional catheters. Despite these advances, patients with copious amounts of thick secretions may not tolerate intubation with an endobronchial tube owing to inadequate secretion removal. The small diameter lumens also impose an added load to spontaneous breathing.

VENTILATORY TECHNIQUES

A variety of methods for the application of DLV have been described. These include (*a*) single ventilators with modified distribution circuits; (*b*) two ventilators in synchronous modes; (*c*) two ventilators in asynchronous mode; (*d*) a conventional ventilator with contralateral continuous positive airway pressure (CPAP); (*e*) a conventional ventilator with contralateral high frequency ventilation; and (*f*) differential CPAP. Often, the system used depends on local resources and treatment preferences.

The simplest system is differential CPAP. This method does not require a ventilator, but rather, two distinct CPAP systems. The CPAP level is titrated to each lung independently, commensurate with the degree of lung injury. This system is obviously limited in that alveolar ventilation must be accomplished entirely by the patient.

Early descriptions of DLV often used a single ventilator with modified distribution circuits. These systems place a "Y" in the inspiratory limb of the ventilator circuit and continue the "two new" inspiratory limbs onto the double-lumen tube. In most cases, a variable flow resistance device is placed in the inspiratory limb providing ventilation to the uninjured lung. This allows the clinician to select V_T delivery to each lung by increasing flow resistance (increased V_T delivery to the injured lung) or decreasing resistance (increased V_T delivery to the uninjured lung). In either case, the final delivered volumes are a product of lung compliance and circuit resistance. Expiratory gas is directed through separate expiratory limbs, each with its own PEEP device. The appropriate PEEP level, commensurate with the degree of lung injury, can then be applied to each lung. This technique is often referred to as *selective PEEP*.

Problems with circuit modification techniques are related to the large number of connections prone to disconnection and leakage. Additionally, any sudden change in impedance of either lung will result in undesirable modifications of V_T delivery. This technique also limits the variables, which may be independently adjusted, to V_T and PEEP.

The most popular and useful technique requires the use of two ventilators.

This allows complete independent adjustment of all ventilator parameters. Early on, considerable controversy was raised over the need to synchronize the delivery of a mechanical breath to each lung. Proponents believed synchronization would improve $\dot{V}_A/\dot{Q}$ matching and that asynchronous DLV would exaggerate $\dot{V}_A/\dot{Q}$ imbalance and would be unsettling for the patient. Most recent evidence suggests that synchronization is unimportant. In fact, in animal studies, ventilation 180° out of phase has resulted in improved cardiac output and a fall in pulmonary vascular resistance. However, this technique has not been tested in humans.

A single ventilator used with contralateral CPAP or high frequency ventilation can also be useful, particularly in the setting of unilateral bronchopleural fistula. Either system is easily set up and maintained, posing no more technical difficulties than conventional use of these techniques.

CHOOSING VENTILATOR SETTINGS

Because we recommend using a dual ventilator system, descriptions of setting ventilatory parameters will be based on this set-up. As a rule, we do not believe that using differential CPAP or contralateral CPAP is advisable in the intensive care unit (ICU). The small diameter of the individual endobronchial tube lumens may impose an inordinate amount of inspiratory work during spontaneous breathing.

Although all ventilatory parameters may be adjusted independently, the most important are V_T and PEEP. Of the two, V_T is most easily set simply by splitting the volume delivered during conventional ventilation in half. A rule of thumb is 5–6 ml/kg to each lung. Some authors have suggested increasing V_T to the injured lung as a method of increasing ventilation and decreasing atelectasis. We caution against this because excessive V_T delivery will overdistend nondependent compliant alveoli and may worsen gas exchange or result in barotrauma. Another strategy for V_T partitioning is by constructing a static compliance curve for each lung. With this technique, V_T is increased until flattening (or inflection point) of the curve occurs, suggesting overdistension. The previous volume is then selected as the optimal V_T. This technique is useful, but requires some sophisticated bedside monitoring equipment and clinical experience to use effectively.

East et al. suggested that optimal V_T delivery could be accomplished by equalization of end-tidal carbon dioxide concentrations (ETCO$_2$). They tested this hypothesis in an animal model of unilateral lung injury and found that the simple technique of equal V_Ts remained the most efficient (highest PaO$_2$, lowest PaCO$_2$). Selecting PEEP levels is somewhat more difficult and subjective. Whenever possible after DLV initiation, PEEP to each lung should be placed at the lowest possible level (we suggest 5 cmH$_2$O). Subsequently, PEEP to the injured lung should be increased incrementally. After each increase in PEEP, arterial blood gases should be measured and static compliance determined. If possible, determination of cardiac output and $\dot{Q}sp/\dot{Q}t$ should also be simultaneously performed. Once an acceptable PaO_2 or $\dot{Q}sp/\dot{Q}t$ is achieved (which will be subject to considerable variation between institutions), the same approach should be taken to determine optimal PEEP of the more compliant lung.

Other techniques to determine optimal PEEP include matching $ETCO_2$ for each lung, matching end-inspiratory pause pressures, or equalizing the dead space to tidal volume ratio (V_D/V_T). All these techniques are more cumbersome and no more effective than monitoring arterial blood gases and static compliance. Because each situation will be different, determination of optimal PEEP will be dependent on individual choice of therapeutic endpoints.

MONITORING

Essential monitoring during DLV includes (*a*) measurement of blood gases; (*b*) static compliance; (*c*) inspired and expired V_T; and (*d*) cuff pressures. With the dual ventilator system, each ventilator should be treated as it would be normally. This should include maintenance of alarms and humidification, recordings of airway pressures (peak, pause, end-expiratory, and mean) and volumes (spontaneous and mechanical).

Endobronchial tubes should receive special attention with respect to position, security, and patency. Evidence of thick secretions should alert the operators to the potential need to revert to a single-lumen tube or more frequent saline installation and suctioning.

DISCONTINUATION OF DIFFERENTIAL LUNG VENTILATION

In most of the cases described within, DLV can usually be discontinued after 48 hours. The exact time to return the patient to the single-lumen tube and to conventional support is unknown. The simplest and most widely used method is based on compliance. When peak airway pressure and PEEP requirements in each lung become similar, the transition can generally be made.

CONCLUSION

The technique of DLV can be accomplished with readily available equipment, which is already known to the critical care staff. The clinical usefulness of DLV is well described and rests on sound physiologic principles. When applied using the criteria presented here, DLV is safe, effective, and superior to conventional techniques.

Suggested Readings

Branson RD. Independent lung ventilation. In: Branson RD, Hurst JM, Davis KD (eds). Problems in respiratory care—alternate modes of ventilation. Philadelphia, JB Lippincott, Vol. 2(1), 1989, pp 48–60.

Branson RD, Hurst JM, DeHaven CB. Treatment of unilateral pulmonary contusion with synchronous independent lung ventilation. Respir Care 29:361–367, 1984.

East TD, Pace NL, Westenskow DR. Synchronous versus asynchronous differential lung ventilation with PEEP after unilateral acid aspiration in the dog. Crit Care Med 11: 441–444, 1983.

Hurst JM, DeHaven CB, Branson RD. Comparison of conventional mechanical ventilation and synchronous independent lung ventilation in the treatment of unilateral lung injury. J Trauma 25:766–770, 1985.

Siegel JH, Stoklosa JC, Borg U, et al. Quantification of asymmetric lung pathophysiology as a guide to the use of simultaneous independent lung ventilation in post-traumatic and septic adult respiratory distress syndrome. Ann Surg 202:425–439, 1985.

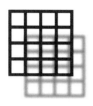

14
Airway Pressure Release Ventilation
M. Christine Stock

Airway pressure release ventilation (APRV) was designed to deliver continuous positive airway pressure (CPAP), to simultaneously mechanically augment alveolar ventilation, and to allow unrestricted spontaneous ventilation. APRV is a CPAP system that allows augmentation of alveolar ventilation by briefly interrupting CPAP.

EQUIPMENT

A brief discussion of equipment requirements is important for any mode of ventilation because success of the modality depends on the choice of appropriate equipment. The APRV circuit is a high-flow CPAP system with a release valve in the expiratory limb (Fig. 14.1) (1). Opening this release valve for 1–2 seconds allows circuit and airway pressures to drop from the CPAP level used for oxygenation support to near-ambient pressure (or to a lower CPAP level) (Fig. 14.2). This brief interruption of CPAP causes airway pressure to fall, and thereby, allows lung volume to decrease. When the release valve closes, airway pressure increases to the higher CPAP level, and lung volume is restored to the augmented functional residual capacity (FRC). Thus, each mechanical breath is created by the brief interruption and restoration of CPAP. Because each breath is delivered by *releasing* (i.e., decreasing) pressure, rather than increasing airway pressure, the peak airway pressure cannot exceed the CPAP level. The lower level to which pressure is released can be ambient pressure or a predetermined supra-ambient pressure, the "release pressure."

APRV can be delivered successfully only with equipment that meets stringent requirements. The continuous gas flow must meet the patient's peak inspiratory flow to allow unrestricted spontaneous ventilation (see Chapter 8, Breathing Circuits for Spontaneous Ventilation and the Work of Breathing). Flows of 90–100 L/minute obviate the need for a demand valve or reservoir bag in the inspiratory limb of the circuit. Many currently marketed demand valves do not supply gas sufficiently rapidly or with low enough inertia to allow unrestricted inspiration; their use can cause increased work and discomfort (2). Thus, only select ventilators can safely and effectively deliver APRV.

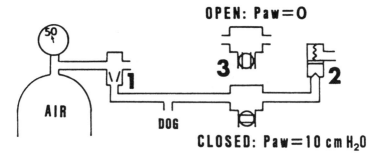

Figure 14.1. Airway pressure release ventilator is schematically depicted. A 50-psi oxygen source drives a Venturi device (*1*) capable of entraining enough room air to deliver 90–100 L/minute. This high gas flow exceeds the peak inspiratory flow needs of the patient. When the switch in the expiratory limb (*3*) is closed, airway pressure (*Paw*) equals the pressure generated by the threshold resistor expiratory valve (*2*). When the switch opens, gas escapes to the atmosphere at near-ambient pressure or to a predetermined, lower continuous positive airway pressure level. See text for further discussion. (Reproduced with permission from Stock MC, Downs JB, Frolicher DA. Airway pressure release ventilation. Crit Care Med 15:462–466, 1987.)

Successful CO_2 elimination depends on rapid increases and decreases in airway pressure. Thus, the humidifier, circuit, tubing, and connections must offer minimal flow resistance: $1-2$ $cmH_2O/100$ L/minute. To effect rapid changes in airway pressure, the release (expiratory) valve in the expiratory limb of the circuit must attain the fully opened or closed position in 10 msec.

The expiratory valve that creates CPAP must be a threshold resistor, so that widely varying gas flows do not influence airway pressure. If a CPAP valve or other ventilator components create resistance to flow, airway pressure will vary with the gas flow in the circuit. If the circuit flow varies markedly throughout the spontaneous ventilatory cycle, the fluctuating airway pressures increase ventilatory work (see Chapter 8). Further, if the patient coughs and greatly increases expiratory flow, exceptionally high peak airway pressures (>200 to 300 mmHg) will result and may cause barotrauma.

Clinical Efficacy

Initial animal studies, published in 1987 (1), demonstrated that APRV successfully ventilated the lungs and oxygenated the arterial blood of dogs with oleic acid-induced acute lung injury while preserving cardiac function. Compared with conventional ventilation with CPAP, APRV improved arterial oxygenation, decreased physiologic dead space ventilation, and lowered peak airway pressures.

The first demonstration of APRV efficacy in humans was performed in patients

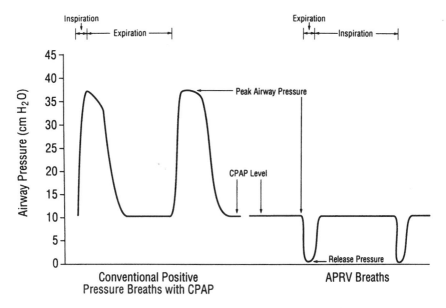

Figure 14.2. Typical airway pressure patterns of conventional positive pressure breaths with continuous positive airway pressure (*CPAP*) and of airway pressure release ventilator (APRV) breaths. In this example, the CPAP levels are identical during both modes of ventilation. During conventional ventilation, the positive pressure breath is delivered above the CPAP level, necessitating that mean airway pressure be greater than the CPAP level. In contrast, during APRV, expiration occurs by releasing airway pressure *below* the CPAP level, thus creating a situation where the mean airway pressure is necessarily less than the CPAP level. Further, the inspiratory-to-expiratory time ratio is reversed during APRV. During conventional positive pressure breaths, inspiration is shorter than or equal to expiration. During APRV breaths, expiratory time should not exceed 1.5–2 seconds, thus creating a situation where inspiratory time is longer than expiratory time when a mechanical ventilatory rate of <20 breaths per minute is employed. This figure also defines the CPAP and release pressure levels during APRV. The difference between the CPAP and release pressure levels is the change in airway pressure and determines the mechanical tidal volume (V_T). Patients with lower lung compliance need a greater CPAP-release pressure gradient to obtain the same V_T compared with patients who have more normal (greater) lung compliance.

following cardiac operations. Compared with conventional ventilation with 5 cmH$_2$O CPAP, APRV successfully ventilated the lungs and ensured satisfactory arterial oxygenation with lower peak airway pressures, similar hemodynamic profile, and similar gas exchange (3). Mechanical ventilation was discontinued by gradually decreasing the number of APRV breaths per minute as the patient increased spontaneous minute ventilation. This APRV weaning method, which is similar to that of intermittent mandatory ventilation (see Chapter 9, Intermittent

Mandatory Ventilation), resulted in successful discontinuation of ventilatory support for all patients. Then, CPAP was decreased from 10 to 5 cmH$_2$O and patients were extubated without complication.

Subsequently, a multi-institutional investigation demonstrated that APRV is a feasible alternative to conventional ventilation to augment alveolar ventilation in patients with acute lung injury of mild-to-moderate severity (4). APRV application required an increase in the mean CPAP level from 13 $\pm$ 3 to 21 $\pm$ 9 cmH$_2$O and a release pressure of 6 cmH$_2$O. After APRV titration, mean airway pressure was no different during APRV than it had been during optimal conventional ventilation. However, APRV supported ventilation with a 55% reduction in peak airway pressure. Further, 11 patients in this study had elevated PaCO$_2$s despite optimal conventional ventilatory support. Of these patients, all but three were successfully ventilated with APRV. Failure of three patients to be ventilated adequately with APRV was due to an inadequate level of CPAP or to inadequate tidal volume (V$_T$). Cane reported a series of patients with severe ARDS who were successfully ventilated with APRV. These patients also experienced significantly lower peak airway pressures during APRV (5).

Animal investigation demonstrated that instituting full ventilatory support with APRV did not disturb hemodynamic function when compared with spontaneous ventilation at a similar CPAP level (6). However, when switching from APRV to full ventilatory support with conventional ventilation and CPAP, stroke volume, cardiac output, and oxygen delivery significantly decreased. Further, conventional ventilation significantly increased oxygen extraction, whereas ventilatory support with APRV resulted in oxygen extraction and delivery similar to that during spontaneous ventilation with CPAP. Thus, the detrimental hemodynamic effects of conventional ventilatory support do not occur with APRV. APRV's hemodynamic pattern was indistinguishable from that during spontaneous ventilation with CPAP.

Ventilatory Parameters

Conventional ventilation requires that the clinician choose V$_T$, ventilatory rate, inspiratory-to-expiratory time ratio, F$_I$O$_2$, and CPAP level. To institute APRV, the choice of parameters is different.

TIDAL VOLUME

Because APRV is pressure-limited, one chooses a maximal airway pressure rather than a V$_T$. The pressure limit during APRV is the CPAP level from which pressure is released. The resultant V$_T$ is determined by the change in airway pressure from inspiration to expiration and the patient's lung-thorax compliance. The peak inspiratory pressure is the CPAP level; the expiratory pressure is the release pressure. Thus, if one chose a CPAP level of 10 cmH_2O, ambient release pressure (0 cmH_2O), and the patient's lung-thorax compliance was 100 ml/ cmH_2O, the V_T would be (100 ml/cmH_2O × 10 cmH_2O) or 1000 ml. Patients with normal lungs usually receive adequate V_Ts from 10 to 15 cmH_2O (3) with ambient release pressures. Alternatively, patients with less compliant lung (ARDS) require higher CPAP levels, ≥20 to 30 cmH_2O (4,5), and supra-ambient release pressures (5–10 cmH_2O). The APRV CPAP level required to ventilate ARDS patients is higher than the CPAP level needed to improve oxygenation during conventional ventilation. However, to obtain comparable arterial oxygenation, mean airway pressure during APRV and conventional ventilation is similar. Even with APRV's higher CPAP level, peak airway pressures are still reduced by ~50%.

INSPIRATORY-TO-EXPIRATORY TIME RATIO

Conventional ventilation usually employs inspiratory-to-expiratory time ratios of ≥1:2 (longer expiration). A ratio that reaches 1:1 defines inverse ratio ventilation (see Chapter 12, Inverse Ratio Ventilation and the Inspiratory/Expiratory Ratio). APRV's short expiratory time necessarily results in inspiratory times that far exceed expiratory times. In contrast to inverse ratio ventilation, which does not permit spontaneous breathing by the patient, APRV (by definition) allows unrestricted spontaneous ventilation. Thus, APRV is to inverse ratio ventilation what IMV is to control mode ventilation.

Expiratory times during APRV are necessarily short to prevent loss of lung volume from the alveoli recruited by CPAP. Expiratory (release) times of 0.5 second worked empirically in early human studies (3). While the expiratory valve is open, exhalation should proceed until expiratory flow stops. Experimental work confirmed the theoretical notion that adequate expiratory time is determined by the expiratory time constant of the patient's lung-thorax (defined as the product of compliance and resistance) (7). When lung compliance is low (e.g., ARDS), less time is needed to empty the lungs completely than when the lung compliance is normal or high. From a practical standpoint, 0.5 second should be adequate release time for patients with normal lungs; thus, those with stiff lungs should tolerate shorter expiratory times. Patients with ARDS may only require 0.25–0.3 second, provided that airway resistance is normal. Ultimately, to prevent gas trapping, one should listen to the chest or measure expiratory flow to assure that exhalation is completed before the delivery of the next breath.

Release of CPAP potentially can cause loss of alveolar volume. Clinicians observe this phenomenon when they attempt to suction the airways of patients receiving high-level CPAP, and see arterial oxygenation decline and pink froth issue forth from the tracheal tube. In addition to clinical observation, animal studies demonstrate no decrease in arterial oxygenation or oxygen delivery, and no increase in physiologic shunt from the short, periodic releases of CPAP that constitute the expiratory phase of APRV (8).

CLINICAL APPLICATION

Although APRV was designed to be used in patients with stiff lungs, it will successfully ventilate and oxygenate patients who have only mild pulmonary impairment or normal lung compliance. Because the technique relies on rapid increases and decreases in airway pressure for its success, patients with increased airway resistance should not be ventilated with APRV until further investigation demonstrates efficacy in these patients. Patients with an overtly prolonged expiratory phase or audible wheezing should be excluded from APRV at present. The remainder of this section is divided into two parts: a description of APRV use in patients with relatively normal lung compliance, and a description of APRV in patients with moderately to severely decreased lung compliance.

Patients with Relatively Normal Lung Compliance

The tidal volume delivered with APRV is determined by the patient's lung-thorax compliance and the change in airway pressure. Normal lung-thorax compliance is 100 ml/cmH$_2$O; thus, a change in airway pressure of 10 cmH$_2$O would produce a V$_T$ of 1000 ml. Most critically ill recumbent patients who do not have overt pulmonary disease rarely have lung-thorax compliance >70 ml/cmH$_2$O. Airway pressure changes of 10–12 cmH$_2$O produce V$_T$s of ~700–800 ml. Thus, a CPAP level of 10–12 cmH$_2$O should be chosen and ambient or near-ambient (no greater than 2 cmH$_2$O) pressure should be chosen as the release pressure. The airway pressure gradient from the CPAP level to the release level will determine the V$_T$.

The expiratory time should not exceed 1.5–2 seconds. This expiratory duration allows prolonged inspiratory times that should enhance inspired gas distribution, decrease dead space ventilation, and enhance arterial oxygenation. Adding inspiratory and expiratory times renders total ventilatory cycle time, which, in turn, determines mechanical ventilatory rate (a total ventilatory cycle time of 10 seconds results in a mechanical ventilatory rate of 6 breaths/minute). If expiratory time is fixed at 1.5–2 seconds, the inspiratory time then determines the rate of mechanical ventilation. Thus, the inspiratory-to-expiratory time ratio is not chosen for the ratio *per se;* rather, the inspiratory time is chosen to set the mechanical ventilatory rate. Mechanical rates should not exceed 15 breaths per minute (a total ventilatory cycle time of 3 seconds). Lower rates are probably more beneficial. If ventilatory rates >12 to 14 breaths per minute seem necessary, increasing the CPAP level in 2 cmH$_2$O increments may be better, thereby increasing V$_T$. F$_I$O$_2$ should

Table 14.1. Data from Apneic Humans Receiving APRV and Conventional Ventilation After Cardiac Operations (X ± SD)

Variable[a]	APRV	Conventional Ventilation
Peak Paw (cmH$_2$O)	11 ± 1	32 ± 4[b]
pHa	7.38 ± 0.04	7.39 ± 0.04
Paco$_2$ (mmHg)	38 ± 4	36 ± 3
Pao$_2$/F$_I$O$_2$ (mmHg)	281 ± 45	263 ± 40
HR (beats/minute)	79 ± 16	79 ± 16
CO (L/minute)	5.2 ± 1.2	5.3 ± 0.9
S$\bar{v}$o$_2$ (%)	67 ± 4	63 ± 10

[a] *Abbreviations: Paw = airway pressure; CO = cardiac output; S$\bar{v}$o$_2$ = mixed-venous oxyhemoglobin saturation.*
[b] *$p < 0.01$ compared to APRV.*

be chosen at the lowest level that achieves an arterial oxyhemoglobin saturation (SaO$_2$) ≥ 0.92. Table 14.1 gives the initial settings for the APRV ventilator for the patient with relatively normal lung-thorax compliance who requires full ventilatory support. Arterial blood gas determinations then should be made. If lung-thorax compliance is relatively normal, F$_I$O$_2$ ≤0.40 should result in satisfactory arterial oxygenation in combination with 10 cmH$_2$O CPAP. If this strategy does not succeed, please see the next section on ventilation of patients with moderate to severe decreases in lung-thorax compliance.

Because the APRV circuit allows unrestricted spontaneous ventilation, the patient should be allowed to contribute as much spontaneous breathing as possible. Thus, one titrates the ventilator to deliver the lowest level of ventilatory support that the patient needs. Starting from a mechanical rate of 12 breaths per minute (expiratory time, 1.5 seconds; inspiratory time, 3.5 seconds), if the PaCO$_2$ is normal or low, then the mechanical ventilatory rate can be decreased by lengthening inspiratory time. The mechanical ventilatory rate should be decreased until either tachypnea or respiratory acidemia occurs. Then, the next highest mechanical ventilatory rate that does not precipitate tachypnea or respiratory acidemia should be used. If hypercarbia or tachypnea persists, the mechanical ventilatory rate should be increased up to but not above 15 breaths per minute (inspiratory time, 1.5 seconds). If this level of ventilatory support is reached without successfully reducing PaCO$_2$ or respiratory rate, the patient's lung compliance is probably lower than originally estimated and the CPAP level should be increased.

Patients with Moderately to Severely Decreased Lung Compliance

A primary goal of therapy for patients with severely decreased lung compliance is to increase FRC without further injuring pulmonary tissue. Hence, an "optimal"

Table 14.2. Initial APRV Settings for Ventilation of Patients with Normal or Mildly Decreased Lung-Thorax Compliance

CPAP level	10–12 cmH$_2$O
Release level	0–2 cmH$_2$O
F$_I$O$_2$	Lowest needed to keep Sao$_2$ ≥ 0.92, usually F$_I$O$_2$ ≤ 0.40
Expiratory time	1.5 seconds
Inspiratory time	Determines mechanical ventilatory rate; start at 2.5 seconds (total ventilatory cycle time = 5 sec; rate: 12 breaths/minute should result in full ventilatory support
Monitor	Arterial blood gases, respiratory rate, respiratory pattern

CPAP level first should be chosen to support arterial oxygenation and to decrease, as much as possible, the elastic work of breathing (see Chapter 19, Acute Respiratory Distress Syndrome). Once "optimum" CPAP is established and F$_I$O$_2$ ≤0.50 to minimize the risk of oxygen toxicity, start mechanical ventilation with APRV at a rate of 10 breaths per minute (expiratory time, 1.5 seconds; inspiratory time, 4.5 seconds). The CPAP level chosen should be ~10 cmH$_2$O above the patient's optimum CPAP level. Release pressure should be ~10 cmH$_2$O, and the CPAP-release pressure gradient should equal the original optimum CPAP level (4).

Thus, if the patient required 15 cmH$_2$O as optimum CPAP, the APRV-CPAP level should be started at 25 cmH$_2$O and release pressure at 10 cmH$_2$O. For most patients, this approach will result in an adequate V$_T$ that can be used with mechanical ventilatory rates <15 breaths/minute (Table 14.2). After these initial settings are chosen, arterial blood gas and spontaneous respiratory rate determinations should be made. The CPAP level should be maintained such that an F$_I$O$_2$ 0.5 can be used. If the PaCO$_2$ is normal or low and if the patient's spontaneous respiratory rate <30, the rate of mechanical ventilation can be decreased (by increasing inspiratory time) until either respiratory rate begins to increase or respiratory acidemia occurs. Then, the next highest mechanical ventilatory rate that did not result in these changes should be employed. If tachypnea persists or if the arterial PaCO$_2$ is high, the ventilatory rate can be increased (by decreasing inspiratory time), but it should not be increased above 15 breaths per minute. If a maximal respiratory mechanical ventilatory rate has been achieved and tachypnea or respiratory acidemia persists, the CPAP level can be increased. This maneuver will increase both the CPAP-release pressure gradient and the V$_T$. These recommendations are based on scientific literature. Other approaches may be useful, but should be studied before they are put to clinical use.

WEANING

Ventilatory failure is likely to resolve before the decrement in FRC is resolved, unless nutritional support has been poor or unless ventilatory muscle fatigue has intervened. Thus, when withdrawing support, ventilation should be reduced first by decreasing the mechanical ventilation rate. The reduction in rate should be done gradually, as the patient tolerates, until the mechanical rate is zero. The CPAP and release pressure levels should be kept constant. When the mechanical ventilatory rate is zero, the patient will be breathing with the CPAP system. Weaning from ventilation should be stopped if the patient's spontaneous respiratory rate increases significantly, if respiratory acidemia occurs, or if the patient begins to use accessory muscles of respiration, particularly the sternocleidomastoid muscles. The mechanical ventilation rate then should be increased back to the level where these changes did not exist and the patient should be given either additional therapy or time to continue healing.

Once the mechanical ventilatory rate is zero, the patient's CPAP level should be decreased commensurate with recovery from acute lung injury (see Chapter 19). When the CPAP level has been weaned to 5 cmH$_2$O, the patient can be extubated if other extubation criteria are met.

SUMMARY

APRV is a ventilatory mode early in its development. It is designed to deliver CPAP and to ventilate the lungs of patients with stiff lungs. Ventilation is accomplished by briefly interrupting CPAP, allowing airway pressure to fall and the lungs to empty passively. It ventilates humans with normal lungs and with mildly impaired lungs without disturbing hemodynamic function. Patients with moderate to severe acute lung injury and ventilatory failure can be ventilated effectively, possibly with less dead space ventilation than conventional ventilation. Mean airway pressure during APRV seems to be the primary determinant of arterial oxygenation. Because APRV is still developmental, further study of its physiology and application will be forthcoming. Most APRV study has been directed toward efficacy. Studies to demonstrate the best airway pressure changes, best ventilation rates, and limitations are either under way or waiting to be done.

ACKNOWLEDGMENT

The author thanks Mrs. Dianne Byrd for editorial assistance.

References

1. Stock MC, Downs JB, Frolicher DA. Airway pressure release ventilation. Crit Care Med 15: 462–466, 1987.
2. Chiang AA, Steinfeld A, Gropper C, MacIntyre N. Demand-flow airway pressure release ventilation

as a partial ventilatory support mode: Comparison with synchronized intermittent mandatory ventilation and pressure support ventilation. Crit Care Med 22:1431–1437, 1994.

3. Garner W, Downs JB, Stock MC, et al. Airway pressure release ventilation (APRV): a human trial. Chest 94:779–781, 1988.

4. Räsänen J, Cane RD, Downs JB, Hurst JM, Jousela IT, Kirby RR, Rogrove HJ, Stock MC. Airway pressure release ventilation during acute lung injury: A prospective multicenter trial. Crit Care Med 19:1234–1241, 1991.

5. Cane RD, Peruzzi WT, Shapiro BA. Airway pressure release ventilation in severe acute respiratory failure. Chest 100: 460–463, 1991.

6. Räsänen J, Downs JB, Stock MC. Cardiovascular effects of conventional positive pressure ventilation and airway pressure release ventilation. Chest 93:911–915, 1988.

7. Martin LD, Wetzel RC. Optimal release time during airway pressure release ventilation in neonatal sheep. Crit Care Med 22:486–493, 1994.

8. Smith RA, Smith DB. Does airway pressure release ventilation alter lung function after acute lung injury? Chest 107:805–808, 1995.

15
Noninvasive Ventilation in Acute Respiratory Failure
Laurent Brochard

Interest in noninvasive ventilation originated with concern for patients with hypoventilatory syndromes (1). Recently, however, randomized controlled trials (2–5) established noninvasive ventilation as an alternative to endotracheal intubation to avoid endotracheal intubation in patients with acute respiratory failure. This notion arose from retrospective initial studies (6,7) and from the difficulties encountered in the routine application of this technique (8). Carefully controlled studies assessing both controlled efficacy and safety of this procedure are required before it can be put into routine clinical use.

The main objective of noninvasive ventilation is to deliver adequate ventilatory support without an endotracheal tube. For patients who receive mechanical ventilation at home, noninvasive ventilation can be used (*a*) as early treatment, (*b*) to prevent deterioration of chronic respiratory insufficiency, or (*c*) as an alternative to tracheotomy. During acute respiratory failure, the main objectives are to avoid complications of endotracheal intubation and to deliver ventilatory support to patients for whom endotracheal intubation is not desirable. Although mechanical ventilation is a lifesaving procedure, its use is complicated by serious morbidity and mortality (9). For instance, endotracheal intubation can precipitate cardiac arrest, cause aspiration of foreign materials into the lungs, laryngeal or tracheal injury, and it can result in long-term adverse sequelae.

Tracheal tubes are implicated in the genesis of nosocomial pneumonia, which is frequently accompanied by bacterial colonization of the pharynx and upper gastrointestinal tract that results in repeated microaspiration of contaminated secretions around the tracheal tube. Nosocomial pneumonia is responsible for prolonged hospital stays and it significantly increases mortality. Tracheal tubes also are associated with a high incidence of nosocomial sinusitis because of abnormal (or no) sinus drainage, especially when the tube resides in the nose. Indirectly, the need for heavy sedation and some of the difficulties in weaning from ventilatory support may be related to the presence of an endotracheal tube.

In other cases, withholding endotracheal intubation and mechanical ventilation may be justified by poor short-term prognosis due to the physiologic or severity of the underlying disease (6,10). In addition, some patients with late-stage disease refuse to be intubated. The decision not to intubate a patient is formed by the patient and/or family and the primary physician. For such patients, noninvasive ventilation may allow adequate support for respiratory distress with a lower risk of complications. In the same way, because the decision whether or not to intubate may be difficult at an early phase of acute respiratory failure, noninvasive ventilation may be used to postpone endotracheal intubation.

TECHNIQUES AND THEIR PHYSIOLOGIC EFFECTS

Perithoracic Ventilation

Several devices generating a perithoracic negative pressure have been proposed for neuromuscular disorders, including iron-lung, cuirass, or poncho-wrap ventilators (11). Most of these devices use conventional respiratory frequency. Recently developed devices synchronize spontaneous respiratory effort and the negative pressure breath. In a tank ventilator (iron-lung), the whole body, except the head and the neck, is submitted to intermittent negative pressure, whereas with the two other techniques only the thorax and the abdomen (poncho) or the thorax alone (cuirass) are exposed to the changes in pressure. The cuirass ventilator also has been used to deliver negative pressure high-frequency oscillations. Lastly, inflatable vests have been used in chronic obstructive pulmonary disease (COPD) patients to deliver positive-pressure high-frequency oscillations (12).

In the 1950s, negative pressure ventilation was anecdotally effective in acute exacerbations of chronic lung disease. More recent reports confirm these observations (13).

Several studies suggested beneficial effects of 6- to 8-hour periods of negative pressure ventilation in COPD patients with mild or moderate decompensation. Most studies concerning negative pressure ventilation during acute respiratory failure describe only short-term effects, have no or questionable control groups, and suggest only a mild efficacy. They do not allow one to conclude that noninvasive ventilation might satisfy the goals defined above.

Reported side effects noted, mainly during chronic use of these techniques, include obstructive sleep apnea and back pain (11). Negative pressure ventilator use is also limited by the scarcity of the equipment and because the apparatus may restrict routine intensive care unit (ICU) procedures.

Interesting effects have been described with external high-frequency oscillations in stable COPD patients. A study by Piquet et al. (12) showed that oscillations delivered during expiration only induced dramatic changes in the patient's breathing pattern with a subsequent decrease in the pressure-time index of the diaphragm. Again, however, the experience with such techniques during acute respiratory failure is extremely limited.

Positive Pressure Ventilation

VENTILATORY MODES

Continuous Positive Airway Pressure

Continuous positive airway pressure (CPAP) has been used for many years in patients with hypoxemic respiratory failure. Improvement in respiratory system compliance has led to a decrease in the work of breathing and to an increase in comfort (14). There also has been an improvement in oxygenation. Delivered via a face mask, this type of therapy may be poorly tolerated by some patients. CPAP has also been used in patients with left ventricular failure to improve both hemodynamics and respiratory mechanics (15). In fact, acute hypercapnic cardiogenic pulmonary edema is the only situation in which a clear benefit of CPAP has been demonstrated in a randomized controlled trial (15). In a study by Bersten et al. (15), CPAP significantly improved several cardiac and pulmonary physiologic parameters and reduced the number of patients requiring intubation.

Classically, CPAP and positive end-expiratory pressure (PEEP) were considered to be contraindicated for patients with COPD for fear of enhancing hyperinflation and thereby worsening abnormal pulmonary mechanics. The notion of dynamic hyperinflation, which might be responsible for the respiratory system's positive elastic recoil at end-expiration in such patients, suggests that perhaps CPAP or PEEP might be beneficial (16,17). When flow limitation causes dynamic hyperinflation, CPAP or PEEP may reduce the mouth-to-alveolar pressure gradient which exists at the beginning of inspiratory muscle activity and thereby also reduce the inspiratory work of breathing (16,17). In nonintubated COPD patients, very few data are available on the effects of CPAP. Miro et al. (18) used a 5 or 10 cmH_2O mask CPAP in seven hypercapnic alert COPD patients. In five patients, CPAP improved gas exchange but had to be withdrawn because of side effects from one patient who was intubated. Another patient was intubated when gas exchange deteriorated. The small number of patients and the absence of control group make these results inconclusive. A more promising combination might be the concurrent use of CPAP and pressure support ventilation (19,20). Appendini et al. (20) demonstrated that the combination of these two types of ventilatory support with a mask in COPD patients had greater efficacy than use of each one alone to reduce inspiratory muscle effort. However, Fernandez et al. (19) found that low levels of external PEEP could be used in only four of 14 patients during acute exacerbation of COPD; the other 10 patients experienced excessive leaks about the mask.

Intermittent Positive-pressure Ventilation

Volume-limited and pressure-limited modes have been used for noninvasive ventilation. Assist-control ventilation can be used with convental settings for breathing frequency and inspiratory flow rate. If ventilation is volume-limited, any leakage around the mask will decrease the volume delivered to the patient. Therefore, some authors have recommended using larger tidal volumes than usually chosen for intubated patients.

Pressure support ventilation also has been used widely for noninvasive ventilation (4,19–24). This ventilatory mode usually decreases the inspiratory work of breathing, increases tidal volume, and reduces spontaneous breathing frequency (25). During noninvasive ventilation, the presence of leaks is roughly compensated by the ventilator because the inspiratory pressure is maintained constant; it may, however, cause problems in the cycling mechanism from inspiration to expiration based on the flow decay. Thus, some authors prefer to use pressure-control ventilation, in which the inspiratory time is preset, or they add conventual positive pressure volume-limited breaths using synchronized intermittent mandatory ventilation to pressure support. This problem may also be solved by using an adjustable flow threshold for cycling (4,21). Thus, the problem of how to make the ventilator compensate for leaks around the mask requires sophisticated knowledge of ventilators and may limit noninvasive ventilation use if sophisticated problem-solvers are not available.

Frequency of Delivery of Ventilatory Support

In most clinical series, noninvasive ventilatory support was delivered intermittently throughout the day (3,5–8,19,21–23). In many studies, ventilation duration was 12 to 16 hours on the first day or, occasionally, almost continuously with periods of 10–20 minutes where the assistance was stopped to allow the patient to drink, expectorate, or rest. On subsequent days, ventilatory assistance was gradually reduced, depending on the clinical status of the patient. Ventilatory assistance was remarkably short in most series: a total of 8 ± 4 hours of ventilation in the study by Fernandez et al. (19), 3 ±1 day in that by Brochard et al. (21), and 4 ± 2 days in the study by Wysocki et al. (22).

PHYSIOLOGIC EFFECTS

In initial reports on noninvasive ventilation, blood gas abnormalities were corrected partially and failures (i.e., patients who eventually required endotracheal intubation) were most often not related to ventilation failure by itself (6,7,24). In an open study, Meduri et al. (6) described the treatment of hypercapnic respiratory distress in 18 patients using essentially pressure support ventilation. In 13 of 18 patients, intubation was avoided and the authors noted that an improvement in $PaCO_2$ and pHa during the first 2 hours was a good predictor of technique success (absence of intubation). Additionally, in a subgroup of seven patients, face mask

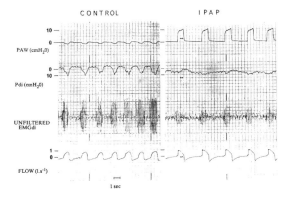

Figure 15.1. Tracings of airway pressure (Paw), transdiaphragmatic pressure (Pdi), electrical activity of the diaphragm (Edi), and flow (V) measured in a chronic obstructive pulmonary disease (COPD) patient admitted for acute exacerbation, during baseline (*left panel*) and during noninvasive ventilation with inspiratory positive airway pressure (IPAP) (similar to pressure support) (*right panel*). Note the dramatic reduction in respiratory muscle activity concomitant with modifications in breathing pattern. N Engl J Med 323:1523–1530, 1990. Used with permission.

ventilation was applied because of postextubation-hypercapnic respiratory distress. Assisted ventilation was delivered noninvasively with immediate efficacy.

Physiologic studies of the effects of noninvasive pressure support or pressure-limited ventilation on breathing pattern and respiratory muscle activity have been reported in patients with chronic respiratory insufficiency (21,26,27). Comparable results were obtained in severe, but stable COPD patients, and in patients admitted for acute exacerbation of their disease. Delivered noninvasively, pressure support assists each spontaneous breath and can reduce the transdiaphragmatic pressure, respiratory muscle pressure-time index, or the diaphragmatic electromyographic activity (Fig. 15.1). This reduction in muscle effort is accompanied by alterations in breathing pattern with increase in tidal volume, reduction in breathing frequency, and, frequently, an increase in minute ventilation. (See, also, Chapter 11, Pressure Support Ventilation). Oxygenation parameters are improved with a concomitant increase in alveolar ventilation.

In six stable hypercapnic patients with COPD, Nava et al. (27) showed that improvement in gas exchange was associated with a substantial reduction in diaphragmatic electromyogram (EMG). Further, Carrey et al. (26) demonstrated a reduced diaphragmatic EMG with nasal positive-pressure ventilation, in normal subjects as well as in patients with obstructive or restrictive chronic lung disease. Brochard et al. (21) also showed reduced diaphragmatic pressure-time index and diaphragmatic EMG activity in nine patients with acute respiratory distress and noninvasive pressure support ventilation. Despite the EMG results, muscular effort may remain substantially elevated in some patients, however, suggesting that some patients only reap modest therapeutic efficacy.

MECHANISMS OF ACTION

The first mechanism of action is simply to oxygenate the patient. This raises the problem of interpretation in open studies with apparent benefits of noninvasive ventilation because similar beneficial results may be obtained by ensuring adequate oxygenation, whatever the equipment. In patients with COPD, however, oxygen may worsen hypercapnia and respiratory acidosis, which may constitute a major limitation for standard treatment. By increasing alveolar ventilation, noninvasive ventilation may allow sufficient oxygenation without raising $PaCO_2$.

In some studies, noninvasive ventilation delivered with pressure support improved alveolar ventilation and decreased $PaCO_2$. In other studies, the main effect on gas exchange was improved oxygenation, obtained by simply raising the inspired oxygen fraction, but without the increased $PaCO_2$ that is often reported with oxygen therapy alone (4,19). This apparent discrepancy may reflect differences in the severity of the patients' illnesses. It is also possible that optimal assistance was not delivered in some patients owing to the urgency of the situation. Fernandez et al. (19) previously reported that pressure support ventilation via a full face mask suppressed oxygen-induced hypercapnia in COPD patients. In patients successfully treated noninvasively, we found that the rate at which $PaCO_2$ decreased was much slower than the increase in oxygenation (4).

As mentioned, noninvasive pressure support ventilation results in partial unloading of the respiratory muscles (see Fig. 15.1) (21,26,27). The mechanism by which beneficial effects are observed, therefore, may be a combination of adequate oxygenation and partial unloading of the respiratory muscles, which allow the patient to put his or her muscles partially at rest while keeping alveolar ventilation initially constant.

INFLUENCE OF THE TECHNIQUE

Ventilatory Mode

The effects of intermittent positive pressure breathing (IPPB) were markedly different from those of pressure support when delivered in nonintubated subjects in a high ventilatory demand situation. Breathing with IPPB may induce extra work owing to the superimposed impedance to the respiratory circuit and to the poor response of the ventilatory device (28). This problem emphasizes the importance of the ventilatory mode and the equipment used when treating patients with ventilatory failure or with high ventilatory demand.

Pressure support ventilation and assist-control ventilation have been the two most frequently used ventilatory modes, with or without PEEP. Vitacca et al. (23) compared the clinical efficacy of the two ventilation modes in a randomized study in 29 COPD patients. The efficacy of the technique was similar in the two groups with regard to the need for endotracheal intubation (12% for pressure support ventilation [PSV] and 23% for intermittent positive pressure ventilation [IPPV]). Interestingly, treatment compliance was better and the side effects were fewer with pressure support ventilation. This observation may be explained by the higher peak mask pressure generated with assist-control ventilation and the lower level of comfort in the presence of high peak airway pressure.

Patient-ventilator Interface

In patients with chronic respiratory failure, noninvasive ventilation usually has been delivered through a nasal mask (1). Commercially available models can be used and high-quality masks of multiple sizes are now available. Customized silicone masks can be individually molded to the patient's nose. Masks are secured to the head with straps.

In the acute care settings, many clinicians use full face masks on their patients (4,19,22). Nasal masks, however, present many advantages compared with full face masks, including better patient comfort, ease of use, and lower internal dead space. During nasal ventilation, however, inadvertent loss of volume through the mouth may cause serious problems. Patients can experience marked patient-ventilator asynchrony during air leakage through the mouth. Carrey et al. (26) showed that during nasal positive pressure ventilation, mouth position was a crucial factor with respect to the technique's success in reducing respiratory muscle activity. Because gas insufflated through the nose may escape through the mouth, mouth closure is mandatory. Many patients with acute respiratory failure do not choose to breathe solely via the nose and are often not cooperative enough to do so on request. Disadvantages of full face mask are the high degree of discomfort or anxiety generated in some patients, the large internal dead space of the mask, and the difficulty in obtaining a perfect fit to the patient's face. Recently, manufacturers are trying to improve the quality of these masks.

We used a specially adapted full face mask in our studies; it is noteworthy that side effects were few and did not cause withdrawal from ventilatory support in any patient (4,21). This was probably explained by the short duration of assistance used in these studies. Pressure-limited ventilation mode use allows the peak pressure to be limited in the mask, a factor which may play a role in the number and degree of leaks, in the risk of gastric inflation, and in the subjective tolerance of the ventilatory support.

CLINICAL RESULTS

Many open studies included patients whose clinical status was severe enough to make the physician estimate that endotracheal intubation was immediately deemed necessary, or that it might be necessary after a few hours of further clinical deterioration. In this manner, most authors reported success rates varying from 51% to 87% in hypercapnic patients, most of them having COPD. Similar results were shown in patients with hypoxemic lung failure. Data obtained in open studies, however, is difficult to interpret.

Wysocki et al. (22) assessed the effects of noninvasive pressure support ventilation in 17 consecutive patients with various types of respiratory distress, due to either hypercapnia or hypoxemia. The overall success rate was 47%. Successes were significantly more frequent in the hypercapnic group. Recently, Wysocki et al (2) reported the results of a randomized controlled trial comparing noninvasive ventilation to conventional therapy in 41 non-COPD patients with various causes of respiratory failure in the ICU. Patients with organ failure other than the lungs were not included. On an intention-to-treat basis, no benefit could be demonstrated in terms of intubation need, length of hospital stay, or mortality. When a subgroup of patients with acute hypercapnic ventilatory failure was examined (e.g., postoperative ventilatory failure or postextubation respiratory distress), significant improvement was found concerning the need for endotracheal intubation and the length of hospital stay, with a trend toward a lower mortality. These results indicated that acute hypercapnic ventilatory failure seemed to be a good indication for noninvasive ventilation.

This notion was confirmed in a randomized, prospective study by Kramer et al. (3) that showed that noninvasive ventilation reduced the need for intubation in patients with acute respiratory insufficiency who were otherwise stable, particularly those with COPD. The time that nurses and therapists spent at the bedside was analyzed and found to be similar whatever the therapeutic approach.

Bott et al. (5) prospectively compared, in a randomized controlled study, two groups of patients admitted for acute exacerbations of COPD. The same medical treatment was applied to all patients, but only one of the two groups received nasal noninvasive positive pressure ventilation. The pH improved significantly (from 7.35 to 7.38) in the group treated with noninvasive ventilation, whereas pH declined in the control group after 1 hour. Visual analog scores over the first 3 days of admission showed less breathlessness in the group treated with noninvasive ventilation. Lastly, survival rates were compared in the two groups. In an intention-to-treat analysis, the difference was not significant. However, when the four patients who did not tolerate noninvasive ventilation were excluded from the analysis, the mortality rate was significantly lower in the treated group (4% vs. 30%, $p <$ 0.05).

We reported our initial experience from a single institution in a series of 13 patients admitted for acute exacerbations of COPD (21). Results obtained in this group were analyzed in a case-control manner, each treated patient being matched with an historical control. A large significant reduction in endotracheal intubation need was observed between the two groups (8% vs. 85%). This reduction was associated with a reduction in the length of ventilatory assistance (3 days vs. 12 days) and in the length of stay in the ICU (7 days vs. 19 days). Recently, we extended our investigation to a multicenter, randomized trial conducted in five European centers (4). Patients were included in the study when admitted for acute exacerbation of COPD with objective criteria for severity based on breathing frequency, pH, and $PaCO_2$. Patients with a clear and treatable cause for decompensation (e.g., pneumonia, need for surgery, pneumothorax, acute myocardial infarction) or patients with other organ failure were not included in the study. A total of 83 patients were randomized either to conventional therapy with oxygen, antibiotics, and bronchodilator or to conservative therapy plus noninvasive pressure support ventilation delivered via a full face mask. Pressure support was delivered with a specially manufactured device, designed to have a highly sensitive flow-triggering system, fast pressurization rate, and low expiratory resistance (ARM 25, Taema, France). On admission, the patients' mean pH in the two groups was approximately 7.27, $PaCO_2$ 70 mmHg, and $PaCO_2$ 40 mmHg while they were breathing room air. Although the two groups were well matched on admission, a marked significant reduction in the need for endotracheal intubation was noted: 25% in the group treated with noninvasive ventilation versus 75% in the conventional group. Significant reductions in the length of hospital stay and in the in-hospital mortality (9% vs. 29%) were found. These results were obtained in a carefully selected group of patients (only 31% of all COPD patients admitted in the centers during the study period could be included), but they demonstrated that major benefits can be expected from noninvasive ventilation in the treatment of carefully selected COPD patients admitted for acute respiratory failure.

COMPLICATIONS OF NONINVASIVE VENTILATION

Complications reported with this technique are usually of minor severity but they may necessitate withdrawal of the technique. Complications include skin pressure lesions and facial pains, dry nose, eye irritation, discomfort, sleeplessness, mask leakage, and gastric distension. Mask intolerance or its poor adaptation to the patient's face may be a major limitation to the use of noninvasive ventilation. In the Meduri et al. study (6), two of 13 patients could not be ventilated adequately because of large leaks and therapy was therefore withdrawn. One patient developed intolerance to the mask after 2 hours of treatment. Lastly, two patients developed mild facial pressure necrosis at the mask contact site, which healed spontaneously in 2 days. Fernandez et al. (19) noted no significant side effects except nose pain among 14 episodes of treatment for acute respiratory failure. In the randomized study by Bott et al. (5), of the 30 patients randomized to the noninvasive ventilation group, four could not be ventilated: two because they could not cooperate, one because he was unable to breathe through his nose, and one because he requested the withdrawal of all active treatment. Comatose patients who cannot protect their upper airways should not receive noninvasive ventilation. Those who cannot spontaneously perform pulmonary toilet and need frequent suctioning may be difficult to treat with this technique.

Gastric distension seems to be uncommon with pressure support ventilation when mask pressure is limited to 20 cmH_2O (21). Therefore, gastric suctioning is not recommended.

An increase in peak mask pressure augments the risks of leakage and of gastric distension. It also necessitates a tight mask fit with an increased risk of pressure-related side effects.

CONCLUSION

Noninvasive ventilation may bring considerable benefits in the treatment of acute hypercapnic ventilatory failure, especially in patients with COPD (3–5,21). Reduction in the need for endotracheal intubation has been demonstrated in selected groups. Several reports also show that noninvasive ventilation in this population may be associated with a reduction both in the length of hospital stay and in mortality.

A number of technique failures have been reported and further efforts are needed to understand their causes. Part of the explanation may be in the equipment used and improvement is clearly needed in the type of assistance delivered to patients. New forms of pressure supported ventilation may bring new benefits.

References

1. Hill N S. Noninvasive ventilation. Does it work, for whom and how? Am Rev Respir Dis 147: 1050–1055, 1993.
2. Wysocki M, Tric L, Wolff M, Millet HBH. Noninvasive pressure support ventilation in patients with acute respiratory failure. A randomized comparison with conventional therapy. Chest 107: 761–768, 1995.
3. Kramer N, Meyer TJ, Meharg J, Cece RD, Hill NS. Randomized, prospective trial of noninvasive positive pressure ventilation in acute respiratory failure. Am J Respir Crit Care Med 151: 1799–1806, 1995.
4. Brochard L, Mancebo J, Wysocki M, Lofaso F, Conti G, Rauss A, Simonneau G, Benito S, Gasparetto A, Lemaire F, Isabey D, Harf A. Noninvasive ventilation for acute exacerbation of chronic obstructive pulmonary disease. N Engl J Med; in press, 1995.
5. Bott J, Carroll MP, Conway JH, Klilty SEJ, Ward EM, Brown AM, Paul EA, Elliott MW, Godfrey RC, Wedzicha JA, Moxham J. Randomised controlled trial of nasal ventilation in acute ventilatory failure due to chronic obstructive airways disease. Lancet 341:1555–1557, 1993.

6. Meduri GU, Abou-Shala N, Fox RC, Jones CB, Leeper KV, Wunderink RG. Noninvasive face mask mechanical ventilation in patients with acute hypercapnic respiratory failure. Chest 100: 445–454, 1991.

7. Meduri GU, Conoscenti CC, Menashe PSN. Noninvasive face mask ventilation in patients with acute respiratory failure. Chest 95:865–870, 1989.

8. Chevrolet JC, Jolliet P, Abajo B, Toussi A, Louis M. Nasal positive pressure ventilation in patients with acute respiratory failure. Difficult and time-consuming procedure for nurses. Chest 100: 775–782, 1991.

9. Pingleton SK. Complications of acute respiratory failure. Am Rev Respir Dis 137:1463–1493, 1988.

10. Benhamou D, Girault C, Faure C, Portier F, Muir JF. Nasal mask ventilation in acute respiratory failure. Experience in elderly patients. Chest 102:912–917, 1992.

11. Ambrosino N, Rampulla C. Negative pressure ventilation in COPD patients. Eur Respir Rev 2: 353–356, 1992.

12. Piquet J, Brochard L, Isabey D, De Cremoux H, Chang HK, Bignon J, Harf A. High frequency chest wall oscillation in patients with chronic airflow obstruction. Am Rev Respir Dis 136: 1355–1359, 1987.

13. Sauret JM, Guitart AC, Rodriguez-Frojan G, Cornudella R. Intermittent short-term negative pressure ventilation and increased oxygenation in COPD patients with severe hypercapnic respiratory failure. Chest 100:455–459, 1991.

14. Katz JA, Marks JD. Inspiratory work with and without continuous positive airway pressure in patients with acute respiratory failure. Anesthesiology 63:598–607, 1985.

15. Bersten A, Holt AW, Vedig AE, Skowronski GA, Baggoley CJ. Treatment of severe cardiogenic pulmonary edema with continuous positive airway pressure delivered by face mask. N Engl J Med 325:1825–1830, 1991.

16. Petrof DJ, Legaré M, Goldberg P, Milic-Emili J, Gotfried SB. Continuous positive airway pressure reduces work of breathing and dyspnea during weaning from mechanical ventilation in severe chronic obstructive pulmonary disease. Am Rev Respir Dis 141:281–289, 1990.

17. Smith TC, Marini JJ. Impact of PEEP on lung mechanics and work of breathing in severe airflow obstruction. J Appl Physiol 65:1488–1499, 1988.

18. Miro AM, Shivaram U, Hertig I. Continuous positive airway pressure in COPD patients in acute respiratory failure. Chest 103:266–268, 1993.

19. Fernandez R, Blanch LP, Valles J, Baigorri F, Artigas A. Pressure support ventilation via face mask in acute respiratory failure in hypercapnic COPD patients. Intensive Care Med 19: 456–461, 1993.

20. Appendini L, Patessio A, Zanaboni S, Carone M, Gukov B, Donner CF, Rossi A. Physiologic effects of positive end-expiratory pressure and mask pressure support during exacerbations of chronic obstructive pulmonary disease. Am J Respir Crit Care Med 149:1069–1076, 1994.

21. Brochard L, Isabey D, Piquet J, Amaro P, Mancebo J, Messadi AA, Brun-Buisson C, Rauss A, Lemaire F, Harf A. Reversal of acute exacerbations of chronic obstructive lung disease by inspiratory assistance with a face mask. N Engl J Med 323:1523–1530, 1990.

22. Wysocki M, Tric L, Wolff M A, Gertner J, Millet H, Herman B. Noninvasive pressure support ventilation in patients with acute respiratory failure. Chest 103:907–913, 1993.

23. Vitacca M, Rubini F, Foglio K, Scalvani S, Nava S, Ambrosino N. Noninvasive modalities of positive pressure ventilation improve the outcome of acute exacerbations in COLD patients. Intensive Care Med 19:450–455, 1993.

24. Pennock B E, Grawshaw L, Kaplan P D. Noninvasive nasal mask ventilation for acute respiratory failure. Institution of a new therapeutic technology for routine use. Chest 105:441–444, 1994.

25. Brochard L, Harf A, Lorino H, Lemaire F. Inspiratory pressure support prevents diaphragmatic fatigue during weaning from mechanical ventilation. Am Rev Respir Dis 139:513–521, 1989.

26. Carrey Z, Gottfried SB, Levy RD. Ventilatory muscle support in respiratory failure with nasal positive pressure ventilation. Chest 97:150–158, 1990.

27. Nava S, Ambrosino N, Rubini F, Fracchia C, Rampulla C, Torri G, Calderini E. Effect of nasal pressure support ventilation and external PEEP on diaphragmatic activity in patients with severe stable COPD. Chest 103:143–150, 1993.

28. Mancebo J, Amaro P, Mollo JL, Lorino H, Lemaire F, Brochard L. Comparison of the effects of pressure support ventilation delivered by three different ventilators during weaning from mechanical ventilation. Intensive Care Med 21; in press, 1995.

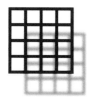

16
Continuous Flow Apneic Ventilation and Other Techniques of Intratracheal Gas Insufflation

R. Brian Smith

Gas exchange during apnea has been extensively studied in animals and humans for many years. Apneic diffusion oxygenation is used clinically to support oxygenation. More recently, there has been renewed interest in ventilation during apnea because a significant amount of CO_2 can be removed by placing the oxygen-carrying catheters into the mainstem bronchi. A stimulus to develop these techniques has been the desire to lower airway pressure during artificial ventilation. Single catheters have been used in the trachea (transtracheal oxygenation, tracheal insufflation of oxygen [TRIO], tracheal gas insufflation [TGI], percutaneous transtracheal ventilation [PTJV]). Techniques using two endobronchial catheters include constant flow ventilation (CFV), continuous flow apneic ventilation (CFAV), and intermittent flow expiratory ventilation.

APNEIC DIFFUSION OXYGENATION

Apneic diffusion oxygenation is used to support oxygenation in paralyzed anesthetized patients undergoing short surgical procedures. Usually these are procedures performed on the airways during laryngoscopy and bronchoscopy. The technique begins with preoxygenation and denitrogenation of the lungs. This takes 3–5 minutes of breathing 100% oxygen using a high flow to eliminate nitrogen. The patient is anesthetized with thiopental and then paralyzed with a muscle relaxant. The patient's lungs are manually hyperventilated to lower arterial carbon dioxide partial pressure ($PaCO_2$). A catheter with a 3–4 mm internal diameter is placed either into the nasopharynx or trachea and the surgical procedure is started. The advantages of apneic diffusion oxygenation are (*a*) there is good oxygenation; (*b*) it is simple to perform; and (*c*) the airway is accessible to the surgeon or endoscopist. The disadvantages are (*a*) there is no protection of the airway from aspiration of gastric contents; (*b*) the $PaCO_2$ will rise as very little is eliminated from the lungs during apnea; and (*c*) the procedure must be short because of the rising $PaCO_2$. The consequences of a high $PaCO_2$, which are well known, are caused by the rise in endogenous catecholamines. They include hypertension, tachydysrhythmias, and raised intracranial pressure. Patient monitoring should include blood pressure, electrocardiogram, pulse oximetry, and when indicated, blood gas analysis.

Probably the first documented clinical use of apneic diffusion oxygenation was in 1946 by Comroe and Dripps (1) in two patients who were comatose and apneic. Insufflation of O_2 into the trachea at 6 L/minute for 3 hours resulted in a $PaCO_2$ of 314 mmHg in a 196-lb man. O_2 saturation was 75% and 65%, respectively, in both patients. No reference was made to the effects of the elevated $PaCO_2$ on the cardiovascular system and it appeared that both patients survived the experiment.

Eger and Severinghaus, in 1961 (2), studied the rate of $PaCO_2$ rise in the alveoli ($PaCO_2$) during anesthesia in apneic humans. They determined the rate of rise from a relatively normal $PaCO_2$ and then from a lowered $PaCO_2$ produced by prolonged hyperventilation. The overall rate of CO_2 rise before hyperventilation was 4.2 mmHg/minute and after hyperventilation it was 3.05 mmHg/minute. They found that the rate of $PaCO_2$ rise versus time may be divided into two sections (Fig. 16.1). The rise during the first 15–45 seconds was rapid and represented an equilibrium of $PaCO_2$ with venous blood. This rapid rise was then succeeded by a slower and near-linear rate of rise of ~3 mmHg/minute. The shape of the graph before and after hyperventilation remained the same. The rate of rise during the first minute of apnea after hyperventilation was 9.6 mmHg/minute compared with 13.4 mmHg/minute without hyperventilation. Heller et al. (3),

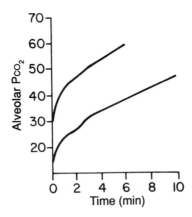

Figure 16.1. Average rates of rise of alveolar Pco_2 before (*upper graph*) and after (*lower graph*) hyperventilation. The length of each graph is determined by the number of minutes during which points are present from all five subjects.

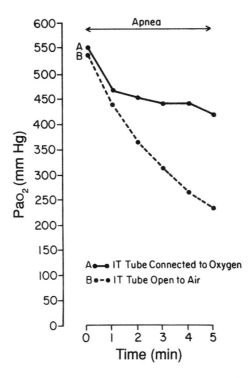

Figure 16.2. The average PaO_2 values during apnea (in mmHg) of seven subjects. The two curves illustrate the difference in rate of fall of PaO_2 depending on whether the airway was attached to a reservoir of O_2 or allowed to remain open to the atmosphere.

in 1964, showed a more rapid decline in PaO_2 in patients during apnea with the endotracheal tube left exposed to air as compared with exposure to O_2. Figure 16.2, shows that after 5 minutes of apnea, the seven patients exposed to O_2, average PaO_2 of 425 mmHg whereas the PaO_2 in those exposed to air was 225 mmHg.

The first evaluation of elevated $PaCO_2$ effects on the cardiovascular system was by Frumin et al. in 1959 (4) who studied eight healthy patients under thiopental anesthesia paralyzed with succinylcholine. After breathing O_2 and undergoing denitrogenation, the patients were kept apneic for 30–55 minutes. Oxygen was administered through an endotracheal tube. The lowest O_2 saturation was 98% and the highest $PaCO_2$ ranged from 130–250 mmHg. The highest blood pressure ranged from 150/80 mmHg to 200/100 mmHg, with an average rise of 26%. In three of these patients, blood epinephrine and norepinephrine levels were measured; both were increased during apnea. All patients recovered from the experiment without complications.

The effects of buffering CO_2 on the hypercapnia associated with apneic diffusion oxygenation (e.g., tris-(hydroxymethyl) aminomethane, THAM) can result in a normal pH and an elevated $PaCO_2$. No measurable stimulation of the sympathoadrenal system and no circulation impairment were shown. These effects have been demonstrated experimentally. There are no clinical applications of buffering CO_2 during apneic diffusion oxygenation in the literature.

Tracheal Insufflation of Oxygen

Jacoby et al., in 1951 (5) used transtracheal oxygen insufflation in apneic dogs by inserting a percutaneous catheter into the trachea. Using flow rates up to 15 L/minute adequate oxygenation was maintained and some carbon dioxide eliminated. In 1985 Slutsky et al. (6), using low flows of oxygen through a transtracheal catheter in dogs, demonstrated survival for as long as 5 hours with $PaCO_2$ levels plateauing between 100 and 200 mmHg.

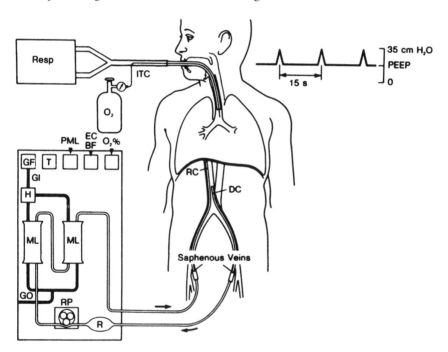

Figure 16.3. Cannulation and perfusion circuit. *DC,* indicates blood drainage catheter; *ECBF,* extracorporeal blood flow; *GF,* gas flow monitor; *GI,* gas inlet; *GO,* gas outlet; *H,* humidifier; *ITC,* intratracheal catheter; *ML,* membrane lung; *O_2%, venous drainage blood oxygen monitor;* *PML,* membrane lung pressure, in-out; *R,* venous reservoir; *RC,* blood return catheter; *Resp,* respirator; *RP,* roller pump; *PEEP,* positive end-expiratory pressure; *T,* ambient temperature control.

Low Flow Extracorporeal Removal of CO_2

More recently, apneic diffusion oxygenation has been combined with a low-flow extracorporeal removal of CO_2 (ECCO$_2$R) in patients with respiratory failure. The rationale of this therapy lies in the reduction in high airway pressure taking place during mechanical ventilation of these patients. Considerable evidence exists that high airway pressures adversely affect the healing process in the lungs. Further developments of this technique have shown that apneic diffusion oxygenation can be performed safely for many days when metabolic CO_2 is removed by an extracorporeal membrane lung (ECCO$_2$R) and 100% O_2 is supplied directly into the trachea, keeping intrapulmonary pressures at 5 cmH$_2$O. Increasing continuous airway pressure to 20 cmH$_2$O was shown to reduce shunts and improve oxygenation, functional residual capacity (FRC), and compliance.

Gattinoni et al. (7) reported ECCO$_2$R use in a series of patients with severe acute respiratory failure of parenchymal origin. Most of the metabolic CO_2 production was cleared through a low-flow venovenous bypass (Fig. 16.3). To avoid lung injury from mechanical ventilation, O_2 was administered continuously into the trachea (apneic diffusion oxygenation) and 3–5 breaths per minute were given at a low peak airway pressure of 35–45 cmH$_2$O. The gas exchange of all these patients was so poor that a 90% mortality rate had been expected before ECCO$_2$R was instituted. Lung function improved in 31 patients (72.8%) and 21 patients (48.8%) survived.

CONSTANT FLOW VENTILATION (CFV)/CONSTANT FLOW APNEIC VENTILATION (CFAV)

Experimental Work

In 1982 Lehnert et al. (8) studied constant-flow endobronchial air ventilation in four apneic dogs (the authors called this constant flow ventilation [CFV]). They found that normal blood gas values could be maintained for as long as 2 hours. A correlation between CO_2 elimination and total gas flow was found. Smith et al. (9) reported on the use of a similar technique, which they called constant flow apneic ventilation (CFAV), in 17 anesthetized paralyzed dogs. Each mainstem bronchus was cannulated with a 2.5-mm internal diameter polyethylene catheter using a fiberoptic bronchoscope. An endotracheal tube was placed in the trachea to hold the catheters in place. Heated humidified air was continuously delivered equally to each catheter. Total flows of air ranged from 8–28 L/minute. Adequate gas exchange in terms of PaO$_2$ and PaCO$_2$ was found after 30 minutes with flows >16 L/minute. A second group of animals was managed similarly and a continuous flow of air was insufflated at the optimal flow of 1.0 L/kg/minute for 5 hours. All animals were adequately oxygenated after 5 hours of CFAV and adequate CO_2

elimination was achieved in all animals. In three additional animals, pulmonary gas distribution was evaluated using Xe^{133} in relation to catheter placement. Results showed significant differences between PaO_2 and $PaCO_2$ values with the catheters in the trachea compared within the bronchi. With the catheters above the carina, gas distribution was limited to the large airways with no peripheral distribution, resulting in a low PaO_2 and an elevated $PaCO_2$. Endobronchial catheters allowed gas distribution to the peripheral airways, and oxygenation and ventilation were normal.

Subsequent experimental work has been reported on the effects of catheter position, catheter size, and gas exit velocity. Because of the large effective minute insufflation flows even for small individuals, attempts have been made to lower the flows by studying the mean gas exit velocity from the catheters (10). Exit velocity of gas matched with two different-sized catheters, 2.5 mm and 1.4 mm, at a mean of 448 cm/kg/minute (the velocity of gas exiting a 2.5-mm catheter at a flow of 1 L/kg/minute) has been studied in dogs. The results are shown in Figure 16.4. No significant differences were noted in pH, $PaCO_2$, and PaO_2 between the two catheters. However, significantly less bronchial insufflation flow (70%) was required to maintain oxygenation and ventilation for the 1.4-mm (internal diameter) catheters. The mean gas exit velocity from the bronchial insufflation catheters may be a more important determinant of gas exchange than the insufflation flow.

Babinski and coworkers showed a difference has been shown in $PaCO_2$ elimina-

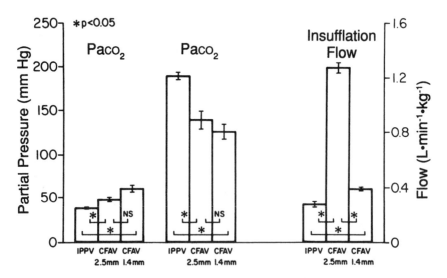

Figure 16.4. Inflation flow, $PaCO_2$ and PaO_2 are presented as mean values ± SEM. The *asterisk* represents statistical significance at $p < 0.05$.

tion when insufflation gas of air is compared with an insufflation gas of oxygen. CO_2 elimination is significantly better when air is used (11). Differences cannot be explained on different physical properties of the gases, such as density and dynamic and kinematic viscosity. Possibly, the superiority with air is related to the "alveolar splinting" with nitrogen. Optimal catheter placement in dogs has been shown to be ~2 cm below the carina. However, similar studies have not been performed in humans.

Because of the possible clinical value of CFAV during thoracic surgery, experimental work has been done using CFAV during thoracotomy in dogs. Adequate CO_2 removal takes place with air and oxygen. However, to obtain an adequate PaO_2, an F_IO_2 of 0.4 is required (12).

Low flow endobronchial insufflation with air was studied as it may be useful in emergencies in which positive pressure mechanical ventilation is not possible (13). Mackenzie et al. (13) used insufflation catheters positioned blindly in the mainstem bronchi of six anesthetized apneic dogs averaging 9.6 kg. They found flow rates of 2.5 L/minute PaO_2 could be maintained >45 mmHg and $PaCO_2$ <65 mmHg. All dogs survived for 2 hours without neurologic sequelae. The authors postulated that this technique could be used in an emergency in the field through a cricothyroidotomy, particularly in situations where oxygen equipment is limited (e.g., mass casualties).

Hachenberg, et al. (14), studied CFAV during experimental left ventricular failure in dogs. Because peak intrathoracic pressure is lower with CFAV than with CMV the authors considered that CFAV may be advantageous in patients with impaired cardiovascular function. Heated humidified oxygen-enriched air (F_IO_2 0.4) was continuously delivered by two catheters positioned with one within each mainstem bronchus at two flow rates of 1.2 and 1.6 L/kg/minute. Conventional mechanical ventilation was used as reference ventilation. Neither ventilatory mode impaired cardiac performance. Acute left ventricular failure (LFV) was induced by proximal occlusion of the left anterior descending coronary artery. CFAV maintained sufficient gas exchanged with LVF. CMV with PEEP was more effective in achieving oxygenation and CO_2 elimination with fewer adverse cardiopulmonary effects.

Hachenberg et al. (15), also studied the effects of CFAV in canine experimental pulmonary emphysema. Their results showed that, in dogs with emphysematous lungs, CFAV maintained sufficient gas exchange. CMV was more effective in terms of oxygenation and CO_2 elimination.

Clinical Investigation

The first clinical evaluation of CFAV was in five adult female patients by Babinski et al. in 1985 (16). The average age was 40.3 years and the average weight was 53.8 kg. The patients were scheduled for elective gynecologic procedures (four abdominal hysterectomies, one vaginal hysterectomy). After induction anesthesia with thiopental (5 mg/kg) and fentanyl (5 μg/kg), and paralysis with pancuronium bromide (0.12 mg/kg), patients were ventilated by face mask with O_2 at an F_IO_2 of 1.0. Two polyethylene catheters (outer diameter, 2.5 mm) were each inserted into the right and left mainstem bronchi. Each catheter had a curved tip measuring 2 cm in length, with the angulation from the axis of 20° for the right side and 30° for the left side. The endobronchial position was checked by fiberoptic bronchoscopy. Subsequently, tracheal intubation was performed using a 7.5 mm outer diameter tracheal tube. CFAV was started when both catheters were connected to the gas delivery system. Humidified O_2 was delivered at total flows between 0.6 and 0.7 L/kg/minute (Figs. 16.5 and 16.6). Arterial blood gases were analyzed every 5 minutes for 30 minutes. Monitoring included ECG, indirect blood pressure, heart rate, temperature, and peripheral nerve stimulation. Adequate oxygenation was maintained in all patients (299 ± 37 mmHg) at 30 minutes. A significant (<0.05) rise in $PaCO_2$ occured at 30 minutes (37.0 ± 4.0 mmHg) compared with the control (54.9 ± 4.0 mmHg). The mean rise in $PaCO_2$ was 0.6 mmHg/minute compared with 3.8 mmHg/minute with apneic diffusion oxygenation. In one patient, no increase was observed in $PaCO_2$ during the 30 minutes of CFAV. These results demonstrate that CFAV can maintain blood gases in a clinically useful range for as long as 30 minutes.

In 1986, Breen et al. (17) used endobronchial catheters just below the carina for CFAV in five patients having nonthoracic surgery. The insufflating gas was 50% N_2O in O_2 at a flow of 1 L/kg/minute. After 30 minutes of CFAV, the $PaCO_2$ had increased to 69.2 ± 14.5 from 35.9 ± 2.9 mmHg, a rate of rise of 1.11 mmHg/minute. The authors included a high airway-pressure relief device

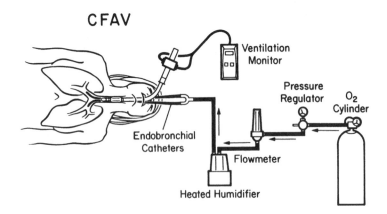

Figure 16.5. Schematic presentation of the gas delivery system during the clinical application of continuous flow apneic ventilation (*CFAV*) in five patients.

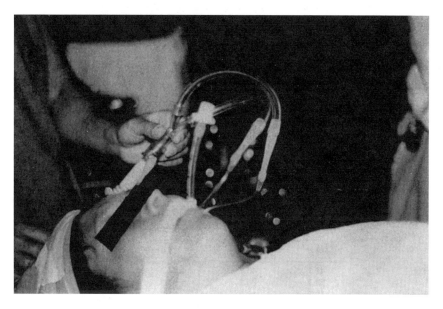

Figure 16.6. Patient with endobronchial catheters in place.

in the system to decrease the likelihood of barotrauma. No complications were related to the procedure in any of the patients, although one patient with a history of epilepsy convulsed in the recovery room.

Breen et al. (17) showed a rise in $PaCO_2$ of 1.11 mmHg/minute in their patients compared with a rise of 0.6 mmHg/minute in the study by Babinski's group. However, a number of differences exist between the studies. The flow used by Breen et al. (17) was 1.0 L/kg/minute compared with 0.6-0.7 L/kg/minute by Babinski et. al. (16). This would favor better CO_2 elimination in the former study. However, in the latter study, the endobronchial catheters were placed deeper in the bronchi, which has been shown in dogs to improve CO_2 elimination. In addition, Breen's group used N_2O/O_2 compared with 100% O_2 by Babinski's group. The role that N_2O plays in CO_2 elimination is unknown in the CFAV system, but its use may have slowed the CO_2 elimination. Controlled studies are needed to evaluate fully the role of this gas in CO_2 transport. The Breen et al. study (13) indicates that the rise in $PaCO_2$ may start to plateau at 20–30 minutes. Plateauing may be extremely important if CFAV is to have long-term clinical applications.

CFAV also was evaluated in seven brain dead patients (average age, 63 years; average weight, 53 kg) by Ebata et al. (18) in Japan in 1988. One hundred percent O_2 was insufflated at varying flow rates through one or two polyethylene catheters (2.1 mm internal diameter) placed at either mainstem bronchi or 2 cm above the

Table 16.1. Paco$_2$ (mm Hg) at Various Catheter Placements

Flow Rates (L/kg·min)	Both Bronchi		Unilateral Bronchus	Trachea	
	1.0	0.5	1.0	1.0	0.6
Before CFAV	40.7	40.5	44.4	45.2	44.4
End CFAV	54.7	60.3	66.3	68.2	73.0
ΔPaco$_2$	13.9	19.8	21.9	23.2	28.7

carina (Table 16.1). In every patient, each procedure was performed for 10 minutes with an interval of PaCO$_2$ maintained at 40–45 mmHg with intermittent positive pressure breathing for 30 minutes between them. The authors confirmed the findings of other workers that CFAV was most effective in CO$_2$ elimination when O$_2$ was insufflated into both bronchi at high flow rates.

CFAV has been used in patients during internal mammary artery harvest for coronary artery bypass. Watson et al. called this continuous endobronchial insufflation of O$_2$ (19). Lung inflation with conventional mechanical ventilation (CMV) impairs the surgical access. They (19) studied seven patients undergoing internal mammary artery harvest. Endobronchial insufflation of O$_2$ was used following medium sternotomy (and opening of the pericardium). Two 2-mm internal diameter catheters were inserted 3 cm into each mainstem bronchus using a bronchoscope. Total flow of humidified O$_2$ was 45 L/minute (half going into each lung). All patients received at least 20 minutes of O$_2$ insufflation. Adequate oxygenation occurred in all patients. An average rise in PaCO$_2$ of 5 mmHg occurred between 5 and 20 minutes (0.3 mmHg/minute) and an average of 19 mmHg from PaCO$_2$ values on CMV. PaO$_2$ was never <129 mmHg and PaCO$_2$ never >65 mmHg. Surgical time was reduced from 23 minutes on CMV to 17 minutes with the endobronchial insufflation of O$_2$. In all patients, the surgeon's access to internal mammary artery harvest was improved in the endobronchial insufflation of O$_2$ group.

Gas transport during CFAV may be related to convective gas movement, cardiogenic oscillation effects, and molecular diffusion. Experimental evidence shows that cardiogenic oscillation and collateral airways both play a role in gas exchange with CFAV. Because of the high flow rates used during CFAV, the directional streaming probably takes place in the area closest to the insufflation jet. Gas enters and leaves the same airway spontaneously. The jet of insufflating gas generates turbulence below the tips of the catheters and the turbulent diffusivity may be part of the gas-transport mechanism. Therefore, the higher the flow of insufflated gas, the further into the periphery of the lungs this turbulence will extend. This may explain, in part, why human patients subjected to CFAV retain CO_2 and dogs do not. The flow used in dogs was 1 L/kg/minute, whereas such a high flow rate was thought to be dangerous in humans and only 0.6–0.7 L/kg/minute was used by Babinski et al. (15).

OTHER TECHNIQUES OF INTRATRACHEAL GAS INSUFFLATION

The effect of tracheal gas insufflation on gas exchange in canine oleic acid-induced lung injury was studied by Nahum et al. (20). They studied paralyzed anesthetized dogs using an intratracheal catheter introduced through one of the lumens of the modified endotracheal tube positioned 1 cm above the carina. With constant end-expiratory lung volume and tidal volume, tracheal gas insufflation did not affect oxygenation.

Larsson (21) described a simple method for improving O_2 removal without increasing airway pressure by eliminating apparatus dead space. In six intravenously anesthetized pigs, gas was insufflated through one lumen of a tracheal double lumen tube allowing expiration through the other during mechanical ventilation. During the mechanical ventilation, additional gas flow of 0.3 L/kg/minute was delivered by the inspiratory lumen during the expiratory phase. This technique resulted in an 18% decrease in $PaCO_2$.

Kolobow et al. (22) described a new pulmonary ventilatory mode called *intratracheal pulmonary ventilation*. A continuous flow of air and oxygen was introduced through a small catheter, the tip of which was positioned at the carina. They mounted a Venturi device on the tip of the catheter (reversed thrust catheter [RTC]) that avoids back pressure and facilitates expiration. In experiments in healthy anesthetized sheep, the intratracheal pulmonary ventilation system with the RTC maintained end-expiratory pressure of the level carina at near zero centimeters of water. The system also reduced tidal volumes by one half at their lowest respiratory rates (respiratory rates from 10 to 120/minute) with a proportional decrease in peak inspiratory pressure. The authors felt that this system with the venturi was advantageous because of the resulting low or zero intratracheal pressure.

Clinical

Constant flow insufflation (CFI) has been used to prevent arterial oxygen desaturation during endotracheal suctioning. Brochard et al. (23) administered CFI to seven patients ventilated for acute respiratory failure. The CFI was administered by a modified endotracheal tube in which small capillaries allowed high velocity jet flow delivery near the tracheal tube end during disconnection from the ventilator. In comparison to apnea alone, CFI prevented a fall in arterial oxygen tension, 16 ± 7 mmHg during CFI versus 117 ± 27 mmHg, during apnea after 90 seconds of disconnection from the ventilator. However, hypercapnia was not reduced. In the second part of the study, CFI was used to prevent arterial oxygen desaturation during endotracheal suctioning. In seven other patients, who were sedated and not paralyzed, endotracheal tube suctioning was performed with or without administration of CFI. In five of the seven patients oxygen desaturation was fully prevented when CFI was used. In all patients, during suctioning when CFI was not used, oxygen desaturation occurred. ($-15.6\% \pm 2.6\%$) In the two remaining patients desaturation was much lower and recovery time was much shorter when CFI was used. Assessment of lung volume by computed tomography scanning in five patients demonstrated that CFI prevented the 27% fall in lung volume induced by tracheal suctioning. The authors proposed that this be a simple method to avoid or minimize arterial oxygen desaturation during disconnection from the ventilator during endotracheal suctioning in severely hypoxemic patients ventilated for acute respiratory failure.

Tracheal gas insufflation was used to decrease dead space and to increase CO_2 clearance during mechanical ventilation (24). Six patients with ARDS meeting extracorporeal membrane oxygenation criteria were studied. All were hypoxemic and hypercapnic on optimal pressure control ventilation; 4 L of O_2 was insufflated continuously via an intratracheal catheter. $PaCO_2$ decreased from 118 ± 32 to 84 ± 26 mmHg. No significant change in $PaCO_2$ or airway pressure was seen. This paper is accompanied by an editorial in which the implications of the study (25) are discussed.

Intermittent-flow expiratory ventilation (intermittent flow expiratory ventilation) is one of the latest developments in limited-excursion pulmonary ventilation (26). The method involves the delivery of fresh gas to the respiratory tree during expiration, thereby flushing out the anatomic dead space and ensuring the gas initially delivered to the alveolus with the succeeding inspiration can participate in gas exchange. By eliminating end tidal gas in the conducting air passages, series dead space is functionally reduced, permitting lowering of the tidal volume and air pressures without the corresponding reduction in CO_2 removal. This effect may benefit patients who have acute lung injury by permitting ventilator settings with lower tidal volumes and peak airway pressure. The intermittent flow expiratory ventilation delivery technique, a successful clinical application, and possible ways to improve intermittent flow expiratory ventilation efficiency are described.

A case report concerning intermittent flow expiratory ventilation use in a patient with acute respiratory distress syndrome (ARDS)(27) describes a 20-year-old woman who developed ARDS following toxic shock syndrome. Her condition gradually deteriorated with escalating barotrauma. Intermittent flow expiratory ventilation allowed sufficient gas exchange without causing barotrauma and the

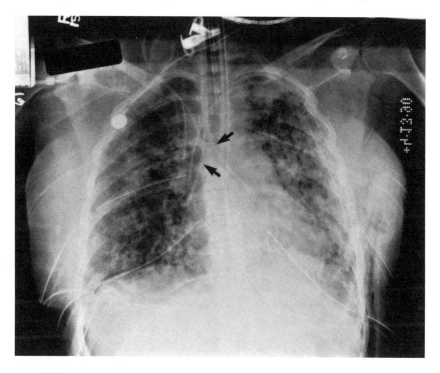

Figure 16.7. The *arrows* show the position of the endobronchial catheters.

patient, who was not expected to survive, eventually left the hospital in good condition. Figure 16.7 shows the endobronchial catheters in place.

SUMMARY

A number of questions must be answered before CFAV can have clinical applicability. Although the optimal catheter position has been found in dogs, it has not been found in humans. The need to reduce the flow because of the barotrauma risk may be resolved by finding the optimal catheter position, size, and gas exit velocity. At present, catheter placement requires fiberoptic bronchoscopy— a cumbersome and time-consuming process. A better catheter design that allows placement without bronchoscopy needs to be developed. In addition, what constitutes an ideal gas mixture and the possible role of nitrogen need further clarification.

The clinical role of other tracheal gas insufflation techniques is still not clear.

The reduction or elimination of apparatus dead space is valuable in many situations during controlled mechanical ventilation.

References

1. Comroe Jr JH, Dripps RD. Artificial respiration. JAMA 130:381–383, 1946.
2. Eger EI, Severinghaus JW. The rate of rise of $PaCO_2$ in the apneic anesthetized patient. Anesthesiology 22:419–425, 1961.
3. Heller ML, Watson TR Jr, Imredy DS. Apneic oxygenation in man: polarographic arterial oxygen tension study. Anesthesiology 25:25–30, 1964.
4. Frumin MJ, Epstein RM, Cohen G. Apneic oxygenation in man. Anesthesiology 20:789–798, 1959.
5. Jacoby JJ, Reed JP, Hamelbert W, et al. Simple method of artificial respiration. Am J Physiol 167:798–799, 1951.
6. Slutsky AS, Watson J, Leith DE, Brown R. Tracheal insufflation of O_2 (TRIO) at low flow rates sustains life for several hours. Anesthesiology 63:278–86, 1985.
7. Gattinoni L, Pesenti A, Mascheroni D, et al. Low-frequency positive-pressure ventilation with extracorporeal CO_2 removal in severe acute respiratory failure. JAMA 256:881–910, 1986.
8. Lehnert BE, Oberdorster G, Slutsky AS. Constant flow ventilation of apneic dogs. J Appl Physiol 53:483–489, 1982.
9. Smith RB, Babinski M, Bunegin L, et al. Continuous flow apneic ventilation. Acta Anaesth Scand 28:631–639, 1984.
10. Bunegin L, Bell GC, Gelineau J, et al. Continuous flow apneic ventilation with small endobronchial catheters. Acta Anaesthesiol Scand 32:603–606, 1988.
11. Babinski MF, Smith RB, Bunegin L, Goldberg I. Effect of nitrogen on carbon dioxide elimination during continuous flow apneic ventilation in dogs. Acta Anaesthesiol Scand 30:357–360, 1986.
12. Babinski MF, Smith RB, Bunegin L. Continuous flow apneic ventilation during thoracotomy. Anesthesiology 65:399–404, 1986.
13. Mackenzie CF, Barnas GM, Smalley J, Moorman R, Baptiste J. Low-flow endobronchial insufflation with air for 2 hours of apnea provides ventilation adequate for survival. Anesth Analg 71: 279–84, 1990.
14. Hachenberg T, Meyer J, Sielenkamper A, Knichwitz G, Haberecht H, Gülker H, Wendt M. Constant-flow ventilation during experimental left ventricular failure. Acta Anaesthesiol Scand 34:206–211, 1990.
15. Hachenberg T, Wendt M, Meyer J, Struckmeier O, Lawin P. Constant-flow ventilation in canine experimental pulmonary emphysema. Acta Anaesthesiol Scand 33:416–421, 1989.
16. Babinski MF, Sierra OG, Smith RB, et al. Clinical application of continuous flow apneic ventilation. Acta Anaesthesiol Scand 29:750–752, 1985.
17. Breen PH, Sznajder JF, Morrison P, et al. Constant flow ventilation in anesthetized patients: efficacy and safety. Anesth Analg 65:1161–1169, 1986.
18. Ebata T, Tsuchiya K, Tsuchida Y, et al. Constant flow ventilation in brain dead patients. Abstracts 9th World Congress of Anaesthesiologists, Vol. II, 1988, p AO945.
19. Watson R, Szarko R, Sequeira A, Mackenzie CF, Mark L. Continuous endobronchial insufflation during median sternotomy. Anesthesiology 73:3A, 1990.
20. Nahum A, Chandra A, Niknam J, Ravenscraft SA, Adams AB, Marini JJ. Effect of tracheal gas insufflation on gas exchange in canine oleic acid-induced lung injury. Crit Care Med 23(2): 348–356, 1995.
21. Larsson A. Elimination of apparatus dead space—a simple method for improving CO_2 removal without increasing airway pressure. Acta Anaesthesiol Scand 36:796–799, 1992.

22. Kolobow T, Powers T, Mandava S, Aprigliano M, Kawaguchi A, Tsuno K, Mueller E. Intratracheal pulmonary ventilation (intratracheal pulmonary ventilation): control of positive end-expiratory pressure at the level of the carina through the use of a novel intratracheal pulmonary ventilation catheter design. Anesth Analg 78:455–461, 1994.
23. Brochard L, Mion G, Isabey D, Bertrand C, Messadi AA, Mancebo J, Boussignac G, Vasile N, Lemaire F, Harf A. Constant-flow insufflation prevents arterial oxygen desaturation during endotracheal suctioning.
24. Belghith M, Fierobe L, Brunet F, Monchi M, Mira JP. Is tracheal gas insufflation an alternative to extrapulmonary gas exchangers in severe ARDS? Chest 107:1416–1419, 1995.
25. Kirby RR. Primum non nocere. Chest 107:1186–1187, 1995.
26. Gilbert J, Larsson A, Smith RB, Bunegin L. Intermittent-flow expiratory ventilation (IFEV): delivery technique and principles of action—a preliminary communication. Biomedical Instrumentation & Technology 25:451–456, 1991.
27. Gilbert J, Bunegin L, Larsson A, Smith RB, Erian R, Solomon D, Rogers J, Otte W. Intermittent flow expiratory ventilation: new technique of limited excursion pulmonary ventilation. Crit Care Med 19:1086–1089, 1991.

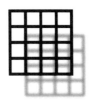

17
High Frequency Ventilation
Jean-Jacques Rouby

There are three different types of high frequency ventilation (HFV): high frequency oscillation (HFO); high frequency positive pressure ventilation (HFPPV); and high frequency jet ventilation (HFJV). HFO has been extensively studied by physiologists, but it remains an experimental method of mechanical ventilation. Until now, only HFPPV and HFJV have received defined clinical applications and occupy a specific place in the wide range of ventilatory support techniques available for anesthesia and critical care. When compared with conventional techniques, their main advantages lie in the fact that they enable adequate gas exchange using small tidal volumes close to the patient's dead-space volume. In the anesthetized patient, this enables a reduction of movements in the operating field and facilitates surgical working conditions. In the critically ill, this enables reduction in peak airway pressure and in the deleterious hemodynamic effects resulting from the increase in intrathoracic pressure. As long as certain technical conditions are respected, such as adequate warming and humidification of the gas mixture delivered to the patient, then HFPPV and HFJV offer attractive alternatives to conventional ventilation in a limited number of indications.

TECHNICAL ASPECTS

HFPPV and HFJV, which are very similar, deliver small tidal volumes (V_Ts between 1 and 5 ml·kg^{-1}) at high frequencies (between 60 and 400·min^{-1}) and require a specific ventilator characterized by a reduced internal volume and noncompliant ventilatory circuits. The use of a conventional ventilator to provide HFV invariably results in an insufficient V_T delivered to the patient because of the gas compression within the internal volume of the ventilator. In HFPPV, a technique developed by Sjöstrand in Sweden in the mid-1970s, a pneumatic valve interrupts a gas flow of air and oxygen supplied to the ventilator at a constant driving pressure. Inspired gases are delivered to the patient through conventional connectors attached to the endotracheal tube and expiration passively occurs through an expiratory valve. V_T decreases with respiratory frequency and increases with inspiratory-to-expiratory ratio (I/E) and is equal to the volume delivered by

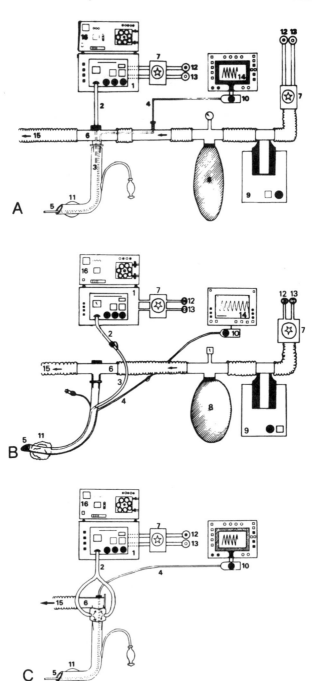

the ventilator (there is no entrainment). Respiratory frequencies ranging from 60–100 breaths·min^{-1} and V$_T$s between 1.5 and 5 ml·kg^{-1} can be used. HFJV, a technique developed by Klain and Smith in the United States in the early 1980s, differs from HFPPV in two aspects: first, the driving pressure of gases is higher and can be modulated; and second, inspired gases are delivered to the patient through different injection systems that produce gas entrainment. Because HFJV is much more widely used than HFPPV, the HFJV system will be described in detail.

Circuit for High Frequency Jet Ventilation

As shown in Figure 17.1, air and oxygen are supplied to the jet ventilator under a high pressure ($\approx$4 atmospheres) and are mixed in a blender where there is a pressure drop of about 1 atmosphere. Therefore, the driving pressure of gases arriving at the jet ventilator is ~3 atmospheres. Gases are then pulsed either by a pneumatic valve or by an electronically controlled solenoid valve in a non-compliant connecting tube fixed to the injection system. There is a 0.5-atmosphere pressure loss within the ventilatory circuits and, therefore, the operating pressure in the connecting tube is ~2.5 atmospheres. Inside the ventilator, there is a second-stage pressure regulator that enables smooth control of driving pressure and, consequently, of operating pressure, from its maximal value to zero. Because most of the injection systems accelerate gases and produce gas entrainment, the V$_T$ delivered to the patient is equal to the jet gas volume delivered by the ventilator (V$_{jet}$) plus the entrained volume (E):

$$V_T \text{ (ml)} = V_{(jet)} + E$$

Therefore, most of the HFJV circuits include an open circuit that provides warmed and humidified gases for entrainment. This additional circuit connected to the injection system via a three-way swivel adapter should be able to deliver a maximal flow of 30 L·min^{-1} at the same F$_I$O$_2$ as the gases delivered by the ventilator. Finally, a safe jet ventilator should have various capabilities, such as:

1. Provide a range of respiratory frequencies between 0 and 400·min^{-1};
2. Enable changes in I/E ratio independent of respiratory frequency;

◄───

Figure 17.1. A. Injection system using an injection cannula. **B.** Injection system using the jetting channel of a special endotracheal tube. **C.** Injection system not associated with gas entrainment. *1*= jet ventilator; *2* = connecting tube; *3* = injection system; *4* = intratracheal catheter; *5* = endotracheal or tracheostomy tube; *6* = three-way swivel adapter; *7* = blender; *8* = balloon reservoir; *9* = conventional humidifier; *10* = pressure transducer; *11* = cuff; *12* = oxygen supply; *13* = air supply; *14* = airway pressure monitoring; *15* = open expiratory line; *16* = jet humidifier.

3. Display the minute ventilation, the jet gas volume delivered by the ventilator, and the operating pressure;
4. Include a system for monitoring mean airway pressure;
5. Include low- and high-pressure alarm systems.

Humidification and Warming of Gases Delivered to the Patient

If HFJV is to be administered to a patient for >2 hours, then adequate warming and humidification of the gas mixture is critical. Some of the failures attributed to HFJV itself are, in fact, failures in the humidification system. The first rule is to avoid "homemade systems" and to recognize the complexity of the problem. The most difficult problem is to provide adequate warming of the gases. Along the injection system, there is a marked reduction in pressure; operating pressure is between 1 and 2.5 atmospheres, whereas mean airway pressure is just a few centimeters H_2O. This pressure drop results in a marked gas cooling within the trachea. Therefore, the temperature of gases within the connecting tube has to be >60°C in order to reach a temperature of 37°C within the trachea. In fact, the only way to achieve adequate warming and humidification of the gases during HFJV is to use a hot vaporizer. A continuous infusion rate of distilled water is vaporized at 100°C and delivered to the connecting tube during each expiratory phase. Electrical resistances embedded in the connecting tube wall avoid gas cooling and condensation so that gas temperature at the entry of the injection system remains >60°C. As during conventional ventilation, 44 mg H_2O must be added to each liter of dry gas delivered by the ventilator to reach 100% relative humidity. The quantity of water ($\dot{Q}_{H_2O}$ in ml/hour) that should be provided to the vaporizer depends on the minute ventilation delivered by the ventilator ($\dot{V}$ in L/minute) (1):

$$\dot{Q}_{H_2O} \text{ (ml/hour)} = 2.64 \ \dot{V}$$

Consequently, any changes in ventilatory settings should be associated with a corresponding change in the rate of humidification. Warming and humidification of the additional gases are achieved by a conventional humidifier. Most of the jet ventilators commercially available are not equipped for adequate warming and humidification of the gases delivered to the patient. The Acutronic ventilator (Acutronic Medical Systems AG, Kreuzstrasse 100 CH-8645 Jona-Rapperswil, Switzerland) is equipped with a particularly reliable and efficient heater and humidifier that has been proved clinically safe for long-term HFJV.

Different Methods of Injection

INJECTION SYSTEMS USING INJECTOR CANNULAS

This type of injection uses short injector cannulas, 4–5 cm in length, with varying internal diameters. As shown in Figure. 17.1*A*, a rigid (metallic) injector cannula can be inserted into a three-way swivel adapter fixed to the tracheostomy or to the endotracheal tube. A semirigid, specially constructed injector cannula can also be inserted percutaneously into the trachea under local anesthesia. This injection system, which is used for laryngeal and vocal cord surgery and in emergency situations when endotracheal intubation is impossible, requires complete permeability of the upper airways and solid fixation to avoid accidental displacement. When decreasing the internal diameter of the injection cannula, the V_T and the HFJV-induced PEEP effect decrease, reducing CO_2 elimination and mean airway pressure (2).

INJECTION SYSTEMS USING A SPECIAL JET ENDOTRACHEAL TUBE

This type of injection requires the presence of a Hi-Lo Jet Endotracheal Tube (NCC, Division Mallinckrodt, Argyle, USA) characterized by two additional channels (Fig. 17.1*B*): the jet insufflation channel, ending 6 cm before the distal tip of the endotracheal tube and the airway pressure-monitoring channel. This type of injection is one of the most convenient for providing HFJV. The connection between the ventilator and the jet insufflation channel is supple, permitting movements of the patient's head. Suctioning without interrupting HFJV is possible, rendering this dangerous maneuver particularly safe in hypoxemic patients. The distal site of injection close to the carina has two important consequences: first, the anatomic dead space is reduced; and second, gas entrainment decreases, representing only 25% of V_T. When compared with injection systems using injector cannulas, this type of injection tends to decrease V_T and "PEEP effect" while maintaining the same level of CO_2 elimination (2).

INJECTION SYSTEMS USING INTRATRACHEAL AND INTRABRONCHIAL CATHETERS

This type of injection, which requires small internal diameter catheters positioned within the tracheobronchial tree, is used for laryngeal surgery, bronchoscopies, and laryngoscopies, as well as tracheal and bronchial surgery. The catheter can be positioned either using oral or nasal approaches, or via a percutaneous transtracheal route. It can also be passed through a conventional endotracheal tube or solidly affixed to a flexible fiberoptic bronchoscope. When using a rigid bronchoscope, a special additional metallic channel fixed on the external wall is used for injection (3). Because the length (>30 cm) and the small internal diameter (<2 mm) of these catheters markedly increase resistance to gas flow, a high driving pressure (>3 atmospheres) is most often necessary to deliver an adequate V_T to the patient.

INJECTION SYSTEMS SUPPRESSING GAS ENTRAINMENT

As shown in Figure 17.1 *C,* this type of injection requires a specially constructed intermediary piece characterized by two orifices facing each other, by which means the injection is performed. Absence of entrainment markedly simplifies the minute ventilation monitoring because the V_T is equal to the jet gas volume, which is generally displayed on the front panel of the ventilator. This type of injection is frequently used when HFJV is combined with conventional ventilation.

EFFECTS ON LUNG VOLUME AND PRESSURES—MEAN AIRWAY PRESSURE MONITORING

It is important to keep in mind that HFV is a positive pressure ventilation. Because of expiratory flow limitation, all types of HFV induce a PEEP effect whose intensity depends on factors related to the ventilatory settings and to the patient him- or herself. As shown in Figure 17.2, HFJV increases functional residual capacity (FRC) and mean lung volume (around which the lungs oscillate). The PEEP effect increases with I/E ratio, driving pressure, and, to a lesser degree, with respiratory frequency (4). At fixed ventilatory settings, the higher the respiratory compliance, the greater the PEEP effect. In other words, patients with normal or elevated respiratory compliance can be markedly overdistended by using inadequate ventilatory settings—I/E ratio >0.43 and driving pressures >2 bars—whereas patients with acute respiratory failure and reduced respiratory compliance can benefit from the PEEP effect (5).

Is there a simple respiratory parameter to monitor that accurately reflects the PEEP effect? If the case is negative, then HFV would certainly appear as an unpredictable and unsafe technique. Lung volume changes cannot be easily monitored in clinical practice. Mean airway pressure, which is the pressure corresponding to the mean lung volume above apneic FRC, is easy to measure. During HFPPV and HFJV, it has been shown that mean airway pressure is a good reflection of mean alveolar pressure (Fig. 17.3). In other words, there is no gradient between the pressure measured in the upper airways and in the distal airways (5,6), so that the HFJV-induced increase in mean lung volume can be inferred from mean airway pressure according to the static respiratory compliance. Consequently, the continuous monitoring of mean airway pressure appears mandatory when high driving pressures or elevated I/E ratios are used. Unfortunately, this does not apply to HFO. Because the expiratory phase is active, some distal bronchi collapse during expiration, creating a pressure gradient between proximal and

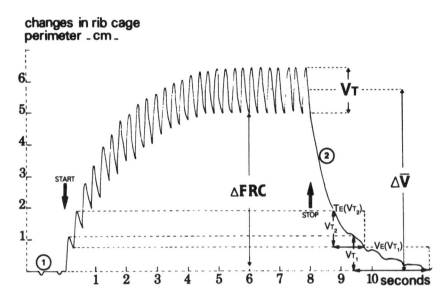

Figure 17.2. Recording of changes in rib cage perimeter—equivalent to changes in lung volume—induced during a short period of HFJV in an anesthetized patient. *Left* and *right arrows* indicate the starting and finishing times of HFJV. Ventilatory settings used are frequency 200·min⁻¹, I/E ratio 0.43, and driving pressure 2.2 atm. ΔFRC = increase in functional residual capacity; $\Delta\bar{V}$ = mean pulmonary volume above apneic functional residual capacity; V_T = tidal volume; V_{T1} = first V_T; V_{T2} = second V_T; T_E (V_{T1}) $T_E(V_{T1})$ = spontaneous relaxation time of V_{T1}; T_E (V_{T2}) = spontaneous relaxation time of V_{T2} ① baseline corresponding to apneic functional residual capacity (with cardiac artifacts); ② passive exhalation curve with cardiac artifacts in its inferior section. (Reprinted with permission from Rouby JJ, Simonneau G, Benhamou D, et al. Factors influencing pulmonary volumes and CO_2 elimination during high-frequency jet ventilation. Anesthesiology 63:473–482, 1985.)

distal airways, and, consequently, mean airway pressure no longer reflects mean alveolar pressure. Finally, the monitoring of mean airway pressure is one of the principal elements of safety during HFPPV and HFJV. To avoid an artifact of negative pressure due to gas entrainment, airway pressure should be measured in the trachea at least 5 cm below the injection site. In patients with normal lungs, mean airway pressure should never exceed 5 cmH₂O. In patients with acute respiratory failure, there is a strong relationship between the increase in mean airway pressure and improvement in arterial oxygenation (4). The addition of a PEEP valve on the expiratory circuit is not necessary and contributes to a decrease in alveolar ventilation (7).

What are the mechanisms of CO_2 elimination during HFV? In patients with normal respiratory function, normocapnia is obtained with V_Ts of 2 ml·kg⁻¹

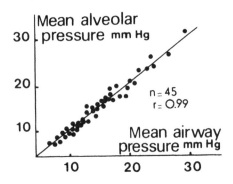

Figure 17.3. Relationship between mean alveolar pressure and mean airway pressure in 15 critically ill patients with acute respiratory failure ventilated with HFJV. Changes in airway pressure are induced by increasing I/E ratio. For each patient, three different I/E ratios are used: 0.25, 0.43, and 0.67. The *dark line* is the identity line. (Reprinted with permission from Rouby JJ, Fusciardi J, Bourgain JL, et al. High-frequency jet ventilation in postoperative respiratory failure: determinants of oxygenation. Anesthesiology 59:281–287, 1983.)

(i.e., V_T close to dead-space volume). This clearly suggests that mechanisms other than convection (e.g., augmented dispersion and pendelluft) play a role in gas transport during HFV. In contrast, in patients with diseased lungs, normocapnia requires higher V_Ts, around 3 ml·kg^{-1}, probably because acute respiratory failure is frequently associated with increased physiologic dead space.

Factors influencing the different components of V_T are well known (6). The jet gas volume delivered by the ventilator increases with I/E ratio and driving pressure and decreases with respiratory frequency. Entrainment increases with driving pressure and decreases with I/E ratio and frequency. When the injection system produces gas entrainment, V_T increases with driving pressure, decreases with respiratory frequency, and does not change with I/E ratio (Fig. 17.4). When the injection system is not associated with gas entrainment, V_T is equal to the jet gas volume delivered by the ventilator.

CLINICAL INDICATIONS OF HIGH FREQUENCY POSITIVE PRESSURE VENTILATION AND HIGH FREQUENCY JET VENTILATION

HFPPV and HFJV have been used in almost all types of surgery and acute respiratory failures with no apparent decisive advantage. However, in a limited number of indications, their superiority over conventional ventilation methods has been clearly established (8).

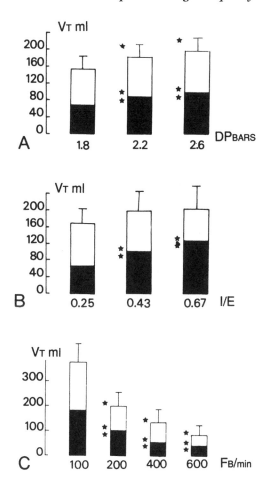

Figure 17.4. Effect of increasing driving pressure (DP), inspiratory/expiratory (I/E) ratio, and frequency (F) on tidal volume (V_T), jet gas volume delivered by the ventilator (■), and entrainment (□) in 15 critically ill patients under HFJV using an injector cannula fixed to the proximal tip of the endotracheal tube (mean ± SD, * $P < 0.05$ compared with control value). (Reprinted with permission from Rouby JJ, Simmoneau G, Benhamou D, et al. Factors influencing volumes and CO_2 elimination during high-frequency jet ventilation. Anesthesiology 63 : 473–482, 1985.)

Indications in Anesthesia

Situations in which HFV enables patients to be ventilated by means of small-diameter injection systems. Ear, nose, and throat surgery, bronchoscopies, laryngoscopies, and laser surgery can be performed without tracheal intubation, using either a percutaneous transtracheal injector cannula or an additional jetting channel fixed to the fiberoptic bronchoscope. Upper airway surgery (e.g., tracheal reconstruction or bronchial resection) can be performed using catheters passed through the endotracheal tube (9). Mean airway pressure measurement is not possible; CO_2 elimination can be monitored using transcutaneous PCO_2.

Surgical resection of aneurisms involving the thoracic descending aorta and requiring a left thoracic incision with retraction and collapse of the left lung. To avoid life-threatening intraoperative deterioration of arterial oxygenation, continuous positive airway pressure (CPAP) administration to the left lung through the left channel of the Carlens tube is generally recommended. However, this type of one-lung ventilation is not always effective in avoiding severe hypoxemia. HFJV applied to the left lung, while conventional ventilation is maintained on the right lung, appears much more efficient in terms of gas exchange. In fact, HFJV enables collapsed alveoli to be recruited rapidly, whereas CPAP-induced alveolar recruitment is slower and passive. To avoid left lung overdistension, which could alter surgical working conditions, mean airway pressure should not exceed 10 cmH_2O.

Situations in which movements of the operating field can be suppressed by HFV. In vocal cord surgery (10), use of a percutaneous transtracheal injector cannula and selection of adequate ventilatory settings, keeps the operating field completely free and keeps the vocal cords immobile, thus providing ideal surgical working conditions for microsurgery.

During lithotripsy, the use of HFJV during extracorporeal shock-wave lithotripsy dramatically minimizes stone movement, reduces the number and intensity of the required shock waves, and enables the use of fewer electrodes. Single-breath measurement of end-tidal PCO_2 provides a satisfactory monitor for CO_2 elimination in partially submerged patients.

Indications in Critical Care

Emergency situations during which tracheal intubation is impossible. The insertion of a transtracheal injector cannula is life-saving for the patient. It must be emphasized that minimal permeability of the upper airways should persist to avoid pulmonary overdistension.

Acute respiratory failure with circulatory shock. HFV represents an interesting alternative to conventional ventilation with PEEP in patients with acute respiratory failure and circulatory shock: arterial pressure and cardiac output are found to be higher in HFV conditions when both techniques are compared at the same level of mean airway pressure and alveolar ventilation (11). HFV appears to respect regulatory mechanisms of arterial pressure better, possibly because of less stimulating pulmonary stretch receptors that normally alter the efficiency of baroreflex regulation of arterial pressure.

Acute ventricular failure. The administration of small V_Ts at high frequencies provides the possibility of increasing intrathoracic pressure selectively during systole by synchronizing HFV on the ECG. In cardiac patients with low cardiac output, synchronous HFJV markedly improves cardiac index and left ventricular function, when compared with intermittent positive pressure ventilation (12). This beneficial effect results from a decrease in left ventricular afterload produced by the elevation of intrathoracic pressure during left ventricular ejection.

Bronchopleural fistulae with large air leak flows. HFV is indicated in the presence of a massive bronchopleural fistula, when conventional ventilation fails to provide adequate gas exchange. It must always be kept in mind that mean airway pressure is the main determinant for both arterial oxygenation and air leak flow. When a large bronchopleural fistula complicates an acute pulmonary disease, severe hypoxemia with CO_2 retention occurs during conventional ventilation because the major part of the V_T is lost through the bronchopleural fistula and because a PEEP cannot be maintained throughout expiration. During HFV, the short expiratory time prevents the lungs from returning to their resting FRC between each ventilatory cycle, thus facilitating alveolar recruitment and increasing mean airway pressure. At this stage, the price to pay for the improvement in gas exchange is an increase in air leak flow. Subsequently, and only if parenchymal pulmonary lesions regress with treatment, mean airway pressure can be diminished progressively, thus enabling a gradual decrease in air leak flow. When a large bronchopleural fistula complicates upper airway surgery in the absence of pulmonary lesions, HFV provides the possibility of using low mean airway pressure and, therefore, of decreasing air leak flow. It must be emphasized that the air leak flow can be decreased only when HFV can ensure adequate gas exchange at a mean airway pressure lower than that of conventional ventilation.

Tracheal lesions secondary to trauma, tracheostomy, or prolonged intubation. When a tracheal lesion complicating tracheostomy, prolonged intubation, or trauma has been surgically repaired and requires mechanical ventilation with a deflated cuff, HFV is superior to conventional ventilation in providing adequate gas exchange. HFV is particularly beneficial in the treatment of tracheal rupture, tracheomalacia, and tracheoesophageal fistula.

Severe acute respiratory failure with elevated peak airway pressure (>50 cmH_2O) and reduced respiratory compliance can benefit from a combination of HFV and conventional ventilation. This promising technique, although not yet evaluated in a large series of patients, can markedly improve arterial oxygenation without increasing airway pressures. A combination of eight V_Ts of 4 ml·kg^{-1} (using an inspiratory time $<10\%$ to avoid elevated peak airway pressure) with HFV markedly improves arterial oxygenation without surpassing a mean airway pressure of 10 cmH_2O. Because pulmonary barotrauma is directly influenced by the level of peak airway pressure within healthy regions of the diseased lung, this combined ventilation appears to be a safer ventilatory support method.

CONTRAINDICATIONS TO HIGH FREQUENCY VENTILATION

Because of the risk of pulmonary overdistension, HFV is contraindicated in the presence of chronic obstructive pulmonary disease and status asthmaticus. In unilateral lung disease, HFV applied to both lungs results in overdistension of the nondiseased lung, with deterioration of gas exchange and hemodynamic instability.

References

1. Doyle HJ, Napolitano AE, Lippman HR, et al. Different humidification systems for high-frequency jet ventilation. Crit Care Med 12:815–819, 1984.
2. Benhamou D, Ecoffey C, Rouby JJ, et al. High-frequency jet ventilation: the influence of different methods of injection on respiratory parameters. Br J Anaesth 59:1257–1264, 1987.
3. Vourc'h G, Fischler M, Michon F, et al. High-frequency jet ventilation vs. manual jet ventilation during bronchoscopy in patients with tracheo-bronchial stenosis. Br J Anesth 55:969–972, 1983.
4. Rouby JJ, Simonneau G, Benhamou D, et al. Factors influencing pulmonary volumes and CO_2 elimination during high-frequency jet ventilation. Anesthesiology 63:473–482, 1985.
5. Rouby JJ, Fusciardi J, Bourgain JL, et al. High-frequency jet ventilation in postoperative respiratory failure: determinants of oxygenation. Anesthesiology 59:281–287, 1983.
6. Perez Fontan JJ, Heldt GP, Gregory GA. Mean airway pressure and mean alveolar pressure during high-frequency jet ventilation in rabbits. J Appl Physiol 61:456–463, 1986.
7. Mal H, Rouby JJ, Benhamou D, et al. High-frequency jet ventilation in acute respiratory failure: which ventilatory settings? Br J Anaesth 58:18–23, 1986.
8. Rouby JJ, Viars P. Clinical use of high frequency ventilation. Acta Anaesthesiol Scand 33(Suppl. 90):134–139, 1989.
9. El-baz N, Jensik R, Faber LP, et al. One-lung high-frequency ventilation for tracheoplasty and bronchoplasty: a new technique. Ann Thorac Surg 34:564–571, 1982.
10. Klain M, Smith B. High-frequency percutaneous transtracheal jet ventilation. Crit Care Med 5: 280–287, 1977.
11. Fusciardi J, Rouby JJ, Barakat T, et al. Hemodynamic effects of high-frequency jet ventilation in patients with and without circulatory shock. Anesthesiology 65:485–491, 1986.
12. Pinsky MR, Marquez J, Martin D, et al. Ventricular assist by cardiac cycle-specific increases in intrathoracic pressures. Chest 91:709–715, 1987.

Suggested Readings

Borg U, Eriksson I, Sjostrand U. High-frequency positive-pressure ventilation (HFPPV): a review based upon its use during bronchoscopy and for laryngoscopy and microlaryngeal surgery under general anesthesia. Anesth Analg 59:594–603, 1980.

Drazen JM, Kamm RD, Slutsky AS. High-frequency ventilation. Physiol Rev 64:505–543, 1984.

Froese AB, Bryan C. High-frequency ventilation. Am Rev Respir Dis 135:1363–1374, 1987.

Sjöstrand U. High-frequency positive pressure ventilation (HFPPV): a review. Crit Care Med 8:345–364, 1980.

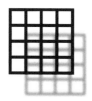

18
Extracorporeal Techniques to Support Ventilation

A. Pesenti • M. Bombino • R. Marcolin
• L. Gattinoni

"Buying time" for the diseased lung to recover has been the dream of extracorporeal respiratory support since its beginning back in the 1970s. The rationale for its use in acute respiratory failure is supported by increasing evidence that conventional mechanical ventilation with high pressure and volume damages the lung.

We briefly review the history of extracorporeal support in adult respiratory failure, focusing on the rationale, indications, and technical requirements of the extracorporeal techniques currently in use.

In 1967, adult respiratory distress syndrome (ARDS) was defined as a clinical entity characterized by severe hypoxemia, bilateral lung infiltrates, and low pulmonary compliance (1). Mechanical ventilation with a high fraction of inspired oxygen (F_IO_2) was required to achieve viable gas exchange. Oxygen toxicity was already a well-recognized problem prompting the introduction of positive end-expiratory pressure (PEEP) as a means to improve oxygenation by increasing functional residual capacity (FRC) and therefore foster a decrease in F_IO_2.

The main goal of extracorporeal support in acute respiratory failure was to maintain viable gas exchange with the lowest F_IO_2. During the last decade increasing evidence indicates that the high pressure and volumes associated with mechanical ventilation have deleterious effects on lung parenchyma. These findings suggested that extracorporeal support may be the only "ideal" substitute to effect pulmonary gas exchange (ventilation plus oxygenation).

EXTRACORPOREAL MEMBRANE OXYGENATION (ECMO)

Hill et al.'s report on the first successful use of ECMO in posttraumatic respiratory failure opened the era of extracorporeal support in adult patients. Following this report, many other centers adopted ECMO for severe respiratory failure unresponsive to conventional mechanical ventilation.

In 1975 the National Heart Lung and Blood Institute (NHLBI) funded a prospective, multicenter randomized trial to evaluate the efficacy of ECMO in the management of ARDS (2).

Inclusion Criteria

To select a population with an expected mortality rate as high as 50% a panel of experts established a set of blood gas values as entry criteria into the study (Table 18.1).

Extracorporeal Technique

CANNULATION AND CIRCUIT

The main rationale of the ECMO study was to provide the maximal oxygenation with the extracorporeal apparatus while decreasing the F_1O_2 requirements to the diseased lungs. The amount of oxygen provided by the extracorporeal device is directly dependent on extracorporeal blood flow. A high flow venoarterial bypass was therefore required.

Venous blood was drained mainly from the right atrium or the inferior vena cava and returned fully saturated to the arterial cannula. Proper positioning of the arterial cannula was a key point in providing oxygen to the coronary circulation; therefore, some centers preferred the use of aortic arch, descending thoracic aorta, or axillary artery cannula rather than femoral artery cannulation.

Venous blood was siphoned to a reservoir and delivered to an artificial lung by a roller nonocclusive pump. Both PVC and silicone rubber tubings were used. The pump chamber was made of extruded polyurethane or silicone. Four types of membrane lung (ML) were in use; gas transfer membranes were either silicone

Table 18.1. ECMO Entry Criteria

Fast entry
PaO_2 <50 mmHg at FIO_2 1.0
PEEP $\geq$5 cmH$_2$O
(three determinations 1 hour apart.)

Slow entry
PaO_2 <50 mmHg at FIO_2 0.6
PEEP $\geq$5 cmH$_2$O
   plus
Shunt fraction $\geq$30% at FIO_2 1.0
(Three determinations 6 hours apart after 48 hours of ICU.)

EMCO, extracorporal membrane oxygenation.

(Sci-Med, Lande-Edwards and Bramson) or a copolymer of silicone and polycarbonate (General Electric Lung) (2).

ANTICOAGULATION

At the time of cannulation a 100 U/kg heparin bolus was given, and the heparin infusion during ECMO was adjusted by frequent determination of the activated clotting time (ACT) to maintain an ACT at 180–200 seconds (2).

Clinical Management

Respiratory guidelines during ECMO were set to maintain a PaO_2 >55 mmHg with the minimum tolerable F_IO_2 ≤0.6. Failure to obtain this goal required the following steps:

- increase extracorporeal bypass flow ECMO flow to maximum
- increase respiratory rate (RR) and tidal volume (V_T)
- increase PEEP up to 15 cmH_2O
- increase plateau inspiratory pressure to 50 cmH_2O
- increase F_IO_2
- use sedation and paralysis
- produce hypothermia (32°C)

The reported clinical results showed that ECMO patients were maintained with lower F_IO_2 compared with control patients. This was accomplished by an extracorporeal blood flow of ~60%–80% of the cardiac output. Throughout the study ECMO patients were ventilated with a V_T of 650 ml on average, an RR about 14/minute, and a PEEP level of 7–12 cmH_2O that generated a peak airway pressure ~50 $cmH_2$0.

Termination of ECMO was considered when PaO_2 was consistently >70 mmHg with F_IO_2 0.6, PEEP 5 cmH_2O, and extracorporeal blood flow 0.5 L/minute. ECMO also could be stopped if there were irreversible central nervous system dysfunction, irreversible cardiac failure, a technical problem with ECMO, uncontrolled bleeding, or lack of evidence of improvement after 5 days on a bypass (2).

Complications

Mechanical failures of the ECMO equipment were reported in 38% of the cases treated. These ranged from pump chamber rupture to oxygenator blood leaks or thrombosis. In no patient did a technical problem cause ECMO termination. Bleeding was the major concern during ECMO. The average daily blood transfusion requirement was 3.6 L (0.6 L in the conventionally treated group). Hemorrhage was listed as the reason for ECMO termination in 16% of the bypass cases (2).

Results

Ninety patients were enrolled into the ECMO study: of the 48 randomized to conventional mechanical ventilation, four survived (8%); of the 42 randomized to receive ECMO plus mechanical ventilation, four survived (10%) (3). After the publication of these results the enthusiasm for the novel ECMO technique faded. Notwithstanding those rather disappointing survival figures, the ECMO study proved that technology was available and safe for long-term extracorporeal respiratory assistance.

EXTRACORPOREAL CO_2 REMOVAL ($ECCO_2R$)

In 1976 the ECMO study was approaching its end when Kolobow et al. (5) started a novel approach to extracorporeal support based on extracorporeal CO_2 removal and apneic oxygenation. The proposed new therapy was based on the different physiologic mechanisms governing O_2 uptake and CO_2 removal (4). Oxygenation is limited by hemoglobin saturation; therefore, it requires high blood flows. The high venous blood CO_2 content warrants its removal even at low blood flow provided an adequately high alveolar ventilation is maintained (Fig. 18.1).

Extracorporeal CO_2 removal ($ECCO_2R$) is based on a low-flow high-ventilation venovenous bypass. Oxygenation is accomplished by the natural lung through a flow of O_2 matching the oxygen consumed (apneic oxygenation; see Chapter 16, Continuous Flow Apneic Ventilation and Other Techniques of Intratracheal Gas Insufflation); lung rest is thus achieved.

Experimental studies, in both spontaneously or mechanically breathing animals, showed a progressive decrease in alveolar ventilation mirroring the increase in CO_2 removal by the artificial lung (Fig. 18.2) (5).

A common side effect of apneic oxygenation was a progressive FRC reduction with a corresponding decay in oxygenation. The introduction of 2–5 breaths/minute (low frequency positive pressure ventilation [LFPPV-$ECCO_2R$]) solved this problem (6). In 1979 this approach was introduced into clinical practice in Milan. After the first successful reports, other European and US centers started to use LFPPV-$ECCO_2R$ in cases of severe respiratory failure. We refer mainly to the data gathered by the Milan group, lacking a registry of all the $ECCO_2R$ cases.

Entry Criteria

At the beginning, we adopted the gas exchange criteria of the ECMO study (see Table 18.1) plus a total static lung compliance <30 ml/cmH$_2$0. Patient age

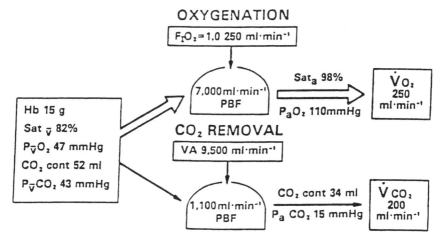

Figure 18.1. Dissociation of oxygenation and CO_2 removal. At normal mixed venous blood, the oxygenation requires normal pulmonary blood flow (PBF) and continuous O_2 supply equal to O_2 consumption (250 ml/minute in this example) without any ventilation. Removal of CO_2 can be accomplished at reduced PBF if matched with sufficiently high alveolar ventilation. (From Gattinoni et al. A new look at therapy of the adult respiratory distress syndrome: motionless lung. Int Anesthesiol Clin 21:98, 1983; with permission.)

and duration of the pulmonary insult did not represent a contraindication to the procedure (7). With time, the entry criteria changed. The ECMO criteria gave a "static" picture of gas exchange derangement in ARDS. PEEP response, positioning, and inhaled nitric oxide response might affect oxygenation and, therefore, they have to be taken into account before considering extracorporeal support.

Extracorporeal Technique

Extracorporeal assemblage is shown in Figure 18.3. Innovations have been introduced during the years regarding the extracorporeal cannulation technique, the use of heparinized microporous artificial lungs, and the use of centrifugal pumps.

CANNULATION

The technique used in our center to realize the venovenous bypass has evolved to make it simpler and to decrease the risk of bleeding. Until 1989 access to the bypass veins was performed at the bedside by a vascular surgeon. In the first

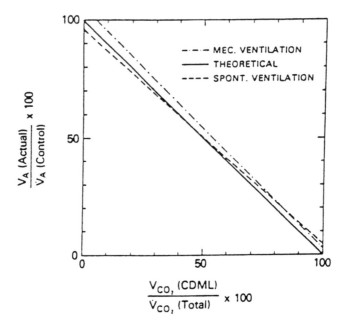

Figure 18.2. Alveolar ventilation (percent of control values) as function of extracorporeal CO_2 removal (percent of total CO_2 production (i.e., VCO_2 of carbon dioxide membrane lung [CDML] plus neutral lungs). The theoretical values are computed assuming $PaCO_2$ and total VCO_2 are constant throughout the procedure. (From Gattinoni et al. A new look at therapy of the adult respiratory distress syndrome: motionless lung. Int Anesthesiol Clin 21:101, 1983; with permission.)

patients treated, the vascular approach was femorojugular; four large catheters were inserted both proximally and distally.

Disadvantages of this kind of cannulation were an increased risk of bleeding and difficult nursing care. These factors prompted the introduction of a double lumen concentric catheter requiring single vein access through the common femoral vein. Distal drainage of the leg was also required. A major advance was the introduction of the saphenosaphenous vein access route. The bleeding risk was greatly reduced owing to the superficial wounds; no need for distal drainage cannulation simplified the technique. A simple ligation of the saphenous veins was performed at the end of bypass. Heparin could be immediately stopped because vein repair was no longer required.

In 1988 the percutaneous cannulation technique was introduced to provide vascular access for $ECCO_2R$. The most common approach in our patients is femorofemoral. Percutaneous cannulation has been a major advance in extracorporeal support technique because bleeding from cannulation sites has been almost eliminated (8).

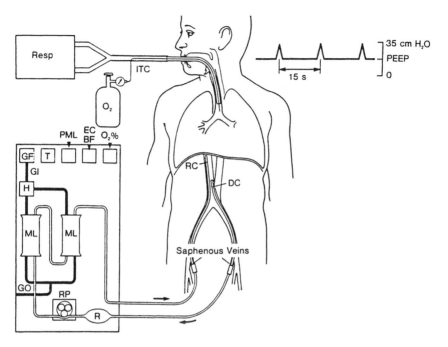

Figure 18.3. Cannulation and perfusion circuit. *DC,* blood drainage catheter; *ECBF,* extracorporeal blood flow; *GF,* gas flow monitor; *GI,* gas inlet; *GO,* gas outlet; *H,* humidifier; *ITC,* intratracheal catheter; *ML,* membrane lung; $O_2\%$, venous drainage blood oxygen monitor; *PML,* membrane lung pressure, in-out; *R,* venous reservoir; *RC,* blood return catheter; *Resp,* respirator; *RP,* roller pump; *PEEP,* positive end-expiratory pressure; *T,* ambient temperature control. (From Gattinoni et al. Low frequency positive-pressure ventilation with extracorporeal CO_2 removal in severe acute respiratory failure. JAMA 256:882, 1986; with permission.)

ARTIFICIAL LUNGS

The Silicone Spiral Coil (Sci-Med) membrane lung showed great safety and good performance in long-term bypasses. Subsequently, heparinized devices were introduced, mainly to decrease the risk of bleeding during major surgery on bypass (9). We now use this heparinized cannula as our first choice. The major disadvantage of this device was plasma leakage, leading to frequent oxygenator changes. Lately a new device (Maxima Plus PRF Oxygenator), characterized by smaller pores, was developed. This new model has performed well with no plasma leakage up to 21 days (10).

EXTRACORPOREAL PUMPS

To date, most of the long-term extracorporeal treatments, both in adults and in newborns, have been performed using a roller pump. With the availability of heparinized lungs, some centers switched to centrifugal pumps, which are available with a heparinized surface (Biomedicus) and do not need a reservoir bag. Monitoring the pressure at the pump head inlet is essential to prevent venous blood degassing and bubble formation. Pressure changes in the venous line will occur whenever the drainage line is occluded or the suction is dangerously high.

Hemolysis, which in our experience was never a problem with the use of the roller pump, is a major disadvantage of centrifugal pumps. Hemolysis is related to deposition of small clots in low-flow zones (mainly around the rotor shaft). Close monitoring of laboratory parameters indicating hemolysis (lactate dehydrogenase, carboxyhemoglobin, free hemoglobin, and so forth), therefore, is recommended with the use of centrifugal devices to time pump head changes.

ANTICOAGULATION

An anticoagulation protocol similar to that used with ECMO was followed with the use of the Sci-Med lungs (11). Different protocols are in use in the centers using heparinized surface systems. These are composed of low–molecular-weight heparin, aprotinin or heparin at a different dosage.

Surface heparinized circuits can be run without systemic anticoagulation. We prefer to maintain a continuous heparin infusion to minimize the risk of clotting in the circuit, in case there is inadvertent cessation or slowing of the blood flow. In case of major bleeding or surgery, heparin infusion can be stopped for hours or days with relative safety. Heparinized surfaces need a normal plasma level of antithrombin III; we routinely replace antithrombin III by slow continuous intravenous infusion (500–1500 U/day).

CLINICAL MANAGEMENT

Patients are kept sedated and paralyzed. When extracorporeal blood flow reaches the maintenance value (20%–30% of cardiac output), ventilatory setting is switched from control mode ventilation (CMV) to intermittent mandatory ventilation (IMV) mode (3–5 breaths/minute). The PEEP level is adjusted to maintain mean airway pressure at the pre-bypass level to avoid the occurrence of frothy edema. A thin intratracheal catheter is inserted to deliver a continuous low flow of oxygen during the long expiratory pause (apneic oxygenation; see Chapter 16).

When gas exchange improves, attempts are made to reestablish assisted spontaneous breathing. Weaning is achieved by reducing F_1O_2 and PEEP and by decreasing CO_2 removal by the artificial lung (partial extracorporeal CO_2 removal) while the ventilatory capability of the patient improves (12).

With the venovenous bypass no modifications in extracorporeal support are required to test the function of the native lung. Shunt fraction reflects the real oxygenation capability of the diseased lung that is perfused with all the cardiac output. Patients are electively prematurely disconnected from $ECCO_2R$ only if irreversible central nervous system dysfunction occurs (7).

Complications

In our experience, a total of 1338 bypass days, extracorporeal assistance has never been stopped for technical reasons. Initially, pump chamber ruptures were frequently observed with the use of roller pumps and silicone rubber tubings; polyurethane pump chambers used later lasted for months.

Hemolysis is the most frequent complication occurring with the use of centrifugal pumps. If one detects evidence of hemolysis, the pump head must be substituted promptly to prevent subsequent renal damage. In our experience the mean duration for the head pump was 7 days. Oxygenators were changed whenever we considered them responsible for coagulation disorders (indicated by platelets consumption or increase fibrin split products) or when a consistent decrease of their performance was detected. Sometimes artificial lungs were also changed if they were potentially a source of systemic sepsis.

Bleeding always has been the major problem with extracorporeal support techniques. This problem is more evident whenever the patient needs surgical intervention, chest tube placement, or thoracotomy. In 1986 we reported an average blood products requirement of 1.8 L/day (7).

The introduction of percutaneous cannulation followed later by heparinized circuits has greatly reduced bleeding. In the last few years, our bypass population showed a dramatic drop of the daily blood requirement to 200–300 ml (see Table 18.2) (8).

The cannulation site was a major site of bleeding before the introduction of percutaneous cannulation. Thoracic bleeding is still the major site of blood loss in our population; 22 patients underwent at least a surgical procedure while on bypass; of the 16 patients who had thoracotomy, five survived. Of 103 patients,

Table 18.2. Transfusion Requirements[a]

	Surgery[b]		No surgery	
	No.	L/day	No.	L/day
Surgical cannulation	11	1.8 ± 1.4	43	0.8 ± 0.4
Percutaneous cannulation	5	1.2 ± 1.1	18	0.4 ± 0.2
Heparinized circuit	6	0.5 ± 0.4	14	0.2 ± 0.1

[a] *Packed red blood cells L/day.*
[b] *Patients undergoing major surgery while on bypass.*

we observed 13 central nervous system (CNS) hemorrhages; of these four patients had an overt concomitant coagulopathy, four had an abnormal brain computed tomography (CT) scan prior to bypass, and one a CNS fungal infection at autopsy. Six of the 13 CNS hemorrhages occurred immediately after bypass connection; the other six occurred during the first 5 days of bypass.

Multiorgan failure due to sepsis is the leading cause of death in our patient population. Twenty-six patients (25%) required extracorporeal support of renal function, of whom two eventually survived.

Results

In 1986 Gattinoni et al. reported 49% survival with LFPPV-ECCO$_2$R in 43 ARDS patients with criteria similar to those used in the ECMO trial (7). This figure was later corroborated by other European and, more recently, US centers with an overall survival rate 40%–50% (Table 18.3) (13). New interest in ECMO prompted comparison of the extracorporeal procedure with the so-called "advanced standard treatment."

In 1994, Morris et al. published the results of a randomized controlled trial performed on an ARDS population in Salt Lake City (14). Survival was not significantly different in the 19 mechanically ventilated patients (42%) compared with 21 patients who received pressure control inverse ratio ventilation followed by LFPPV-ECCO$_2$R (33%). Nevertheless, the overall survival in this ARDS population was better than that of the older ECMO study.

In the "new therapy" group, two patients never underwent LFPPV-ECCO$_2$R, one of them survived. Of the 19 patients having bypass operations, seven were disconnected from therapy because of major bleeding; five of these seven eventually survived. Most strikingly, only six bypass patients eventually survived, five were those disconnected due to bleeding. Although it would appear that bleeding during bypass is a good prognostic factor, this notion is clearly untenable.

Table 18.3. Extracorporeal Support for Adult Respiratory Failure (1980–1994)

	Cases (No.)	Survival (%)
Europe	489	51
US	135	49
Japan	57	48
TOTAL	681	50

From Bartlett RH. Extracorporeal life support (ECLS) for adult respiratory failure: the North American experience. Int J Artif Organs 18:620–630, 1995.

EXTRACORPOREAL RESPIRATORY SUPPORT ROLE IN THE TREATMENT OF ARDS IN THE NINETIES

Rationale

To "rest" the diseased lung while buying time for the healing processes, is the main goal of extracorporeal respiratory support. New insights on the deleterious effects of mechanical ventilation have been gathered in recent years. The ARDS lungs are not homogeneously affected by the disease process, as proved by CT-scan studies. Normally, ventilated areas are interspersed between nonaerated collapsed areas, mainly in the posterobasal portion of the lungs in the supine patient. The normal appearing lung is often reduced to 10%–20% of its usual capacity; this so-called "baby lung" has to provide for the entire gas exchange (15).

Supernormal ventilatory volumes have been commonly used to maintain "normal" blood gases. These volumes will be directed mainly toward the more compliant but relatively small residual healthy areas causing local hyperventilation known to affect lung function and structure adversely (16). To avoid hyperventilation of the "baby lung," retargeting of $PaCO_2$ values has been recently proposed. Permissive hypercapnia reduces but does not abolish completely the volotrauma to the residual healthy lung. Extracorporeal respiratory assistance remains the last resort to completely support alveolar function.

Which Kind of Extracorporeal Assistance?

ECMO and $ECCO_2R$ are the two available techniques to support lung function in ARDS; their main features are summarized in Table 18.4 for comparison.

"Ideal" lung support must provide viable gas exchange while preserving the lung structures. Lungs affected by ARDS have a better chance to heal if they are well nourished and not mechanically stressed. Lung rest is accomplished by apneic oxygenation plus LFPPV while venovenous bypass removes CO_2 thereby main-

Table 18.4. ECMO vs. $ECCO_2R$

	ECMO	*$ECCO_2R$*
Bypass	Venoarterial	Venovenous
ECBF	High	Low
Lung ventilation	"Normal"	Low frequency Apneic oxygenation
Lung perfusion	Decreased	Preserved
Cardiac assist	Yes	No

ECMO, extracorporeal membrane oxygenation; $ECCO_2R$, extracorporeal CO_2 removal.

taining normal lung perfusion. Lung rest was accomplished during the ECMO trial, because the diseased lung was continuously mechanically ventilated, and it was hypoperfused due to the venoarterial approach. Lung tissue necrosis possibly caused by ischemia and alkalosis was indeed a common finding in ECMO patients at necropsy (17).

Logistic and Personnel Problems

A well-trained clinical team with sufficient experience is mandatory in providing long-term extracorporeal assistance. Personnel able to overcome possible technical problems must be available in the hospital around the clock. Work shifts should be kept short to avoid human fatigue, which can lead to errors and misjudgments. Prompt availability of consultants (e.g., thoracic and general surgeons, hematologists, and others), easy access to hospital facilities (e.g., CT), and well-organized laboratory and blood bank services are mandatory during perfusion. Therefore, the extracorporeal support is a complex and multidisciplinary approach that requires dedicated and selected centers.

CONCLUSIONS

The main goal of extracorporeal respiratory assistance is to support lung function while allowing the natural healing process to evolve and the therapies (i.e., antibiotics, nutrition, and so forth) to be effective. The required support may last weeks or months, as reported by several teams in the last few years. During these very long bypass experiences, the function of the natural lung can be almost totally lost (shunt fraction near 100%), which requires higher extracorporeal blood flow to maintain viable oxygenation. Nevertheless, ultimate survival is possible even in these patients. The concept of "irreversible respiratory failure," a potential contradiction for ECMO, must be disputed. Ethical issues arise regarding the elective termination of an extracorporeal support. Recently, some authors tried to define irrecoverable pulmonary parenchymal damage leading to extracorporeal life support withdrawal. Criteria include pulmonary artery pressure >75% of systemic pressure, pulmonary fibrosis by open lung biopsy, absence of aeration on chest radiograph, and poor compliance (18). So far, no consensus exists regarding criteria that define irreversible lung damage. At this time, we limit premature, elective termination of bypass to the cases of irreversible brain damage.

In conclusion, the rationale of extracorporeal support is founded on good pathophysiologic grounds, based on the clinical and experimental evidences of the lung damage determined by pressures and volumes of conventional mechanical ventilation. The extracorporeal technique still needs innovations and refinements to increase its safety—mainly to decrease the risk of bleeding complications. At this time, extracorporeal assistance is restricted to a few specialized centers and to selected cases of severe acute respiratory failure. A complete understanding of the interactions between the extracorporeal apparatus and the body as a whole are still lacking. Future experimental studies directed to explore the effects of the extracorporeal device at the cellular and organ levels are advisable.

References

1. Ashbaugh DG, Bigelow DB, Petty TL, et al. Acute respiratory distress in adults. Lancet 2: 319–323, 1967.
2. National Heart Lung and Blood Institute, Division of Lung Diseases. Extracorporeal support for respiratory insufficiency: A collaborative study in response to RFP-NHLI-73-20. Bethesda, MD: National Heart Lung and Blood Institute 1979; 1–390.
3. Zapol WM, Snider MT, Hill JD, et al. Extracorporeal membrane oxygenation in severe acute respiratory failure. A randomized prospective study. JAMA 242:2193–2196, 1979.
4. Gattinoni L, Pesenti A, Kolobow T, et al. A new look at therapy of the adult respiratory distress syndrome: motionless lung. Int Anesthesiol Clin 1983; 21:97–117, 1983.
5. Kolobow T, Gattinoni L, Tomlinson T, Pierce J. Control of breathing using an extracorporeal membrane lung. Anesthesiology 46:138–141, 1977.
6. Gattinoni L, Kolobow T, Tomlinson T, et al. Low frequency positive pressure ventilation with extracorporeal carbon dioxide removal (LFPPV-ECCO$_2$R): an experimental study. Anesth Analg 55:470–477, 1978.
7. Gattinoni L, Pesenti A, Mascheroni D, et al. Low frequency positive-pressure ventilation with extracorporeal CO$_2$ removal in severe acute respiratory failure. JAMA 256:881–886, 1986.
8. Gattinoni L, Pesenti A, Bombino M, et al. Role of extracorporeal circulation in adult respiratory distress syndrome management. New Horizons 1:603–612, 1993.
9. Bindslev L, Eklund J, Norlander O, et al. Treatment of acute respiratory failure by extracorporeal carbon dioxide elimination performed with a surface heparinized artificial lung. Anesthesiology 67:117–120, 1987.
10. Musch G, Verweij M, Bombino M, et al. Small pore size microporous membrane oxygenator reduces plasma leakage during prolonged extracorporeal circulation: a case report. Int J Artif Organs; in press.
11. Uziel L, Cugno M, Fabrizi I, et al. Physiopathology and management of coagulation during long-term extracorporeal respiratory assistance. Int J Artif Organs 13:280–287, 1990.
12. Marcolin R, Mascheroni D, Pesenti A, et al. Ventilatory impact of partial extracorporeal CO$_2$ removal (PECOR) in ARF patients. Trans Am Soc Artif Intern Organs 32:508–510, 1986.
13. Bartlett RH, DeLosh T, Tracey T. Extracorporeal life support (ECLS) for adult respiratory failure: the North American experience. Int J Artif Organs 18:620–630, 1995.
14. Morris AH, Wallace CJ, Menlove RL, et al. Randomized clinical trial of pressure support-controlled inverse ratio ventilation and extracorporeal CO$_2$ removal for adult respiratory distress syndrome. Am J Respir Crit Care Med 149:295–305, 1994.
15. Gattinoni L, Pesenti A. ARDS: the nonhomogeneous lung. Facts and hypothesis. Intensive and Critical Care Digest 6:1–3, 1987.
16. Dreyfuss D, Soler P, Basset G. High inflation pressure pulmonary edema. Respective effects of high airway pressure, high tidal volume and positive end expiratory pressure. Am Rev Respir Dis 137:1159–1164, 1988.
17. Ratliff JL, Hill JD, Fallat RJ, et al. Complications associated with membrane lung support by venoarterial perfusion. Ann Thorac Surg 19:537–539, 1975.
18. Anderson H III, Steimle C, Shapiro M, et al. Extracorporeal life support for adult cardiorespiratory failure. Surgery 114:161–173, 1993.

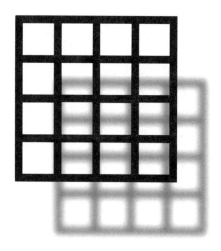

Section III
Disease-Oriented Ventilatory Support

19
Adult Respiratory Distress Syndrome

Roy D. Cane • Carrie L. Gill-Murdoch

The term adult respiratory distress syndrome (ARDS) was proposed in 1967 to describe a clinical constellation of signs and symptoms associated with a variety of insults that followed a consistent and predictable clinical course (1). The features of this syndrome include noncardiogenic pulmonary edema, hypoxemia, and diffuse microatelectasis. Anatomic descriptions of lung abnormalities in situations commonly associated with ARDS were first described during World War II. These descriptions have always documented the morphologic disarrangement of both epithelial and endothelial cells in the lung. In the last 28 years, significant study of ARDS has led to increased understanding of the disease process. Unfortunately, no major breakthroughs in direct therapy have been achieved and the morbidity and mortality associated with this condition remain relatively unchanged.

PREVALENCE

The actual prevalence of ARDS is unknown. Annual case reports number 150,000 in the United States. The heterogeneity of the disease processes that lead to ARDS and the lack of specific definitions of ARDS render it almost impossible to get accurate prevalence data. Similarly, mortality rates are hard to define. Reported mortality is ~50% with a range from 10% to 90% (2). Despite lack of hard data, ARDS undoubtedly contributes significantly to morbidity and mortality of critically ill patients on a worldwide basis.

DEFINITIONS

Defining ARDS is problematic because the clinical presentation embraces a continuum of gas exchange and chest radiographic abnormalities. The term acute lung injury (ALI) has been applied to a wide spectrum of pulmonary pathologic processes that result in consistent abnormalities of gas exchange and chest radiography. ARDS is considered the most severe form of ALI.

A 1992 American/European Consensus Conference on ARDS proposed the following definitions for ALI and ARDS (3).

Acute lung injury is described by the following clinical criteria:

1. The condition should be of acute onset.
2. The deficit in oxygenation should result in a $PaO_2/F_IO_2 \leq 300$ mmHg irrespective of PEEP therapy.
3. A frontal chest radiograph should show bilateral infiltrates.
4. The pulmonary artery occlusion pressure should be ≤ 18 mmHg without any evidence of left atrial hypertension.

The diagnosis of ARDS depends on the presence of all of the above criteria defining ALI, except that the degree of deficit in oxygenation is greater; in ARDS, the PaO_2/F_IO_2 should be ≤ 200 mmHg regardless of PEEP therapy.

We use the term *ALI/ARDS* to discuss aspects of the whole spectrum of lung injury. ARDS is used to denote a severe degree of ALI associated with significant morbidity and difficulty with ventilatory support.

PATHOGENESIS

Injury to specific cellular elements in the lung produces lung parenchymal changes that result in certain clinical criteria. The capillary endothelial cells appear to be the most susceptible to injury (4,5). Endothelial cell damage results in increased transduction of water and protein into the lung interstitium and the development of noncardiogenic pulmonary edema (6). This noncardiogenic edema produces bilateral patchy interstitial infiltrates on a chest radiograph in the dependent lung regions, a moderate reduction in lung compliance, and a mild to moderate degree of hypoxemia. The hypoxemia is partially responsive to increases in inspired oxygen concentration. This clinical picture is consistent with a diagnosis of ALI. Injury to the alveolar epithelium leads to alveolar instability and alveolar flooding resulting in diffuse microatelectasis. Alveolar type 1 cells are more susceptible to injury than are type 2 cells; however, both cell types can be damaged. This diffuse microatelectasis, in conjunction with the noncardiogenic edema, leads to further reduction in lung compliance, worsening hypoxemia with loss of responsiveness to increases in inspired oxygen concentration, and bilateral infiltrates on a chest radiograph of a mixed alveolar and interstitial pattern. This constellation of more severe clinical signs is consistent with the diagnosis of ARDS. The reparative phase of the injury is characterized by proliferation of alveolar type 2 cells with the development of a columnar epithelial lining of the alveoli. These type 2 cells are believed to differentiate subsequently into type 1 cells.

Once the initiating factor has been corrected, lung function can start to improve in as little as 3–4 days. Failure of resolution appears to be related to persistence of the initiating cause and further lung damage secondary to iatrogenic factors (e.g., positive airway pressure development of nosocomial pneumonia or combinations of these factors).

RISK FACTORS

Multiple clinical circumstances and causative factors have been described as risks for the development of ALI/ARDS. It is not clear whether these descriptions are appropriate because of previous laxity in defining ALI/ARDS. Despite this diversity, certain risk factors are consistently associated with the development of ALI/ARDS. A European/American Consensus Conference characterized risk factors into two groups (3). One group termed *direct injury risk factors,* included conditions associated with direct pulmonary parenchymal involvement in the primary disease process that predisposed to lung injury. The other group characterized as *indirect injury risk factors,* were primary conditions associated with nonpulmonary lesions. The major risk factors in these classifications are:
1. Direct injury risk factors
   a. Aspiration
   b. Diffuse pulmonary infections (e.g., bacterial, viral, pneumocystis carinii infections)
   c. Near drowning
   d. Toxic gas inhalation
   e. Lung contusion
2. Indirect injury risk factors
   a. Sepsis syndrome with or without clinically significant hypotension defined as a systolic blood pressure of <90 mmHg with or without evidence of infection outside the lung
   b. Severe nonthoracic trauma
   c. Massive transfusion from emergency resuscitation
   d. Cardiopulmonary bypass

MECHANISMS OF ACUTE LUNG INJURY

The underlying mechanisms of cellular injury are not well understood. Over the years many investigators have described various cellular and humoral elements that appear to play roles in the genesis of lung injury. Although it is generally accepted that these cellular and humoral mediators are responsible for the lung injury, no consensus exists on the actions of specific factors or the sequence of events in the pathogenesis of lung cell damage. The mediators released by neutrophils and macrophages are believed to be responsible for direct cellular toxicity, increases in vascular permeability, chemotaxis of circulating cellular components, and fibrosis. The inflammatory cascade initiated with injury also appears to amplify the host response and the injury. Some of the specific actions of both cellular and humoral elements are discussed below.

Cellular Elements

NEUTROPHILS

Many activated neutrophils collect in the lung during the early stages of ALI/ARDS (7,8). These cells are believed to release toxic oxygen radicals, elastases, and products of arachidonic acid metabolism, which damage pulmonary microvascular endothelial cells and lead to increased vascular permeability, hemorrhage, and parenchymal injury (7). Although neutrophils have been strongly implicated in ALI/ARDS, neutropenic patients also develop lung damage, which suggests that other equally important factors are involved (9).

MACROPHAGES

Macrophages have been shown to release tumor necrosis factor (TNF) in response to endotoxin in sepsis (10). Additionally, alveolar macrophages secrete a variety of chemotactic substances that sequester neutrophils in the lung (11). The early chemotactic action of the macrophages causes neutrophil aggregation that, in turn, is thought to initiate the inflammatory response of the lung (11). The macrophages continue to produce cytokines even after the initiating events have ceased (5). Macrophages also regulate fibroblast function and may play a role in the fibrosis seen in later stages of ARDS (5).

Humoral Elements

CYTOKINES

Elevated levels of TNF in plasma, bronchial secretions, and bronchoalveolar lavage samples have been reported in septic patients (8). TNF promotes release of interleukin 1 (IL1). Administration of TNF to experimental animals produces physiologic changes similar to those associated with septic shock, namely hypotension and metabolic acidosis. IL1, produced by a variety of cells throughout the body, is a nonspecific sepsis mediator and an endogenous pyrogen. IL1 acts on the microvascular endothelium to increase endothelial permeability. Other cytokines, in particular IL2, IL4, IL6, and IL8, have all been implicated in the inflammatory response and in ALI/ARDS. Their roles, although not well understood, include increases in vascular permeability and neutrophil chemotaxis. These cytokines promote increased arachidonic acid metabolism (5). Meduri et al. (12) studied the relationship between initial and later plasma cytokine levels and outcomes in ARDS patients. Nonsurviving patients showed higher initial plasma concentrations of TNF-α, IL-1β, IL-6, and IL-8, which remained persistently elevated over the 10-day study period. Survivors generally had lower initial cytokine concentrations that rapidly declined. These data suggest that persistence of the inflammatory response heralds a poor outcome.

PLATELET ACTIVATING FACTOR

Platelet activating factor, released by platelets, macrophages, and neutrophils, induces pulmonary hypertension, bronchoconstriction, and negative inotropy. Although the role of platelet activating factor in ALI/ARDS is not clear, it is a potent mediator of vascular permeability and increases arachidonic acid metabolism (13).

COMPLEMENT

ALI/ARDS is associated with activation of the complement cascade. C3a and C5a, potent neutrophil stimulants, have been isolated in bronchoalveolar lavage fluid from patient with ALI/ARDS (14). C3a and C5a may facilitate phagocytosis, enhance neutrophil and monocyte activation and chemotaxis, augment vascular permeability, and are direct cytotoxins.

ARACHIDONIC ACID METABOLITES

Arachidonic acid metabolism via the cyclo-oxygenase pathway yields prostaglandins and thromboxane A2 and, via the lipo-oxygenase pathway, leukotrienes. Prostaglandins, thromboxane A2, and leukotrienes promote pulmonary hypertension, increased vascular permeability, and bronchoconstriction (13).

OXYGEN RADICALS

Normal cellular metabolism of oxygen to water involves tetravalent electron transfer. A small amount of oxygen escapes the tetravalent electron transfer and undergoes univalent reduction, producing highly reactive metabolites: superoxide (O_2^-), hydrogen peroxide (H_2O_2), singlet oxygen (O^-), and hydroxyl (OH^-) ions, collectively termed *oxygen free radicals* (15). Free radical scavenging enzyme systems normally neutralize these radicals. Any increased production of these reactive oxygen metabolites leads to destructive and unregulated reactions capable of damaging cell membranes and mitochondria, inactiving cytoplasmic and nuclear enzymes, and consequently causing cellular damage and death. Oxygen free radicals are produced by a variety of mechanisms including activation of cellular elements, namely platelets and phagocytes, especially neutrophils. Oxygen free radical formation also is promoted by high inspired oxygen concentrations and reperfusion of hypoxic tissues (15,16).

CLINICAL MANAGEMENT

No specific therapies for ALI/ARDS have shown efficacy. Ideally, the precipitating cause of the ALI/ARDS should be identified and vigorously treated to minimize perpetuation of the lung insult. Care should be taken to avoid exposure of the patient to any factors likely to cause further lung damage. Excessive positive airway pressure and high inspired oxygen concentrations may aggravate the lung injury.

Pharmacologic treatment with antiinflammatory agents and cytokine antagonists has not been effective; better understanding of the roles of cytokines may lead to improved treatment strategies. The role of steroids in management of ALI/ ARDS is controversial. For many years steroids were given to patients with ALI/ ARDS. However, no compelling data support steroid use in ALI or in the early phase of ARDS. Steroids actually may increase mortality in ARDS associated with sepsis (17). Recent studies, however, have shown improvement in lung function after steroid therapy during the later proliferative phase of ARDS (18). Further study is required to delineate fully the role of steroids in the management of ARDS.

The mainstay of management of ALI/ARDS is support of cardiopulmonary function, particularly as related to oxygenation, ventilation, and pulmonary vascular resistance.

Oxygenation

VENTILATION-TO-PERFUSION RATIOS AND INSPIRED OXYGEN CONCENTRATIONS

In a normal lung, ventilation-to-perfusion ratios ($\dot{V}_A/\dot{Q}$) change very little from inspiration to expiration. In ALI/ARDS the expiratory $\dot{V}_A/\dot{Q}$ is less than the inspiratory $\dot{V}_A/\dot{Q}$. At low $\dot{V}_A/\dot{Q}$, the oxygen flow rate from an alveolus into the blood can exceed the tidal ventilation to that alveolus. Under these circumstances, adequate volumes of stable gas, namely, alveolar nitrogen, help to maintain the alveolar volume (19). Breathing oxygen-augmented gas decreases alveolar nitrogen concentrations and, thus, allows for a reduction in alveolar volume and further decrease in $\dot{V}_A/\dot{Q}$. If alveolar volume falls below a critical level, alveolar collapse and regions of $\dot{V}_A/\dot{Q} = 0$ will develop. Lung units with an inspiratory $\dot{V}_A/\dot{Q} < 0.1$ are unstable when breathing oxygen concentrations of 35% and 50% in dogs with externally restricted lung (20). The multiple inert gas elimination technique was used to assess changes in $\dot{V}_A/\dot{Q}$ in postcardiac surgical patients with mild ALI when breathing increasing concentrations of oxygen (21). Breathing increasing concentrations of inspired oxygen from room air up to 40% resulted in a progressive increase in perfusion to lung regions with $\dot{V}_A/\dot{Q} > 0.1$. This effect appears to have been due to hypoxic pulmonary vasoconstriction (HPV) stimulated by either low alveolar and/or mixed-venous PO_2 ($P_{\bar{V}}O_2$). The $P_{\bar{V}}O_2$ in these patients was <40 mmHg on F_IO_2 from 0.21 to 0.4. Mean $P_{\bar{V}}O_2$ in these patients on 40% oxygen was 36.5 ± 3.7 mmHg, a sufficient level to continue HPV activation. Perfusion to lung regions with $\dot{V}_A/\dot{Q} < 0.005$ increased as inspired oxygen concentration was increased from 60% to 100% (21). As $P_{\bar{V}}O_2$ >40 mmHg levels were achieved on these high oxygen concentrations, this redistribution of perfusion was thought to be due to loss of HPV (22). The PaO_2 of 12 postcardiac surgical patients who breathed 50% oxygen for 16 to 24 hours was shown to be significantly lower than a similar group of 13 patients who breathed room air (66 ± 7 vs. 60 ± 5) (23). Thus, this evidence indicates that breathing augmented inspired oxygen concentrations may not be entirely beneficial in patients with ALI/ARDS. The effect on $\dot{V}_A/\dot{Q}$ of breathing high inspired oxygen concentrations in patients with ARDS needs to be studied further.

ALVEOLAR HYPEROXIA AND ACUTE LUNG INJURY

Small mammals exposed to 100% oxygen for several days manifest ALI/ARDS. These animals demonstrate rapid depletion of the enzymes involved in oxygen reduction and, therefore, accumulate oxygen free radicals when hyperoxic (24). Primates with normal lungs have adequate enzyme reserves that prevent oxygen free radical accumulation in hyperoxic conditions (25). However, preexistent cellular damage may diminish this reserve so that hyperoxic conditions may result in oxygen free radical accumulation. Lung endothelial cells are affected earlier and to a greater extent than epithelial cells by these oxygen free radicals. The type 2 cell in primates is the last parenchymal cell to demonstrate abnormal function secondary to hyperoxia (25). The extent and relative importance of oxygen radical induced lung damage in the overall pathophysiology of the critically ill patient with lung damage is unknown. The safe inspired oxygen concentration is also unknown.

OXYGEN THERAPY IN ALI/ARDS

Because of the potential hazards, the lowest oxygen concentration that maintains adequate arterial oxygenation should be used. The oxygenation deficit in ALI is mild to moderate and usually responds to an F_IO_2 between 0.21 and 0.4. ARDS is associated with more severe hypoxemia secondary to increased amounts of lung with extremely low $\dot{V}_A/\dot{Q}$ ($\dot{V}_A/\dot{Q} < 0.005$). Augmenting the inspired oxygen concentration is seldom sufficient to maintain adequate PaO_2. Positive airway pressure may improve the underlying $\dot{V}_A/\dot{Q}$ and enable maintenance of arterial oxygenation with a lower F_IO_2 (*vide infra*).

Ventilation

Spontaneous ventilation is desirable as hemodynamic function and ventilation perfusion relationships are usually better than with mechanical positive pressure ventilation. If patients with ALI/ARDS are to maintain effective spontaneous breathing, the work of breathing must be maximally efficient. The increase in lung water and decrease in lung volume associated with ALI/ARDS lead to reduced lung compliance, which results in increased work of breathing. The initial step in support of ventilatory function should be to reduce the work of breathing by improving lung compliance or by reducing inspiratory muscle load.

REDUCED RESPIRATORY SYSTEM COMPLIANCE AND WORK OF BREATHING

Any alteration in the volume-pressure relationship of the lung can alter the work of breathing. A normal volume-pressure curve for the lung-thorax system is shown in Figure 19.1. As a result of a small pressure change, normal tidal breathing from functional residual capacity (FRC) occurs along the volume-pressure curve as indicated by the arrow. The elastic work of inspiration can be estimated by the stippled area under the curve. Figure 19.2 shows the volume-pressure curves for normal lung, thorax, and lung-thorax. When the distending pressure of the lung-thorax is zero (i.e., ambient airway pressure), the lung volume is at FRC. At FRC the distending pressure of the lung is equal but opposite to that of the thorax. Any alteration in the volume-pressure relationships for the lung or the thorax will alter the lung-thorax curve and change FRC. The likely alteration of lung volume-pressure curve associated with ALI/ARDS is shown in Figure 19.3. Because the volume-pressure relationships of the lung and thorax can be altered in many ways in ALI/ARDS, a family of right-shifted lung-thorax curves can result. Each will have a reduced FRC (Fig. 19.4). A shift in the volume-pressure curve not only decreases FRC, but can increase the work of breathing. When FRC is decreased, the required pressure change to achieve the same VT will be increased and the work also is increased (Fig. 19.5). When this occurs, the patient will decrease tidal volume and increase respiratory rate in an effort to minimize work. Although the institution of mechanical ventilation will reduce or eliminate work of breathing, an increase in FRC and compliance may provide an alternative means of decreasing work of breathing. Restoration of FRC can be accomplished with continuous positive pressure breathing (CPAP) and an increase in distending pressure (Fig. 19.6). Because injury severity varies from patient to patient, positive

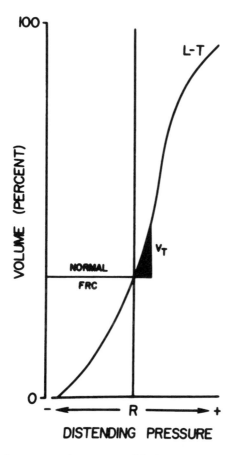

Figure 19.1. Normal pressure-volume curve of the lung-thorax (*L-T*). Volume as a percent of total lung capacity is plotted as a function of distending pressure (*R*). At ambient airway pressure, R equals zero. During inspiration, R is increased and lung volume (*V$_T$*) increases from normal functional residual capacity (*FRC*). As a result of a small pressure change, normal tidal breathing from FRC occurs along the pressure-volume curve, as indicated by the *arrow*. The elastic work of inspiration can be estimated by the stippled area under the curve. (Reprinted with permission from Downs JB, Douglas ME. Physiologic effects of respiratory therapy. In: Shoemaker W, Ayers S, Grevnik A, et al. (eds). Textbook of critical care, 2nd ed. Philadelphia, WB Saunders 1989, p 602.)

pressure breathing must be individualized, titrated for each patient, and reassessed frequently. Application of an airway pressure sufficient to restore FRC to a more favorable portion of the volume-pressure curve, reduces the required change in transpulmonary pressure. In other words, compliance will improve and work of breathing is reduced.

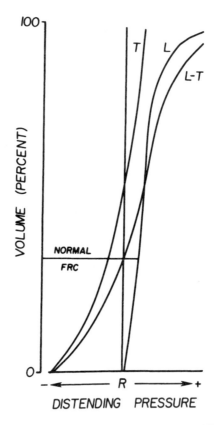

Figure 19.2. Normal pressure-volume curves of the thorax (*T*), lung (*L*), and lung-thorax (*L-T*). Volume as a percent of total lung capacity is plotted as a function of distending pressure (*R*). Lung-thorax R is zero when airway pressure is ambient; distending pressure of the lung is, therefore, equal, but opposite, to that of the thorax. These equal counterforces determine and maintain FRC. (Reprinted with permission from Downs JB, Douglas ME. Physiologic effects of respiratory therapy. In: Shoemaker W, Ayers S, Grevnik A, et al. (eds). Textbook of critical care, 2nd ed. Philadelphia, WB Saunders 1989, p 602.)

REDUCTION IN INSPIRATORY MUSCLE LOAD

Mechanical ventilatory support will reduce inspiratory work load. Mechanical ventilatory support can be characterized by the degree minute ventilation support; full ventilatory support where the required minute volume is delivered by the ventilator versus partial ventilatory support where the patient's spontaneous ventilatory efforts contribute to the required minute ventilation. Mechanical ventilation does not ameliorate the pathophysiologic derangements of ALI/ARDS, although

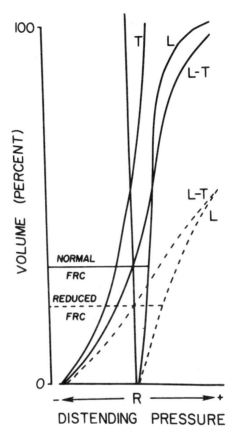

Figure 19.3. Normal (*solid lines*) and abnormal (*dotted lines*) pressure-volume curves of the thorax (*T*), lung (*L*), and lung-thorax (*L-T*). The distending pressure (R) is zero when airway pressure is ambient. The abnormally right-shifted pressure volume curve of the lung, which is characteristic of respiratory failure, results in a new L-T pressure-volume curve and a reduction in functional residual capacity (*FRC*). (Reprinted with permission from Downs JB, Douglas ME. Physiologic effects of respiratory therapy. In: Shoemaker W, Ayers S, Grevnik A, et al. (eds). Textbook of critical care, 2nd ed. Philadelphia, WB Saunders 1989, p 602.)

it can correct respiratory acidosis and eliminate excessive work of breathing. Full support of ventilation does not provide any physiologic advantage compared with a level of partial ventilatory support that adequately reduces work of breathing and augments alveolar ventilation. Partial ventilatory support obviates a need for deep sedation, muscle paralysis, and induction of respiratory alkalosis. Moreover, spontaneous ventilation facilitates $\dot{V}_A/\dot{Q}$ matching. Techniques that permit spon-

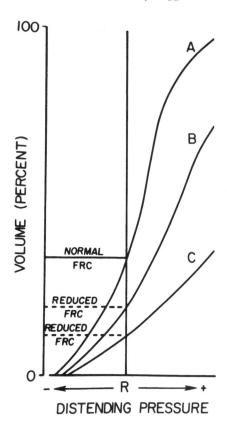

Figure 19.4. Volume as a percent of total lung capacity is plotted as a function of distending pressure (*R*). R is zero when airway pressure is ambient. Curve A represents a normal pressure-volume relationship for the lung-thorax. Curves B and C are shifted to the right. Each curve results in a reduced functional residual capacity (*FRC*). The pressure-volume relationships of the lung and thorax can be altered in an infinite number of ways during respiratory failure, resulting in a family of right-shifted lung-thorax curves. Each curve will have a lower FRC than the curve on its left. (Reprinted with permission from Downs JB, Douglas ME. Physiologic effects of respiratory therapy. In: Shoemaker W, Ayers S, Grevnik A, et al. (eds). Textbook of critical care, 2nd ed. Philadelphia, WB Saunders 1989, p 602.)

taneous breathing activity are likely to maintain ventilatory muscle strength and coordination when compared with total ventilation control. The adverse hemodynamic effects of positive pressure ventilation can be minimized by administering an adequate level of partial ventilatory support and allowing some spontaneous breathing activity to persist.

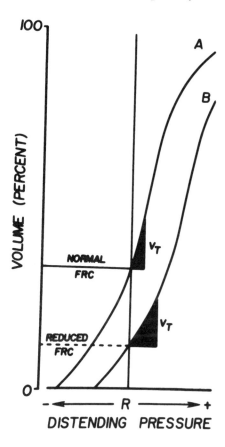

Figure 19.5. Pressure-volume curves of the lung-thorax. Volume as a percent of total lung capacity is plotted as a function of distending pressure (*R*). R is zero when airway pressure is ambient. Curve A represents a normal pressure-volume relationship and B represents a right-shifted curve. (Reprinted with permission from Downs JB, Douglas ME. Physiologic effects of respiratory therapy. In: Shoemaker W, Ayers S, Grevnik A, et al. (eds). Textbook of critical care, 2nd ed. Philadelphia, WB Saunders 1989, p 602.)

SUPPORT OF VENTILATORY FUNCTION WITH POSITIVE AIRWAY PRESSURE

We recommend support of ventilatory function by initial titration of CPAP applied by face mask or endotracheal tube. The required CPAP level is one that tends to normalize the breathing pattern (respiratory rate <25/minute with V_T of ~5 ml/kg) and reduce the physiologic stress as evidenced by a decrease in heart rate, systolic hypertension, diaphoresis, and complaints of dyspnea. For most patients with milder degrees of ALI, CPAP is usually sufficient to enable maintenance of spontaneous ventilation. If the work of breathing on CPAP still exceeds

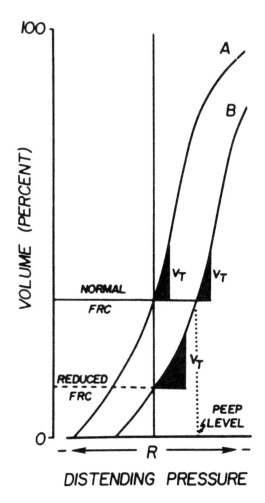

Figure 19.6. These pressure-volume curves of the lung-thorax are equivalent to those in Figure 19.5. When distending pressure (*R*) is increased by positive airway pressure (*PEEP*), FRC can be normalized. When FRC is increased, the work of breathing may be reduced to nearly normal. (Reprinted with permission from Downs JB, Douglas ME. Physiologic effects of respiratory therapy. In: Shoemaker W, Ayers S, Grevnik A, et al. (eds). Textbook of critical care, 2nd ed. Philadelphia, WB Saunders 1989, p 602.)

the functional reserves of the patient, as in the more severe degrees of ALI/ARDS and ARDS, partial ventilatory support plus CPAP should be provided. The partial ventilatory support mode chosen for the patient with ALI/ARDS is largely a matter of physician preference. Recent data concerning airway pressure induced lung damage suggest ways to choose and apply the different mechanical ventilation modes.

MECHANICAL VENTILATORY TECHNIQUES AND ALI/ARDS

Nearly all the different forms of mechanical ventilation can be used to support ventilatory function in patients with ALI/ARDS. A major concern related to mechanical ventilation in patients with significant restriction of lung function secondary to a non-homogeneous pathologic process is the risk of ventilator-induced lung injury. Thus, choice of a mode or technique should be based on consideration of how positive pressure ventilation may injure the lung.

Positive Pressure Ventilation and Lung Injury

The methodologies of most studies documenting positive pressure ventilation induced lung injury are very similar and the discussion of one suffices as a model for the group. The work of Tsuno et al. (26) provides an example. Healthy piglets were placed on full mechanical ventilatory support using a tidal volume (V_T) of 13 ml/kg, a respiratory rate of 20 breaths/minute, and 3–5 cmH$_2$O of PEEP. This resulted in a peak inspiratory pressure (PIP) of <18 cmH$_2$O. These animals were then randomly assigned to one of two groups. The animals in group A, controls, were maintained on the above settings for 48 hours. Group B served as the experimental set wherein mean airway pressure (Paw) was modified by increasing the V_T from 13 ml/kg up to a mean of 65.5 ± 7.6 ml/kg until the PIP reached 40 cmH$_2$O. After 48 hours on this level of ventilatory support, this group was further subdivided into subsets. The animals in subset B1 were sacrificed immediately. In subset B2, ventilatory support was changed back to the baseline intermittent mandatory ventilation (IMV) setting for 3–6 more days before sacrifice. As no significant difference was found between these subgroups, they will be considered as a single group. The respiratory function and pulmonary microanatomy of the two groups were then compared. Group A demonstrated very little change in either pulmonary mechanics or architecture. In Group B, however, marked decreases in oxygenation and ventilatory mechanics were observed. Microscopic examination revealed pathologic changes similar to those seen in human ARDS. From these findings, the authors concluded that the elevated airway pressure in the experimental animals "may affect the underlying process of acute lung injury and may contribute to the specific lung pathology seen in ARDS."

Airway Pressure Versus End Inspiratory Lung Volume and Lung Injury

The fact that positive pressure ventilation may contribute to such pathology seems beyond dispute. The question remains, however, exactly which component of the ventilatory technique is responsible for those changes. In most of these studies (e.g., the Tsuno et al. example given above), an elevated Paw was achieved in the experimental group by raising the V_T, usually to clinically irrelevant levels (up to 65 ml/kg in the report discussed above to >100 ml/kg in another) (27,28). Paw was, in fact, a dependent variable in that situation and as such may not itself actually have influenced the abnormalities observed. As at the alveolar level, there is very little if any gas flow volume and intraalveolar pressure is determined by lung compliance and overall distending pressure applied to the lung. High intraalveolar pressures would be generated by supraphysiologic V_T in animals with normal lung compliance or normal V_T in animals with reduced compliance. Thus, the pathophysiologic changes consistently demonstrated in these animal models probably resulted primarily from the supraphysiologic V_T, although pressure and volume are both important.

Dreyfuss et al. (29) studied the relative importance of volume and pressure in the genesis of lung injury by initially comparing extravascular lung water and ultrastructural lung changes in groups of rats receiving positive pressure ventilation in different combinations of high and low volumes and pressures designated HiV, LoV, HiP, and LoP. In the control animals, traditional positive pressure ventilation with a V_T of 13 ml/kg was employed, which produced a PIP of 7 cmH$_2$O (LoV-LoP). The second group received positive pressure ventilation with V_T increased to achieve a PIP of 45 cmH$_2$O (HiV-HiP). To accomplish this high PIP, an average V_T of 40 ml/kg was necessary. In the third group, 10 cmH$_2$O PEEP was added to a similar HiV-HiP PPV protocol and V_T reduced (average of 25 ml/kg) to maintain the same 45 cmH$_2$O PIP while using PEEP. The fourth group received positive pressure ventilation with a V_T of 19 ml/kg used in combination with an elevated airway pressure of 45 cmH$_2$O (LoV-HiP). This paradoxic LoV-HiP situation was established by thoracoabdominal strapping of the animals with a rubber band, thus, making Paw the independent variable in this group. The final group was ventilated using a V_T of 44 ml/kg generated by a negative inspiratory pressure device, a veterinary iron lung. This was to investigate the effect of high volume alone (HiV-LoP).

The authors found that lung structure was normal in the control animals and in those in the LoV-HiP group. That is, large cyclic changes in airway pressure with conventional V_T between 13 and 19 ml/kg did not affect pulmonary microarchitecture. In contrast, pulmonary edema and structural lung injury similar to that seen in ARDS were observed in all the HiV groups. Thus, only large changes in lung volume, not airway pressure, produced pulmonary pathology in this model. Dreyfuss and Saumon (30) studied the relative influence of end-inspiratory lung volume, V_T, and FRC on the genesis of lung injury as reflected by pulmonary edema developing in rats ventilated with varying combinations of V_T, PEEP levels, and extrathoracic negative pressure. In addition, they examined the influence of hemodynamic factors in the development of pulmonary edema associated with mechanical ventilation. They found that development of pulmonary edema was related to end-inspiratory lung volume and did not depend on any specific level of PEEP or V_T. Moderate levels of PEEP and V_T, individually innocuous, resulted in pulmonary edema when used in combination. PEEP effect was a function of the FRC change, not of the pressure level. The genesis of a critical end-inspiratory volume with externally applied negative pressure (no positive pressure applied to the airway) also was associated with pulmonary edema. The degree of pulmonary edema was less in animals ventilated with PEEP when compared with similar ventilation with zero PEEP. This apparently beneficial effect of PEEP was probably due to a PEEP-induced drop in cardiac output as the degree of edema increased when the PEEP-induced fall in systolic blood pressure was restored by dopamine infusion. They conclude that end-inspiratory lung volume is the major determinant of ventilation-induced edema. Furthermore, that hemodynamic status plays an important role in modulating the amount of edema that develops during lung overinflation.

Concern with the role of positive airway pressure and inflating volumes in the pathogenesis or perpetuation of ALI/ARDS has prompted a shift away from high volume, low rate ventilatory support patterns to various alternative techniques and approaches characterized by minimal ventilatory excursions.

MINIMAL EXCURSIONARY VENTILATION

If increased pulmonary volume, specifically alveolar hyperinflation, is a causative factor in structural lung injury attending positive airway pressure then a reduction in cyclical volume expansion during positive pressure ventilation should ameliorate this problem. Use of conventional volume controlled modes of ventilation with smaller V_T (5–7 ml/kg) and higher ventilator rates are becoming more common. The modes of pressure support ventilation (PSV) and pressure-control ventilation produce variable V_T. The V_T is a function of the applied airway pressure gradient, total respiratory system compliance, and inspiratory time. If the patient's lung compliance deteriorates, the V_T will decrease. Thus, with these modes set to produce a V_T of 5–7 ml/kg the risk of lung overinflation if lung mechanics deteriorate is less than with volume-controlled modes.

In addition to volume controlled positive pressure ventilation using small V_T, PSV, and pressure-control ventilation, minimal excursionary ventilation can be achieved by several other means.

Permissive Hypercapnia

The simplest method of minimal excursionary ventilation is that of permissive hypercapnia or controlled hypoventilation wherein V_T and, hence, total minute ventilation is reduced, accepting the consequent $PaCO_2$ rise provided the pH remains in an acceptable range (pHa >7.2). In Europe where this approach has been taken most aggressively, $PaCO_2$ as high as 90 mmHg has been reported (31). This strategy has improved clinical outcomes in both status asthmaticus and ARDS (32–35).

Elimination of Dead Space

Another approach is the elimination of dead space by the insufflation of fresh gas directly into either the trachea or the bronchus (36,37). Because the dead space volume is flushed out, effective alveolar ventilation for a given V_T should increase. V_T and, therefore, the potential for iatrogenic injury can be reduced while maintaining effective CO_2 elimination.

High Frequency Ventilation

Perhaps the greatest experience with minimal excursionary ventilation techniques is in the field of high frequency ventilation (see also, Chapter 17). Several different options exist but the common denominator is the delivery of fresh gas using a markedly increased ventilatory frequency, with a decreased V_T. Although promising in animal models, the application of these modalities to human patients has been somewhat disappointing (38–40). High frequency oscillation has been used extensively in neonates, but the results are contradictory and the role of this modality remains controversial (41–46). Most experience with these techniques in adults has been with high frequency jet ventilation and, again, no clear application has emerged (46).

Airway Pressure Release Ventilation

Airway pressure release ventilation (APRV) (see also, Chapter 14) can minimize lung volume expansion. In this mode, the inflation pressure is that CPAP level associated with the best lung compliance and oxygenation for that individual patient (46–49). In the usual circumstance, this optimal performance is found near the volume corresponding to the normal FRC. Pulmonary volume is maximal at this point during the APRV cycle. When the release valve opens, gas exits from the lung and lung volume decreases. In terms of lung volume changes, APRV is exactly the opposite of traditional positive ventilation in which ventilation is supported by increasing lung volume above FRC. Thus, APRV allows for ventilatory support in the absence of large volume changes above the optimal resting volume. The advantage of volume reduction ventilatory support is that the potential for alveolar hyperinflation with each tidal ventilation, and thus iatrogenic lung injury, is minimized. Other benefits include improved matching of ventilation and perfusion and a lesser degree of hemodynamic compromise (49,50). The feasibility of this ventilatory support technique has been demonstrated by a number of investigators, including a multicenter clinical trial, but, as with other ventilatory support options, controlled outcome data demonstrating a particular inherent advantage are lacking (47–51).

Combined Pressure Support Ventilation and Expiratory Pressure Release

Räsänen has suggested that the sequential use of a low level of positive inspiratory airway pressure (PSV) in combination with expiratory pressure release may actually prove to be the optimal method of mechanical ventilatory support (52). With this sequence of pressure-assisted inflation and deflation, lung volume would vary somewhat in a sinusoidal fashion above and below FRC, instead of cycling completely either way. The adverse effects of large volume and pressure changes with either method could be minimized and the potential for iatrogenic lung injury may be reduced. A system linking inspiratory PSV with expiratory synchronized airway pressure release has already been described (53). The PSV component was used to synchronize expiratory airway pressure release and to overcome the resistive work imposed by the breathing circuit, but not primarily as part of the ventilatory support. This combination of techniques holds significant theoretic appeal.

Constant mean airway pressure ventilation, an application of Räsänen's concept, has been shown to be effective in providing partial ventilatory support in a porcine, oleic acid model of ALI/ARDS. The theoretic advantages with respect to ventilator-induced injury need to be studied (54).

Extracorporeal Gas Exchange

Extracorporeal membrane oxygenation (ECMO) (see also, Chapter 18) was the first attempt at continuous support that bypassed the lungs. Widely used in the 1970s, it has not been shown to offer any improvement in outcome over conventional ventilatory support in the treatment of severe respiratory dysfunction (55).

Extracorporeal CO_2 removal (ECCO$_2$R) using a membrane lung with venovenous bypass in combination with support of arterial oxygenation via the native lung has been shown to be efficacious in both animal and human studies (56,57). Gattinoni et al. (57) have had significant experience using this technique. CO_2

was removed via the membrane lung in the extracorporeal circuit. Three to five mechanical breaths per minute with PEEP of 15–25 cmH$_2$O and augmented F$_1$O$_2$ were applied to the native lung to maintain arterial oxygenation and prevent atelectasis.V$_T$ was set to ensure that the PIP was maintained <45 cmH$_2$O. Using this technique in patients with severe pulmonary pathology, the authors demonstrated a marked reduction in mortality when compared with historical controls, from >90% to ~50% (57). This study, though preliminary and uncontrolled, demonstrates that extracorporeal techniques can provide support with minimal ventilatory excursions.

The concept of minimal ventilatory excursion for reducing iatrogenic lung injury has recently gained credence. Perhaps strategies employing complete pulmonary rest will prove even more efficacious. Whatever specific ventilatory technique is employed, the support should be delivered in a way that minimizes alveolar overdistension as hyperinflation, rather than the elevated airway pressure itself, is the most likely cause of positive pressure ventilation induced structural lung injury.

PULMONARY VASCULAR RESISTANCE

Recent attention to reducing the pulmonary hypertension associated with ALI/ARDS by inhalation of nitric oxide (NO) has shown some promise. Preliminary data suggest that inhaled NO, a potent pulmonary vasodilator, is associated with significantly improved pulmonary oxygen transfer and earlier improvement in overall lung function in ALI/ARDS (58,59). The effects of NO in ALI/ARDS may involve more than pulmonary vasodilatation. Neutrophils in bronchoalveolar lavage (BAL) fluid of patients with ARDS receiving NO showed decreased spontaneous production of H$_2$O$_2$ and other molecules responsible for neutrophil adhesion when compared with BAL samples from ARDS patients who did not receive NO (60). Furthermore, BAL concentrations of IL-8 and IL-6 were lower in ARDS patients receiving NO than in the control patients. These data suggest that NO may reduce lung inflammation in ARDS. Aerosolized prostacyclin (PGI2) has been shown to improve arterial oxygenation and reduce venous admixture in patients with ARDS (61). PGI2 efficacy was similar to NO. Further study of transbronchial vasodilator therapy is required.

OUTCOME

Routine histologic evaluation of lung tissue from survivors of ALI/ARDS is essentially precluded on ethical grounds. However, Lakshminarayan et al. (62) obtained lung tissue from three survivors at 4 and 14 weeks and at 9 months after ARDS. Biopsy at week 4 revealed combined interstitial and organized pneumonitis. Histologically, at week 14, a presumably old emphysematous component and areas of interstitial fibrosis were noted. Finally, the biopsy at 9 months showed patchy interstitial fibrosis, alveolar type 2 hyperplasia cells, and focal increases in alveolar macrophages and interstitial lymphocytes. These findings seem to correlate with indirect evidence obtained from clinical, radiologic, and pathophysiologic findings in ARDS.

Although the mortality associated with ARDS is high, it is generally believed that few adverse long-term sequelae are seen in survivors. Pulmonary function tests in survivors show return to normal function within 5–7 months (63). When defects are detected, a restrictive pattern often exists as evidenced by a reduced forced vital capacity and diffusing capacity. Some investigators have reported abnormalities in lung volumes, expiratory flow rates, and gas exchange (62,64).

Despite significant advances in the clinical care of patients with ARDS, survival rates remain essentially unchanged at ~50%. Although fewer patients actually die of respiratory failure, many succumb to multisystem organ failure. Approximately 50% of patients with unresolving ARDS develop multisystem organ failure with the kidney being the second most common organ to fail. ARDS with concomitant hepatic failure has almost 100% mortality (5).

References

1. Ashbough DG, Bigelow DB, Petty TL. Acute respiratory distress in adults. Lancet 2:320, 1967.
2. Fowler AA, Hemman RF, Zerbe GO, Bensen KN, Hyers TM. Adult respiratory distress syndrome; progress after onset. Am Rev Resp Dis 132:472–478, 1985.
3. Bernard GR, Artigas A, Brigham KL, Carlet J, Falke K, Hudson L, Lamy M, LeGall JR, Morris A, Spragg R. Report of the American-European consensus conference on ARDS: definitions, mechanisms, relevant outcomes and clinical trial coordination. Intensive Care Med 20:225–232, 1994.
4. Cunningham AJ. Acute respiratory distress syndrome—two decades later. The Yale J Biol Med 64:387–402, 1991.
5. Demling RH. Adult respiratory distress syndrome: Current concepts. New Horizons 1(3): 388–401, 1993.
6. Bachofen M, Weitel ER. Alteration of the gas exchange apparatus in adult respiratory insufficiency associated with septicimia. Am Rev Resp Dis 116:589–615, 1977.
7. Wiener-Kronish JP, Gropper MA, Matthay MA. The adult respiratory distress syndrome: Definition and prognosis, pathogenesis and treatment. Br Anaesth 65:107–129, 1990.
8. Goldsberry KT, Hurst JM. Adult respiratory distress syndrome and sepsis. New Horizons 1(2): 342–347, 1993.
9. Strieter RM, Lynch JP, Basha MA, Standiford TJ, Kasahara K, Kunkel SL. Host responses in mediating sepsis and adult respiratory distress syndrome. Semin Respir Infect 5(3):233–247, 1990.
10. Roten R, Market M, Feihl F, Schaller M-D, Tagan M-C, Perret C. Plasma levels of tumor necrosis factor in the adult respiratory distress syndrome. Am Rev Respir Dis 143: 590–592, 1991.
11. Dehring DJ, Wismer BC. Intravascular macrophages in pulmonary capilaries of humans. Am Rev Respir Dis 139:1027–1029, 1989.

12. Meduri GU, Headley S, Kohler G, Stentz F, Tolley E, Umberger R, Leeper K. Persistent elevation of inflammatory cytokines predicts a poor outcome in ARDS. Chest 107:1062–1073, 1995.
13. Fink A, Geva D, Zung A, Konichezky S, Eliraz A, Bentwich Z. Adult respiratory distress syndrome: Role of leukotriene C4 and platelet activating factor. Crit Care Med 18:925–990, 1990.
14. Robbins RA, Russ WD, Thoriask R, Rasmussen JK, Kay HD. Activation of the complement system in the adult respiratory distress syndrome. Am Rev Resp Dis 135:651–658, 1987.
15. Riserg B, Smith L, Örtenwall P. Oxygen radicals and lung injury. Acta Anaesthesiol Scand 35(Suppl. 95):106–118, 1991.
16. Griffith MD, Garcia JG, James HL, Callahan KS, Iriana S, Holiday D. Hyperoxic exposure in humans. Chest 101:392–397, 1992.
17. The Veterans Administration Systemic Sepsis Study Group (1987). The effects of high dose glucocorticoid therapy on mortality in patients with clinical signs of systemic sepsis. N Engl J Med 317:659–665, 1987.
18. Meduri GU, Chinn AJ, Leeper KV, Wunderink RG, Tolley E, Winer-Muram HT, Khare V, Eltkorky M. Corticosteroid rescue treatment of progressive fibroproloiferation in late ARDS: patterns of response and predictors of outcome. Chest 105:1516–1527, 1994.
19. Baker AB, McGinn A, Joyce C. Effect on lung volumes of oxygen concentration when breathing is restricted. Br J Anaesth 70:259–266, 1993.
20. Cane RD, O'Lenic T, Downs JB. Ventilation:perfusion relationships are adversely affected by breathing oxygen concentrations below 50%. Anesthesiology 81(3A):A273, 1994.
21. Marshall BE, Clarke WR, Costarino AT, Chen L, Miller F, Marshall C. The dose response relationship for hypoxic pulmonary vasoconstriction. Respiratory Physiology 96:231–247, 1994.
22. Murdoch CG, Gill P, Cane RD, Downs JB, Smith DB, Novitsky D. Changes in perfusion, not ventilation, mediate V_A/Q responses to augmented F_IO_2. Crit Care Med 24:A28, 1996.
23. Douglas ME, Downs JB, Dannemiller FJ, Hodges MR, Munson ES. Change in pulmonary venous admixture with varying inspired oxygen. Anesth Analg 55:688–695, 1976.
24. Steinberg H, Greenwald RA, Moak SA, DiPak DK. The effect of oxygen adaptation on oxyradical lung injury to pulmonary epitelium. Am Rev Resp Dis 128:94, 1983.
25. Mason FJ. Phospolipid syntesis in primary colutes of type II alveolar cells. Am Rev Resp Dis 115:352, 1977.
26. Tsuno K, Miura K, Takeya M, Kolobow T, Morioka T. Histopathologic pulmonary changes from mechanical ventilation at high peak airway pressures. Am Rev Respir Dis 43:1115–1120, 1991.
27. Kolobow T, Moretti M, Fumagilli R, Mascheroni D, Prato P, Chen V, Joris M. Severe impairment in lung function induced by high peak airway pressure during mechanical ventilation—an experimental study. Am Rev Respir Dis 135:312–315, 1987.
28. Dreyfuss D, Basset G, Soler P, Saumon G. Intermittent positive-pressure hyperventilation with high inflation pressures produces pulmonary microvascular injury in rats. Am Rev Respir Dis 132:880–884, 1985.
29. Dreyfuss D, Soler P, Basset G, Saumon G. High inflation pressure pulmonary edema—respiratory effects of high airway pressure, high tidal volume, and positive end-expiratory pressure. Am Rev Respir Dis 137:1159–1164, 1988.
30. Dreyfuss D, Saumon G. Role of tidal volume, FRC, and end-inspiratory volume in the development of pulmonary edema following mechanical ventilation. Am Rev Respir Dis 148:1194–1203, 1993.
31. Zapol W. Volotrauma and the intravenous oxygenator in patients with adult respiratory distress syndrome [Editorial]. Anesthesiology 77:847–849, 1992.
32. Darioli R, Perret C. Mechanical controlled hypoventilation in status asthmaticus. Am Rev Respir Dis 129:385–387, 1984.
33. Hickling K, Henderson S, Jackson R. Low mortality associated with low volume, pressure limited

ventilation with permissive hypercapnia in severe respiratory distress syndrome. Intensive Care Med 16:372–377, 1990.

34. Feihl EF, Perret C. Permissive hypercapnia: How permissive should we be? Am J Respir Crit Care Med 150:1722–1737, 1994.

35. Roupie E, Dambrosia M, Servillo G, Mentec H, El Atrous S, Beydon L, Brun-Biusson C, Lemaire F, Brochard L. Titration of tidal volume and induced hypercapnia in acute respiratory distress syndrome. Am J Respir Crit Care Med 152:121–128, 1995.

36. Nahum A, Burke W, Ravenscroft S, Marcy T, Adams A, Crooke P, Marini J. Lung mechanics and gas exchange during pressure control ventilation in dogs: augmentation of CO_2 elimination by an intratracheal catheter. Am Rev Respir Dis 146:965–973, 1992.

37. Gilbert J, Bunegin L, Larsson A, Smith R, Erian R, Soloman D, Rogers J, Otte W. Intermittent flow expiratory ventilation: new technique of limited excursion pulmonary ventilation. Crit Care Med 19(S):1086–1089, 1991.

38. Hamilton P, Onayemi A, Smyth J, Gilan J, Cutz E, Fraese A, Bryan A. Comparison of conventional and high-frequency ventilation: oxygenation and lung pathology. J Appl Physiol 55: 131–138, 1983.

39. Nielsen J, Sjostrand V, Edgren E, Lichtwarck-Aschoff M, Svensoon B. An experimental study of different ventilatory modes in piglets in severe respiratory distress induced by surfactant depletion. Intensive Care Med 17:225–233, 1991.

40. Meyer J, Hachenberg T, Tippert G, Mollhoff T, Wendt M. High frequency ventilation in experimental pulmonary emphysema. Intensive Care Med 17:377–382, 1991.

41. Clark R, Gerstmann D, Null D, deLamas R. Prospective randomized comparison of high-frequency oscillatory and conventional ventilation in respiratory distress syndrome. Pediatrics 89: 5–12, 1992.

42. Keszler M, Donn S, Bucciarelli R, Alverson D, Hart M, Lunyen V, Modanla HD, Noguchi A, Peerman SA, Puri A, Smith D, Stavis R, Watkins MN, Harris TR. Multicenter controlled trial comparing high-frequency jet ventilation and conventional mechanical ventilation in newborn infants with pulmonary interstitial emphysema. J Pediatr 119:85–93, 1991.

43. The HFI Study Group. High-frequency oscillatory ventilation compared with conventional mechanical ventilation in the treatment of respiratory failure in preterm infants. N Engl J Med 320:88–93, 1989.

44. Carlo W, Siner B, Chatburn R, Robertson S, Martin R. Early randomized intervention with high-frequency jet ventilation in respiratory distress syndrome. J Pediatr 117:765–770, 1990.

45. HFI Study Group. High-frequency oscillatory ventilation compared with conventional intermittent mechanical ventilation in the treatment of respiratory failure in preterm infants: neurodevelopmental status at 16 to 24 months of post-term age. J Pediatr 117:939–946, 1990.

46. Slutsky A. High-frequency ventilation [Editorial]. Intensive Care Med 17:375–376, 1991.

47. Rasanen J, Cane RD, Downs JB, Hurst JM, Jousela I, Kirby RR, Rogove HJ, Stock MC. Airway pressure release ventilation during acute lung injury—a prospective multicenter trial. Crit Care Med 19:1234–1241, 1991.

48. Cane RD, Peruzzi W, Shapiro B. Airway pressure release ventilation in severe acute respiratory failure. Chest 100:460–463, 1991.

49. Valentine D, Hammond M, Downs J, Sears N, Sims W. Distribution of ventilation and perfusion with different modes of mechanical ventilation. Am Rev Respir Dis 143:1262–1266, 1991.

50. Räsänen J, Downs J. Are new ventilatory modalities really different? [Editorial]. Chest 100: 299–300, 1991.

51. Garner W, Downs J, Stock M, Rasanen J. Airway pressure release ventilation: a human trial. Chest 94:779–781,1988.

52. Räsänen J. IMPRV—synchronized APRV or more? [Editorial]. Intensive Care Med 18:65–66, 1992.

53. Rouby JJ, Benameur M, Jawish D, Cherif A, Andreev A, Dreux S, Viars P. Continuous positive airway pressure (CPAP) vs intermittent mandatory pressure release ventilation (IMPRV) in patients with acute respiratory failure. Intensive Care Med 18:69–75, 1992.
54. Bakke FA, Downs JB, Smith R, Räsänen J. Constant mean airway pressure ventilation (CMAPV), a physiologically designed ventilatory mode. Crit Care Med 1996; 24:A101
55. Zapol W, Snider M, Hill J, Fallat RJ, Bartlett RH, Edmunds H, Morris AH, Peirce EC, Thomas AN, Procter HJ, Drinker PA, Pratt PC, Bagniewski A, Miller RG. Extracorporeal membrane oxygenation in severe acute respiratory failure. JAMA 242:2193–2196, 1979.
56. Gattinoni L, Kolobow T, Tomlenson T, Iapichino G, Samaja M, White D, Pierce J. Low-frequency positive pressure ventilation with extracorporeal carbon dioxide removal (LFPPV-ECCO$_2$R): An experimental study. Anesth Analg 57:470–477, 1978.
57. Gattinoni L, Pesenti A, Mascheroni D, Marcolin R, Fumagali R. Low-frequency positive pressure ventilation with extracorporeal CO$_2$ removal in severe acute respiratory failure. JAMA 256: 881–886, 1986.
58. Rossaint RK, Falke J, Lopez F, Slama K, Pison V, Zapol W. Inhaled nitric oxide for the adult respiratory distress syndrome. N Engl J Med 328:399–405, 1993.
59. Payen DM, Gatecel C, Plaisance P. Almitrine effect on nitric oxide inhalation in adult respiratory distress syndrome. Lancet 3;34:1664, 1993.
60. Chollet-Martin S, Gatecel C, Kermarrec N, Gougerot-Pocidalo M-A, Payen D. Alveolar neutrophil functions and cytokine levels in patients with the adult respiratory distress syndrome during nitric oxide inhalation. Am J Resp Crit Care Med 153:985–990, 1996.
61. Walmrath D, Schneider T, Schermuly R, Olschweski H, Grimminger F, Seeger W. Direct comparison of inhaled nitric oxide and aerosolized prostacyclin in acute respiratory distress syndrome. Am J Resp Crit Care Med 153:991–996, 1996.
62. Lakshminarayan S, Standford RE, Petty TL. Prognosis after recovery from adult respiratory distress syndrome. Am Rev Resp Dis 13:7–16, 1976.
63. Peters JI, Bell RC, Prihoda TJ, Harris G, Andrews C, Johanson WG. Clinical determinants of abnormalities in pulmonary function in survivors of the adult respiratory distress syndrome. Am Rev Resp Dis 139:1163–1168, 1989.
64. Klein JJ, van Haeringen, Sluiter HJ. Pulmonary function after recovery from the adult respiratory distress syndrome. Chest 69(3):350–355, 1976.

20
Chronic Obstructive Pulmonary Disease and Asthma

Eric G. Honig

Respiratory failure due to obstructive lung disease differs from failure due to trauma or acute lung injury in several ways. The physiologic failure is one of ventilation and CO_2 removal. Hypoxia is more easily managed than the shunt hypoxia of acute lung injury. Mechanically, lung volume is increased rather than decreased, although effective compliance may be reduced at the higher lung volumes caused by hyperinflation and air-trapping. Expiratory times are prolonged owing to significantly increased airway resistance. Inadequate time for exhalation results in increased volumes of trapped gas, further hyperinflation, barotrauma, and the potential for iatrogenic lung injury. The primary focus of management of patients with respiratory failure due to obstructive lung disease should be more toward improvement of deranged mechanics than to defense of gas exchange.

ACUTE SEVERE ASTHMA

Incidence

The prevalence of asthma has increased in the United States and comparable industrialized nations for the past 15–20 years. Asthma mortality has similarly increased. In the United States, African-Americans, women, children, and the urban poor have been identified as at particular risk for asthma. The reasons for the increase in morbidity and mortality are not entirely clear, but declining air quality, especially in cities, is felt to play an important role (1,2). Considerable concern exists about the role of beta adrenergic agonists in the rising morbidity from asthma. Epidemics of asthma mortality in England in the 1960s and New Zealand in the 1970s suggested a dose-dependent association between asthma mortality risk and the regular use of beta agonists. The epidemiologic evidence is less impressive when the data are controlled for severity of disease, and mortality risk is significantly reduced when inhaled corticosteroids are included in the medical regimen. Bench studies suggest a possible dissociation between the bronchodilating effects of beta agonists and their mast cell stabilizing properties that permit increased and prolonged exposures to airway irritants. The strength of the evidence is not sufficient to mandate the deletion inhaled beta adrenergic agonists from the list of agents used to control chronic asthma (3). These concerns do not apply to the short-term use of beta agonists in the treatment of acute severe asthma.

Although asthma mortality is increasing, status asthmaticus requiring mechanical ventilation is a relatively unusual event (4) because near fatal or fatal asthma is often a sudden, catastrophic asphyxic event that may cause death even before the patient reaches medical attention. The appropriate focus should be on the identification of high risk patients and intensive medical management, especially with inhaled antiinflammatory agents. The best treatment of status asthmaticus is to treat it 3 days before it occurs (5). Less than 3% of asthmatics requiring mechanical ventilation in one series received adequate doses (>800–1000 μg/d) of inhaled corticosteroids (6). This is in keeping with our own experience. Patients at risk for potentially fatal asthma characteristically have had previous episodes of severe asthma that required intubation and mechanical ventilation or hospitalization. They often require oral corticosteroids for symptomatic control, tend to run low peak expiratory flow rates, and may have had prior episodes of pneumothorax or pneumomediastinum associated with a previous exacerbation of their asthma. They are heavy users of beta agonists for symptomatic relief. Their estimated mortality risk over 5 years is 7% compared with 1–7/100,000 for more stable asthmatics (7).

Bronchodilators

Respiratory failure due to acute severe asthma that requires mechanical ventilation has become the exception rather than the rule. Intensive bronchodilator therapy usually can reverse severe bronchospasm.

Aggressive bronchodilator therapy remains the mainstay of therapy for acute severe asthma. Delivery of bronchodilator medication by metered dose inhalers (MDI) with added spacers has been shown to be as effective as by nebulizers, is more economical in terms of medication and personnel costs, and is the current approach of choice.

Although objective monitoring of response to bronchodilators with spirometry or peak flow measurement is frequently recommended, it is less often done in actual practice. In the absence of objective measurements, bronchodilator therapy should be titrated to desirable clinical endpoints—the relief of dyspnea and wheezing and against side effects.

BETA AGONISTS

Beta adrenergic agonists have been shown to be the most effective agents for the treatment of acute severe asthma. Most patients can be managed by the inhaled

Table 20.1. Beta Adrenergic Agonists

Drug	MDI + Spacer	Nebulized	Frequency
Albuterol	4 puffs	2.5 mg	q 20–60 min
Metaproterenol	3 puffs	15 mg	q 20–60 min

route, but when response is unsatisfactory, subcutaneous administration may be effective. Intravenous beta agonists should be used with caution in patients over 40 years of age or in those with known heart disease, and they should be regarded as an approach of last resort.

Recommended drugs and dosages are shown in Table 20.1. Good results have been reported with continuously nebulized albuterol. If subcutaneous treatment is needed, either epinephrine (0.3 mg) or terbutaline (0.25 mg) is usually employed. Terbutaline may cause more tachycardia than epinephrine when given subcutaneously. Tachycardia is often seen with beta agonist therapy, and intensive beta agonist therapy may cause worsening of ventilation-perfusion relationships and more severe hypoxemia. Beta agonists, especially when used parenterally, may cause hypokalemia by interfering with the Na-K (adenosine triphosphatase [ATPase]) pump system. Serum potassium should be watched closely when intensive beta therapy is used. Lactic acidosis has been reported with beta agonist therapy. Tachyphylaxis to beta agonists has not been reported in the acute care setting.

Anticholinergics

The role of anticholinergic agents in the management of acute severe asthma is poorly defined. In general, there seems to be little added benefit to anticholinergic agents when maximal doses of a beta agonist are used. Anticholinergic agents can be added when response to beta agonist therapy is unsatisfactory, when chronic obstructive lung disease coexists with asthma, or for beta blocker induced asthma (8). Three anticholinergic agents are available in the United States: atropine sulfate, ipratropium bromide, and glycopyrrolate. Systemic absorption and a narrow therapeutic window have led to the preferred use of the latter two agents, both quartenary ammonium compounds (Table 20.2).

Table 20.2. Anticholingergic Bronchodilators

Drug	MDI + Spacer	Nebulized	Frequency
Ipratropium bromide	4–10 puffs	0.5 mg	q 20 min by MDI q 60 min by neb
Glycopyrrolate		2 mg	q 120 min

For convenience, either ipratropium and glycopyrrolate may be mixed with a beta agonist in the same nebulizer. Although the quartenary anticholinergics are well-tolerated, they should be used with caution in the setting of angle-closure glaucoma and in patients with symptomatic prostatism. A paradoxical constrictor response to ipratropium, which may be related to diluent or preservative, has been reported in 4%–20% of patients. Although anticholinergics may cause mouth dryness, they have not been found to dry and thicken mucous secretions in patients with asthma.

Theophylline

Although theophylline was for many years a first line agent, emergency room-based studies in the 1980s firmly established that theophylline was less potent than beta agonists. Meta-analysis failed to demonstrate an objective advantage to adding theophylline to maximal beta adrenergic therapy. Nevertheless, theophylline has not disappeared from the pharmacopeia, perhaps because of its nonbronchodilator properties as a centrally acting respiratory stimulant and as an enhancer of diaphragmatic contractility. Theophylline has a narrow therapeutic window. Toxicity includes nausea and vomiting, tachycardia and arrhythmias, and seizures. Theophylline levels should be titrated to 10 to 15 μg/ml, although toxicity may be seen at levels <10 μg/ml; levels >20 μg/ml may be well-tolerated by some. Theophylline is best reserved for patients who are poorly responsive to inhaled bronchodilators.

If the patient is not receiving a theophylline preparation on presentation, or if initial theophylline level is <2 μg/ml, a loading dose of 5 mg/kg theophylline (6 mg/kg aminophylline) may be safely administered by slow infusion followed by a continuous infusion of 0.4 mg/kg/hour (0.5 mg/kg/hour aminophylline). If the admission theophylline level is unknown or is already therapeutic, the loading dose should be omitted. Oral elixir theophylline is as effective as the parenteral form and may be used instead of infusions. Half-life for theophylline is ~12 hours, but may be as short as 8–9 hours in smokers. Theophylline levels drawn earlier than four half-lives after a step change in the dosage should be interpreted as an incomplete process. If a patient becomes theophylline toxic, administration should be held for one to two half-lives and then resumed at a dose decreased by 25%–30%.

Steroids

Objective evidence from emergency room studies supports the important role of corticosteroids in the management of acute severe asthma. Corticosteroids reduce inflammatory activity and decrease microvascular permeability, working through messenger RNA and changes in protein synthesis. Steroids appear to

Table 20.3. Corticosteroid Preparations

Drug	Route	Relative Potency	Dose
Prednisone	Oral	4	60 mg initially then 60–120 mg daily in divided doses
Methylprednisolone	Oral	5	As above
Hydrocortisone	Intravenous	1	2 mg/kg bolus then 0.5 mg/kg/hr
Methylprednisolone	Intravenous	5	60–80 mg q 6–8h

potentiate response of the beta receptor to adrenergic agonists, but because of the molecular basis for their action, may take 6 hours or more to demonstrate a significant response. Systemic steroid administration on arrival in the emergency room may reduce the need for hospitalization; it appears to decrease both the risk of death associated with the episode and the likelihood of a relapse after emergency room discharge.

Although there is general acceptance of systemic corticosteroid use in acute severe asthma, there is less agreement about the appropriate dose. Commonly used preparations and doses are shown in Table 20.3. From available evidence, it would appear that 30 mg of a prednisone equivalent administered every 4 hours is the minimal effective dose, but it remains to be established whether higher doses produce significantly better outcomes. Oral prednisone is as effective as intravenous hydrocortisone or methylprednisolone, although the parenteral route is generally chosen for patients at risk for intubation. Although inhaled corticosteroid preparations give no additional benefit to systemic preparations, some clinicians elect to continue their use so as not to confuse patients about their importance in asthma maintenance care. Patients should be switched to an oral steroid preparation at the earliest possible moment and then continued on the equivalent of 60–80 mg/day prednisone for 7 to 10 days. Unless patients were previously steroid dependent, they may be rapidly tapered off prednisone at that time.

Antibiotics

Few episodes of acute severe asthma are caused by infection and even fewer are bacterial in origin. Therefore, antibiotics are not routinely needed. Purulent sputum may reflect eosinophils and allergy rather than neutrophils and infection. Wright's staining sputum may prove helpful for differentiation. Chest radiographs are rarely helpful in the management of asthma exacerbations unless strong clinical suspicion exists for an active process. They are helpful in only 1%–5% of cases.

Oxygen

Disturbances in oxygenation are usually relatively mild in acute severe asthma. O_2 needs are generally modest. True shunt is unusual, and only 5% of patients show a PaO_2 <55 mmHg. Humidified oxygen should be provided, titrated to produce near normal saturation. CO_2 retention does not complicate oxygen administration to acute asthmatics.

Other Modalities

Several other therapeutic modalities have been applied in cases of severe asthma refractory to standard therapy. Although successful on occasion, none of these modalities have been sufficiently useful to recommend their routine use, and further study is needed to define an appropriate role for most.

$MgSO_4$

Magnesium sulfate ($MgSO_4$) may relax smooth muscle and may interfere with acetylcholine release at the neuromuscular junction. Several small studies have demonstrated bronchodilator activity in asthmatics or protection against antigen challenge. In acute severe asthma, intravenous $MgSO_4$, given as 10–12 mmol (10–20 g) over 20 minutes or a 1–2 g bolus, has failed to show clinically significant benefit when peak expiratory flow rate (PEFR) is <200 L/minute or when there is poor response to albuterol. Side effects of magnesium administration include hypotension, flushing, mild sedation, and decreased deep tendon reflexes. Serum Mg^{++} should be monitored if $MgSO_4$ is administered.

HeO_2 (HELIOX)

Helium has a lower density than air and its use leads to lower resistive pressure drops across narrowed airways. The resulting reduction in the work of breathing may help a severely ill asthmatic postpone intubation until a corticosteroid effect becomes apparent and the decreased resistance may decrease high inflation pressures in the ventilated asthmatic patient. Helium is customarily mixed with oxygen as 80:20 helium:oxygen. HeO_2 has been employed as a temporizing measure in patients with pH <7.2, or a $PaCO_2$ >50 mmHg. It has been used in ventilated patients with peak inflation pressures ≥75 cmH$_2$O. The average duration of use for heliox in asthma has been ~ 6 hours. Heliox should be employed before resorting to inhalational anesthetics (9,10).

INHALATION ANESTHETICS

Halogenated fluorocarbon inhalation general anesthetics have been used in extremely severe refractory patients who are already mechanically ventilated. Halothane, enflurane, and isoflurane have modest bronchodilating properties that facilitate relaxation, and they may be effective in decreasing peak inflation pressures. These agents rarely are needed in the clinical setting. Of the three gases, isoflurane may offer the best combination of efficacy and safety.

BRONCHOSCOPY

Because widespread mucus plugging may play a prominent role in the pathophysiology of an acute asthma attack, therapeutic bronchoscopic lavage with or without acetylcysteine has been anecdotally reported to be of benefit in a few refractory cases by relieving plugging. In our experience, bronchoscopy is rarely necessary. Because of its irritant potential, acetylcysteine use should be restricted to 48–72 hours only.

Indications for Ventilation

Only about 5% of patients with acute severe asthma will require intubation and mechanical ventilation. The decision to ventilate a patient is a clinical one. It should be based on deteriorating status, impending or actual cardiac or respiratory arrest, decreasing level of consciousness, cyanosis, a silent chest, worsening paradox, or diaphoresis. Orthopneic patients often require intubation as do patients with a respiratory rate >30 breaths/minute, a heart rate >120 beats/minute, or a pulsus paradoxus >12 mmHg. Response in the first 2 hours to the medical regimen outlined above may have predictive utility. The clinical trend is probably more important than the initial findings. Objective measurements of airflow may be helpful, but spirometric efforts may paradoxically worsen bronchospasm or precipitate respiratory arrest. This reaction can be blocked with intravenous atropine. Arterial blood gases should be checked initially; serial blood gases are usually not needed. An increasing $PaCO_2$ correlates with severe obstruction with FEV_1 <25% predicted, but does not absolutely predict the need for intubation. Metabolic acidosis is seen in 28% of patients. This is most often lactic acidemia, due either to respiratory muscle activity or to beta adrenergic agonists.

MANAGEMENT OF VENTILATION

In the acute asthmatic state, airway resistance is markedly increased and time constants for expiration are significantly prolonged. When a patient breathes at high respiratory rates and minute volumes, there may be insufficient time for complete exhalation before the next inspired breath. This leads to progressive hyperinflation. Dynamic functional residual capacity (FRC) will be established at a lung volume above the static FRC of the respiratory system, often on a flatter portion of the lung's pressure-volume curve. The degree of dynamic hyperinflation is proportional to tidal volume, and inversely related to the ratio of expiratory time (T_E) to the time constant for expiration. The recoil pressure associated with the increased FRC is auto-PEEP, which constitutes an added mechanical load against which the patient must work to initiate inspiratory airflow. The reduction in effective compliance at these higher lung volumes adds a further elastic load to the patient's work of breathing. Elevated alveolar pressure at end-inspiration poses a significant risk for barotrauma.

The goal of mechanical ventilation in acute severe asthma is to provide a physiologically adequate minute volume, while minimizing the risk of dynamic hyperinflation, auto-PEEP, and barotrauma. Mechanical considerations, especially the optimization of expiratory time, should take precedence over the normalization of blood gases. Ventilation to eucapnia often leads to dynamic hyperinflation and should not be regarded as an appropriate objective.

Ventilator Settings

Mechanically ventilated asthmatics should initially be placed in the controlled ventilation mode (CMV). Initial settings should provide a tidal volume of 8–10 ml/kg, a rate of 8–14 breaths/minute, with an inspiratory flow rate of 80–100 L/minute. Minute volume should be kept <115 ml/kg/minute. These settings generally result in a moderate respiratory acidosis with a pH ~ 7.2, and they usually avoid an unacceptable degree of hyperinflation, defined as an end-inspiratory volume >20 ml/kg (4). Further adjustments should be made to minute volume and T_E based on arterial blood gases and examination of the patient. Prolongation of T_E may be accomplished by reduction of frequency or tidal volume, or by increases in inspiratory flow rate or the inspiratory-to-expiratory (I/E) ratio. Closer examination of the relationships among volume, flow, and T_E demonstrates that increases in the I/E ratio or reductions in tidal volume are relatively inefficient in prolonging T_E. Increases in inspiratory flow can be somewhat helpful at higher minute volumes, but the most efficient maneuver to prolong T_E is to decrease the respiratory rate or minute volume ($\dot{V}_E$). (Fig. 20.1). Use of a square wave form will shorten inspiratory time and prolong TE. A square wave will increase peak inspiratory pressure but it does not affect alveolar pressure. Low compliance tubing permits a lower set tidal volume to produce a given delivered tidal volume. Increases in inspiratory flow rates will produce higher peak inflation pressures, but these are not reflected in significantly increased alveolar pressure or in increased risk of barotrauma.

Extrinsic PEEP is an option that should be used with caution. Applied PEEP at levels up to 85% of the auto-PEEP level may reduce the work of breathing, relieving airflow obstruction by strutting open narrowed airways, and by counteracting the inspiratory threshold load imposed by auto-PEEP. If too much external PEEP is applied, however, alveolar volume may increase, worsening hypererinfla-

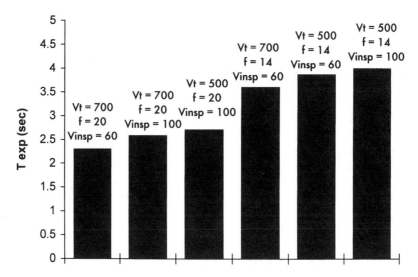

Figure 20.1. Comparison of effects of increasing inspiratory flow rate, decreasing tidal volume, and decreasing minute volume on expiratory time.

tion. Auto-PEEP and applied PEEP are additive in terms of their effects on cardiac preload (11–15).

Delivery of Bronchodilators

Intensive bronchodilator therapy should continue even after the asthma patient is placed on mechanical ventilation. Bronchodilator delivery via the ventilator is less efficient than via spontaneous breathing. Significant losses occur in the ventilator and endotracheal tubing, but therapeutic results can be achieved with higher doses given either by nebulizer or by metered dose inhaler (MDI). The scientific basis for delivery of aerosols to ventilated patients is still being worked out, and optimal doses remain to be determined. The best approach is to titrate to effect and against toxicity. The gradient between peak inflation pressure and plateau pressure can be used to titrate bronchodilator doses to achieve at least a 15% improvement. The best site for delivering bronchodilators is above the Y-connection into the inspiratory limb. A longer inspiratory time gives better delivery but at the cost of decreased T_E and increased dynamic hyperinflation. Deposition is improved by low tidal and minute volumes and by a longer inspiratory pause. Humidifiers in the ventilator circuit decrease deposition and should be bypassed during bronchodilator delivery.

Ventilator delivery via MDI is ~50% that for a spontaneously breathing patient. Holding chambers appear to produce better delivery of active drug than in-line devices, but optimal chamber size and design remain to be determined. When a chamber is used, the MDI should be actuated at end-expiration. Actuation should begin with inspiration for in-line adapters. A 2- to 3-second inspiratory pause should be used if possible. A therapeutic albuterol dose via MDI is 4–20 puffs (360–1800 μg), given up to every 20 minutes and is equivalent to 2.5–10 mg nebulized albuterol.

Delivery via small volume nebulizers is extremely variable, varying four- to fivefold depending on the device and position in the ventilator circuit. Nebulizers are less efficient than MDI delivery, needing doses ten times those for an MDI to achieve the same physiologic effect. Nebulizers do have the advantage of delivering medication on a continuous basis. Clinical efficacy is improved by using larger solution volumes (4 ml) and higher gas flow rates in the range of 8 L/minute (16–19).

Fluids

Asthmatics in particular are subject to hypotension following intubation for acute respiratory failure. Hypotension may be seen in up to 35% of cases and may be potentiated by intravenous sedatives. Volume replacement with infusion of crystalloid is usually sufficient treatment. Caution must be exercised not to overhydrate because the wide swings of pleural pressure in severe asthma may contribute to the development of pulmonary edema.

Controlled Hypoventilation

In mechanical ventilation for asthma and acute respiratory failure in chronic obstructive pulmonary disease (COPD), avoidance of ventilator-associated injury should take precedence over normalization of blood gases. The level of ventilatory support should be titrated to a tolerable level of respiratory acidosis. Recent studies seem to reflect a reduction in mortality in ventilated acute severe asthma, although it is not entirely clear whether deliberate hypoventilation can be credited for this improvement (20). Indeed, review of available data fails to demonstrate a significant reduction in barotrauma or hypotension with this approach. More work is needed to clarify this issue. It has been demonstrated that hypercapnia is usually well-tolerated up to $PaCO_2$ 90 mmHg, particularly when evolution is slow. If the patient cannot be safely ventilated to normocapnia because of high minute volumes, auto-PEEP, dynamic hyperinflation, or excessive alveolar pressure, minute volume may be reduced, allowing $PaCO_2$ to rise by 10 mmHg/hour to a maximum of 80–90 mmHg. PaO_2 should be kept >50 mmHg. Heavy sedation and paralysis may be needed because of increased drive. Elevated intracranial pressure represents an absolute contraindication to controlled hypoventilation.

Although papilledema due to hypercapnia is relatively uncommon, funduscopic examinations should be followed.

Deliberate acidosis should be reversed slowly to avoid post-hypercapnic alkalosis. The common practice is to attempt to correct pH when pH falls below 7.15–7.20. The goal is partial, rather than complete correction of pH. When controlled hypoventilation leads to significant respiratory acidosis, choices for correction are sodium bicarbonate, TRIS (THAM, tromethamine), and carbicarb.

Sodium bicarbonate is the agent most commonly used to compensate for respiratory acidosis. The bicarbonate to be administered is calculated based on the bicarbonate deficit and the bicarbonate space, which is 50% of body weight. Administration of bicarbonate presents a sodium load and does not account for urinary HCO_3 loss or for newly generated CO_2.

TRIS (THAM, tromethamine) does not generate CO_2. It presents no sodium load, but poses potential problems with hypoglycemia, hypotension, and left shifting of the oxyhemoglobin dissociation curve. TRIS requires intact renal function. The dose for TRIS at 0.3M is calculated as the desired change in bicarbonate multiplied by body weight in kilograms. A typical dose is 200–500 ml given over 30 minutes.

Carbicarb is composed of Na carbonate and bicarbonate, each at 0.33 M concentration, and has a higher pK (9.6) than the bicarbonate system. Buffering is mostly by Na carbonate, generating bicarbonate. Carbicarb has not been tested clinically.

ALTERNATIVE TECHNIQUES

High frequency ventilation is absolutely contraindicated because the prolonged expiratory time constants predispose to hyperinflation and barotrauma in the presence of such a rapid respiratory rate.

ADJUNCTIVE MEASURES

Sedation and Paralysis

Sedation and muscular relaxation are recommended during the initial stages of mechanical ventilation, allowing the patient to sleep and to rest the respiratory muscles (Table 20.4). Sedatives should not be used to correct dyssynchrony with the ventilator unless attempts at ventilator adjustment have failed to produce better patient-ventilator interaction. Sedatives should be titrated to drowsiness and response to voice or light touch. The most commonly used sedative agents include the benzodiazepines lorazepam and midazolam, propofol, fentanyl, and haloperidol. In choosing a sedative agent, one should distinguish among the states that are being treated: delirium, pain, anxiety and discomfort. Haloperidol antago-

Table 20.4. Commonly Used Sedatives in the Intensive Care Unit

Drug	Class	Dosage	Time Factors	Metabolism
Fentanyl	Opioid	10–100 µg bolus 0.02–0.5 µg/kg/min 120–240 µg/kg/hr usual	Onset <60 sec Duration 60–240 min $T_{1/2}$ 200 min	Liver, biotransformation, biliary and renal excretion
Lorazepam	Benzodiazepine	1–4 mg q 2–4 hr 0.25–0.5 µg/kg/min 1–2 mg bolus	Onset 2–20 min Duration 4–6 hr $T_{1/2}$ 10–20 hr	Glucuronide conjugation, inactive metabolites excreted via kidney, no accumulation in renal failure
Midazolam	Benzodiazepine	0.03–0.07 mg/kg bolus 0.05–0.1 mg/kg/hr	Onset 2–20 min Duration 30–60 min $T_{1/2}$ 1–2 hr	Hepatic biotransformation; three minimally active metabolites renally excreted
Propofol	Substituted phenol	5 µg/kg/min over 10 min, then 5–50 µg/kg/min	Onset 40 sec Duration 10 min $T_{1/2}$ 1–3 days	Hepatic conjugation, excreted by kidney
Haloperidol	Butyrophenone	0.5–2 mg up to 10 mg IV push; allow 10–20 minutes, then double-dose q 20 minutes to desired effect; repeat last dose as needed; hourly requirements may be converted to infusion	$T_{1/2}$ 3 wk	

nizes dopamine-mediated neurotransmission, leads to better organized thought processes, and is best used to treat delirium. Haloperidol may cause tardive dyskinesia and carries a risk for neuroleptic malignant syndrome and torsades de pointes. Fentanyl is the only one of these agents that also provides analgesic properties. Benzodiazepines are best used for anxiety and generalized discomfort. Lorazepam and midazolam are similar in their pharmacologic profiles, but midazolam is much more expensive. Prolonged use of benzodiazepines may cause tissue accumulation and prolonged depressive effects. Propofol has the advantage of a rapidly titratable level of sedation but may be associated with a lowered seizure threshold (21).

Fentanyl can be reversed with naloxone, and the benzodiazepines can be reversed with flumazenil. When reversal agents are used, the airway should remain protected at all times because airway reflexes recover later than level of consciousness. Rapid reversal always carries the risk of extreme agitation or even seizures.

Neuromuscular blocking agents should be employed for paralysis only when necessary and then as briefly as possible. Indications for paralysis include asynchrony with the ventilator or excessively high inflation pressures. Neuromuscular blockers should never be administered until adequate sedation has been obtained. The nondepolarizing agents *cis*-atracurium or vecuronium are drugs of choice for paralysis. Vecuronium should be avoided in patients with renal failure. Both agents can be administered as a bolus or as continuous infusions. If continuous infusions are used, paralyzing drugs should be held every 4–6 hours to discourage drug accumulation. The paralysis level should be monitored with a nerve stimulator set to train-of-four. Abolition of three of four twitches is considered an appropriate level of paralysis.

MONITORING

The safe ventilatory management of the acute asthmatic calls for the balancing of gas exchange considerations against the risk of hyperinflation and barotrauma. The important determinants of dynamic hyperinflation, tidal volume, and expiratory time should be optimized and followed carefully. Changes in frequency, tidal volume, wave form, and inspiratory flow rates will be reflected in changes in measured airway pressures. Barotrauma, however, has been shown to correlate most closely with trapped gas volume, and with alveolar, rather than airway pressure.

Peak inflation pressure (PIP) is described by the equation:

$$PIP = V_T/C + Vinsp \times R + (PEEP + \text{auto-PEEP})$$

Although high peak pressures are commonly encountered in ventilated asthmatics, most of the measured pressure is related to airway resistance rather than to elevated alveolar pressure. PIP correlates poorly with barotrauma in obstructive pulmonary diseases and no reliable threshold value can be identified. Likewise, the presence or level of auto-PEEP has not been shown to predict the development of barotrauma. Plateau pressure (Pplat) measures airway pressure at the end of inspiration and better reflects alveolar pressure. Peak pressure falls to a plateau exponentially and this process may be prolonged in the presence of airflow obstruction. When measuring Pplat, sufficient time should be allowed to permit a true plateau to be reached. Airway pressure traces on ventilators equipped with graphics modes can be especially helpful for judging plateau adequacy. Pplat somewhat overestimates alveolar pressure. It is advisable to keep Pplat <35 cmH$_2$O to maintain alveolar pressure >30 cmH$_2$O. Pplat, like PIP, may not correlate well with the incidence of barotrauma. Pplat may also vary in reliability because of variations in lung compliance. End-inspiratory lung volume (VEI) has been shown to correlate well with complications of mechanical ventilation. VEI is determined by measuring the amount of air exhaled during a 60-second apnea added to the delivered tidal volume. VEI should be kept >20 ml/kg. This is best accomplished by prolonging TE as much as possible, which is most efficiently achieved by reducing minute ventilation, especially at low breathing frequencies (22) (Fig. 20.2).

Both VEI and auto-PEEP may underestimate the actual degree of hyperinflation and air-trapping if airway closure prevents the free communication of alveoli with the airway opening. Measurement of lung volumes by impedance pneumography or examination of pressure-volume traces may provide alternative evidence of the presence of hyperinflation. In hyperinflation, the pressure-volume trace will show an end-inspiratory flattening manifesting as a "beak" in the curve.

Weaning

Asthma patients should be supported on mechanical ventilation until the bronchospastic process begins to remit. Characteristically, improvement is slow for most of the course, followed by a precipitous improvement in airflow and dyspnea, and a reduction in audible wheezing. As bronchospasm remits, the patient may be switched from CMV to partial support ventilatory modes, such as assist-control (A/CMV), intermittent mandatory ventilation (IMV), synchronized intermittent mandatory ventilation (SIMV), or pressure support ventilation (PSV). IMV and PSV are preferable to A/CMV because of a lower risk for hyperinflation, auto-PEEP, and barotrauma.

With further improvement, patients may be evaluated for weaning, the progressive withdrawal of ventilatory support. Forty percent can be extubated after 24 hours, 70% by 48 hours, and 85% by 5 days. The remainder may take up to 3 weeks to resolve to the point at which extubation is possible. Although clinical judgment usually suffices, a combination of objective measures has been approxi-

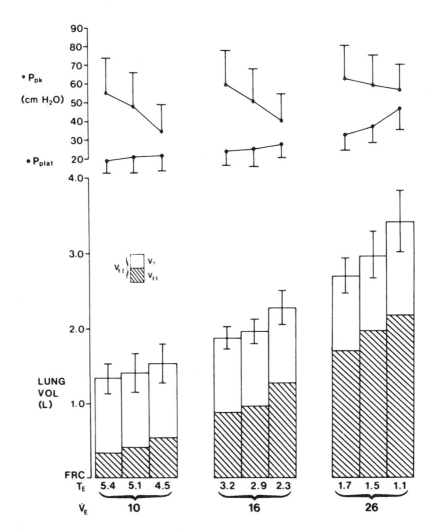

Figure 20.2. Effects of changing $\dot{V}_E$ and T_E at constant tidal volume. Note opposite effects on Ppeak and Pplat as T_E falls at three different levels of minute ventilation (*upper panel*). Note increasing end-inspiratory volume (V_{EI}) and trapped gas volume (V_{EE}) as T_E falls and as $\dot{V}_E$ increases *(lower panel)*. (Reprinted with permission from Tuxen DV, Lane S. The effects of ventilatory pattern on hyperinflation, airway pressures, and circulation in mechanical ventilation of patients with severe air-flow obstruction. Am Rev Respir Dis 136:872–879, 1987.)

mately 75% accurate in predicting weanability, including maximal inspiratory pressure ≤ -25 cmH$_2$O, breathing frequency ≤ 35 breaths/minute, vital capacity ≥ 10 ml/kg body weight, and arterial oxygen saturation $>90\%$ on an F$_1$O$_2$ of $\leq 40\%$ (23,24).

Once asthmatics "break," they can usually be quickly weaned. Because of this, the method used, whether T-piece, IMV, pressure support, or a combination thereof, is relatively unimportant. The respiratory muscles should be reloaded as rapidly as the patient tolerates.

Complications

The major complications associated with mechanical ventilation for acute severe asthma relate to the mechanical consequences of airflow obstruction and are manifested as auto-PEEP and other forms of barotrauma. Acute myopathy associated with corticosteroids and neuromuscular blocking agents is a newly recognized complication of the management of asthmatic respiratory failure.

Auto-peep

Because bronchospasm increases airway resistance several times above normal, time constants for exhalation are significantly prolonged in acute severe asthma. If the asthma patient is breathing spontaneously at high rates or is ventilated at high rates, insufficient time is available for the lung to empty before the next mechanical breath is delivered. This leads to an end-expiratory volume above the mechanical functional residual capacity (FRC) of the respiratory system and is termed *dynamic hyperinflation.* The elastic recoil pressure associated with the elevated volume at end-expiration is manifested as auto-PEEP (intrinsic PEEP, PEEPi, occult PEEP). Virtually 100% of patients ventilated for acute severe asthma or for exacerbations of chronic obstructive lung disease have measurable levels of auto-PEEP that may be as high as 15–20 cmH$_2$O.

Auto-PEEP is a consequence of reduced expiratory airflow, and will occur in the setting of increased airway resistance, increased compliance as is seen in emphysema, and a shortened expiratory time (TE). Continuing inspiratory muscle activity during expiration, as is sometimes seen with ventilator dyssynchrony, can add to auto-PEEP.

Auto-PEEP is associated with dynamic hyperinflation and an increased risk of barotrauma. Auto-PEEP acts in the same way as externally applied PEEP to increase intrathoracic pressure and interfere with venous return to the heart. The consequence is hypotension and a fall in cardiac output. Hypotension due to auto-PEEP may develop within 1–2 minutes of assumption of a rapid breathing pattern and may be reversed as quickly by stopping or slowing the ventilator. Auto-PEEP markedly increases the work of breathing by placing the lung higher on its pressure-volume curve in a region of lower compliance, and by posing an inspiratory threshold load on the respiratory muscles. Airflow cannot be triggered by the patient until a negative pressure equal to set trigger sensitivity plus auto-PEEP is generated. This accounts for the observation of patients expending considerable muscular effort without triggering the ventilator, and may contribute significantly to prolonged ventilator dependence (25–27).

Auto-PEEP can be measured by (*a*) imposing an end-expiratory hold on the ventilator and measuring airway pressure at end-expiration, (*b*) the change in esophageal pressure necessary to produce inspiratory airflow, (*c*) comparing Pplat before and after a prolonged apnea, (*d*) by determining the level of applied PEEP that begins to produce an increase in lung volume. Auto-PEEP can be detected by examination of flow-volume curves on graphics-capable ventilators. Expiratory flow fails to return to zero before the next inspiration begins. Newer generations of microprocessor-driven ventilators are beginning to offer measurements of auto-PEEP as part of their monitoring option packages. Strategies for dealing with dynamic hyperinflation and auto-PEEP were discussed above.

BAROTRAUMA

Pneumothorax, pneumomediastinum, pulmonary tension cysts, subcutaneous emphysema, and pulmonary interstitial emphysema are manifestations of barotrauma, or pressure-induced lung injury that may be seen in any disease process. Barotrauma occurs when alveolar pressures are significantly greater than the surrounding pressure in the interstitial space (28,29). Barotrauma is most commonly caused by alveolar overdistention, but hypovolemia and alveolar capillary underfilling may also contribute to the process. Patients with obstructive pulmonary diseases may be at particular risk for regional overdistention because of the uneven distribution of airway resistance. Recently published series suggest the incidence of pneumothorax in acute severe asthma is 10%–15% and other forms of barotrauma occur in about 12% of cases (4,6,20). Strategies for minimizing alveolar overdistention are the same as those for reducing auto-PEEP discussed above.

ACUTE MYOPATHY

Recent reports have called attention to the occurrence of severe myopathy in patients ventilated for acute severe asthma. The degree of weakness ranges from asymptomatic elevations of serum CK to profound muscular weakness and prolonged ventilator dependence. The myopathy is of acute onset, and involves both proximal and distal muscles differentiating it from pure steroid myopathy, which is subacute and proximal only. Type I and type II fibers are both involved, which distinguishes this form of acute myopathy from critical illness neuropathy, which affects type II fibers only, and is sensorimotor. The incidence, when asymptomatic CK elevations are considered, may be as high as 36%. The syndrome has been attributed to the combined use of corticosteroids and nondepolarizing neuromuscular blocking agents. The amount and duration of neuromuscular blocking agents used appear to be important factors. Although the syndrome was initially attributed to the steroid-ring agents pancuronium and vecuronium, cases have been reported involving atracurium as well. The risk of myopathy can be minimized by using the lowest doses and shortest duration of steroids and neuromuscular blocking agents possible, by monitoring the level of paralysis by muscle stimulator, and by brief drug holidays when continuous infusions of paralyzing agents are used (30,31).

Outcome

Reported mortality from acute severe asthma ranges from 0% to 38% (4,6). Most of these deaths represent anoxic brain injury sustained in the preintubation phase in acute asphyxic presentations. Over the past 10 years, reported mortality has been <10%. Where pressure-limiting strategies have been employed, the aggregate mortality from six series comprising 286 episodes was 2.7% (20).

COPD

Many of the management principles discussed above for acute severe asthma are applicable to the care of patients with acute on chronic respiratory failure (ACRF) associated with chronic obstructive pulmonary disease. The two conditions differ largely in the time course and degree of clearing that may be expected as a result of treatment.

Precipitants

As opposed to acute asthma, infection is the most common identifiable precipitant of ACRF, accounting for some 20%–50% of cases. Most infections appear to represent spread to the lower respiratory tract from endogenous flora. The most common bacterial organisms include *Streptococcus pneumoniae,* beta lactamase positive *Haemophilus influenzae, Branhamella catarrhalis, Legionella* species, and enteric gram-negative rods, but viral infection may also be at fault in some instances. It is sometimes difficult to determine who really has an infection. Other precipitants include congestive heart failure, myocardial infarction, or pulmonary thromboembolism.

Medical Management

As in the acute asthmatic episode, aggressive inhaled bronchodilator therapy combined with corticosteroids is used to forestall the need for intubation and mechanical ventilation. The COPD patient, however, may present additional challenges in clinical judgment. The basic principles of management are to correct life-threatening hypoxemia, correct life-threatening acidosis, treat underlying precipitants, and treat and prevent complications.

BRONCHODILATORS

No fundamental differences are found in the bronchodilator management of acute severe asthma and COPD. Evidence suggests that beta adrenergic agonists or anticholinergics alone produce maximal bronchodilator effect and that using a second agent adds little unless there is a poor response to the first drug. No consensus exists to whether beta agonists or anticholinergics should be the primary agent. Doses and routes of delivery are the same as discussed above. Because COPD tends to affect an older population than asthma, parenteral beta agonists should be employed only as a last resort measure and then only with great caution.

STEROIDS

Systemic corticosteroids are considered part of standard ACRF medical management, although their use is based on a single trial published in 1980 (32). Methylprednisolone is given intravenously at 0.5 mg/kg every 6 hours. Alternative preparations and dose regimens have not been systematically studied but switching to oral preparations as early as possible with subsequent tapering appear reasonable (32).

ANTIBIOTICS

As a group, patients with ACRF have been shown to benefit from antibiotic therapy. When subgroup analysis is applied, benefit is most clear in those patients with strongest evidence of infection, defined as increased dyspnea, increased sputum volume and purulence with neutrophils and an identifiable organism present on Gram's stain of sputum, and in those patients with fever, leukocytosis, or infiltrates on the chest roentgenogram. Coverage should be adequate for the most common organisms listed above and should cover atypical organisms as well. Dosing frequency, side effect profiles, and cost-effectiveness should also be considered. Amoxicillin, trimethoprim sulfa, second-generation cephalosporins, or a macrolide agent are all reasonable first choices (33).

OXYGEN

To correct life-threatening hypoxemia in ACRF, only small increases in F_IO_2 are generally necessary. If F_IO_2 requirements are >40%, superimposed disease such as congestive heart failure or pneumonia should be suspected. The chest roentgenogram should be used to determine if another process is present that may call for higher doses of O_2. In response to oxygen administration, most COPD patients will increase their $PaCO_2$ by 10–15 mmHg but then stabilize. The elevation of $PaCO_2$ may result from hypoventilation due to blunted hypercapnic and hypoxic drives, increased CO_2 production, and an increased dead space. Correction of hypoxemia may further exacerbate hypercapnia via the Haldane effect, which shifts the carbon dioxide dissociation curve to the right in the presence of increased oxygen (34,35). Patients presenting with pH <7.35 and PaO_2 <50 mmHg are at highest risk for CO_2 retention. Establishing a PaO_2 of 55–65 mmHg should avoid excessive hypercapnia in most instances. Initial F_IO_2 levels should range between 24% and 30% by mask or 3–5 L/minute by nasal cannula and patients should be observed closely for progressive CO_2 retention. Because masks are sometimes uncomfortable and poorly tolerated by patients, nasal cannulas should be provided at mealtimes.

OTHER MODALITIES

Patients who do develop significant CO_2 retention with oxygen administration may be given a trial of respiratory stimulants, either theophylline or doxapram. Theophylline should be titrated to a level of 12–15 μg/ml; doxapram has been used successfully at infusion rates of 2 mg/minute with patients who fail to respond to initial interventions with $PaCO_2$ <50 mmHg and H^+ concentration is >55 nmol/L (36).

NUTRITION

COPD patients may be severely malnourished, and prompt attention should be paid to nutritional repletion. Serum albumin, prealbumin, transferrin, cholesterol, and 24-hour urine for urea nitrogen assessments allow an evaluation of the patient's protein-calorie status. Total resting energy needs may be estimated by the Harris-Benedict equation. The enteral route should be used for feeding whenever possible. Although special low carbohydrate-high fat formulations may reduce $\dot{V}CO_2$, avoidance of caloric overfeeding is probably more important in averting excessive metabolic loads.

INDICATIONS FOR VENTILATION

Intubation and ventilation for ACRF is indicated for failure of response to medical management and for $PaCO_2$ >50 mmHg with evidence of obtundation. Before committing to a course of intubation and ventilation, issues such as the patient's quality of life, prognosis, wishes, and values should be explored as thoroughly as time permits. When doubt exists, however, intubation should proceed. If the intervention is subsequently inappropriate or against the patient's wishes, ventilatory support may be withdrawn. Noninvasive ventilation offers an alternative approach to the support of the ACRF patient (see below)(36,37).

Management of Ventilation

BASIC CONSIDERATIONS

The prolonged time constants associated with ACRF call for the same balance of dynamic hyperinflation with gas exchange as with the acute asthmatic. Hyperinflation poses more of a problem in liberation from ventilation than it does in safely ventilating the ACRF patient, and weaning may be a much more prolonged process than for the acute asthmatic. Unlike asthma, high PIP levels are unusual. If PIP is high or CO_2 removal is difficult, coexisting problems (e.g., pneumothorax, pulmonary edema, or mucus plugging) need to be considered.

ALTERNATIVE TECHNIQUES

Noninvasive Ventilation

Tracheobronchial toilet is more efficient through an intact glottis than through an endotracheal tube. Complications increase with the duration of mechanical ventilation and weaning is often a difficult proposition in ACRF. For these reasons, alternative approaches to intubation should be considered whenever possible. Accumulating experience indicates that most ACRF patients, 56%–92%, can be successfully supported through an acute episode by noninvasive ventilation. Where successful, noninvasive ventilation is associated with shorter intensive care unit (ICU) stays and fewer complications. Mask ventilation requires close cooperation between the patient and the respiratory therapist, especially in the first 30–60 minutes. Failure is more likely in anxious, uncooperative, pursed lip breathing patients. Mask ventilation should be avoided in patients with high aspiration risk, impaired swallowing, hemodynamic instability, severe hypoxia, or acute abdominal problems. Nasogastric tubes, which increase the risk of gastric distention, should be avoided. Aspiration of gastric contents is a rare complication. Full face masks should be carefully fitted for each patient and they give better results than nasal masks. Duoderm patches and benzoin improve the seal of the mask and minimize skin necrosis, while allowing small air leaks. Patients selected for noninvasive ventilation should be placed in a semi-Fowler position at 45°. Ventilation can be delivered with a bi-level positive airway pressure (BiPAP) device with inspiratory positive airway pressure (IPAP) set to 15 cmH$_2$O and expiratory positive airway pressure (EPAP) to 8–10 cmH$_2$O. Volume-cycled ventilators may also be used with initial settings of pressure support 10–20 cmH$_2$O (usually 12–15), with CPAP 3–5 cmH$_2$O, and F$_1$O$_2$ 0.4–1.0 as needed. Pressure support should be titrated to produce a tidal volume ≥7 ml/kg and a breathing frequency <25/minute with SaO$_2$ >90%. Small air leaks can be tolerated and are of concern only when tidal volume is compromised. Leaks can be minimized by reducing CPAP or pressure support levels. If leaks are severe, flow triggering should be used, adjusting base flow to maintain desired PEEP levels. Alternatively, pressure control or volume control modes (IMV, A/CMV) can be tried. The success or failure of mask ventilation is usually readily apparent within 2 hours of initiation. Successfully treated patients will show a significant decrease in PaCO$_2$ and increase in pH. Patients may be allowed 15-minute holidays for comfort and for eating. Weaning is accomplished by gradually withdrawing the level of support (38–40).

Tracheal Gas Insufflation

Tracheal gas insufflation (TGI) (see also, Chapter 17, High Frequency Ventilation) has been described as an adjunct to CO$_2$ clearance in the setting of hypercapnia. Oxygen is delivered by continuous flow at 10 L/minute through a 2.2 mm outer diameter catheter threaded through the endotracheal tube to 1 cm above the carina. Ventilator tidal volume is titrated against catheter flow to produce a constant total tidal volume. TGI produces, on average, a 15% reduction in PaCO$_2$ with best results when PaCO$_2$ is high. TGI causes slight increases in PIP, but no increase in mean airway pressure. Airway humidification, and a reliable pressure release mechanism are technical problems that must be resolved before this modality can enjoy wider clinical use (41).

Chronic Home Ventilation

There are approximately 6800 chronic ventilator-dependent patients in the United States. Annual cost of care for each of these patients has been estimated at $250,000–$550,000. Home ventilation programs appear to decrease that cost to about $20,000 yearly. Home ventilation should be considered for the chronic ventilator-dependent patient with adequate financial, educational, motivational, and family resources to manage care at home. Because the family must act as competent respiratory therapists and adequate backup must be available in the home in case of mechanical or power failure, home ventilation is not suitable for every patient. Home ventilation should, at least, be considered on an individual basis in the event of prolonged ventilator dependence.

WEANING

Weaning patients with ACRF from mechanical ventilation is a more prolonged and difficult proposition than weaning the acute asthmatic. Patients with COPD are often malnourished and weaker compared with asthmatics, coexisting pathology is often present, and their underlying disease is less completely reversible. These individuals are less able to deal with any residual hyperinflation that may put their diaphragms at mechanical disadvantage. Particular attention needs be paid to nutritional repletion and to minimizing hyperinflation. The principles of determining readiness for weaning are the same as for the acute asthmatic but weaning progress may be slow. Few data exist to suggest the best available weaning modality for ACRF patients, but it would be expedient to avoid any method likely to produce high respiratory rates predisposing to dynamic hyperinflation and further prolonging the weaning process. One study suggested that a combination of IMV and pressure support is better than IMV alone in weaning patients with ACRF (42).

COMPLICATIONS

Problems of varying severity are commonly encountered. Zwillich et al. (43) reported 400 separate complications among 354 episodes of assisted ventilation over a 5-month period. They called particular attention to tube malfunction, right mainstem intubation, and alveolar hypoventilation as significant correlates of mortality. Several other concerns are particularly germane to ventilation in obstructive diseases.

AUTO-PEEP

Auto-PEEP is a major risk in ACRF of COPD. Because lung compliance tends to be high, most airway pressure is transmitted to pleural space, causing more interference with venous return and hypotension. A sudden onset of hypotension in a ventilated patient with obstructive lung disease is often due to auto-PEEP, but it may also raise the question of tension pneumothorax. Auto-PEEP can be quickly identified as the cause of the problem by giving 100% O_2 and disconnecting the ventilator for 30–45 seconds or reducing the rate to 2–3 breaths/minute for a similar time (Fig. 20.3). Blood pressure will rapidly return to baseline if hyperinflation is relieved. Problems with auto-PEEP are typically associated with high minute volumes, high tidal volumes, and high respiratory rates. All of these conditions should be avoided where possible.

There is more experience regarding the use of applied PEEP to unload respiratory muscles and decrease airway resistance in patients with ACRF than in acute severe asthma (44). Although favorable outcomes have been described using PEEP levels held to ≤85% of measured auto-PEEP or to levels that do not produce a measurable increase in lung volume or VEI, no controlled studies have demonstrated that applied PEEP reduces mortality or shortens weaning in the setting of

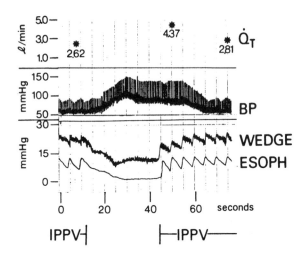

Figure 20.3. Discontinuation of positive pressure ventilation leads to rapid reversal of hypotension and improved cardiac output in patient with significant auto-PEEP. Note time scale. (Reprinted with permission from Pepe PE, Marini JJ. Occult positive end-expiratory pressure in mechanically ventilated patients with airflow obstruction. The auto-PEEP effect. Am Rev Respir Dis 126:166–170, 1982.)

ACRF. Otherwise, the recommended approaches are the same as for asthma discussed above.

TUBE TRAUMA

Nearly two thirds of all endotracheally intubated patients experience some adverse effect from their tube, although most of these problems are relatively self-limited (45). Up to 50% of respiratory failure patients may require reintubation, 13% after self-extubation. Right mainstem intubations are seen in 7%–9% and cuff leaks in 15%. Of all patients, 60% will be symptomatic at extubation, three quarters of these experience hoarseness and 40% have sore throats. Purulent sinusitis may be a cause of pain or occult fever in most nasotracheally intubated patients. No firm data are available to guide the clinician to when to replace an endotracheal tube with a tracheostomy. The tracheostomy tube has the advantage of (*a*) sparing the larynx from tube-related injury; (*b*) patient comfort by freeing the oropharynx; and (*c*) a small reduction in airway resistance. The disadvantage of the tracheostomy relates to the surgical procedure and to infectious and bleeding problems. The decision to proceed with tracheostomy should balance the risks and benefits with assessment of the patient's progress and prognosis for liberation from mechanical ventilation. Tracheostomy becomes the approach of choice when continued progress cannot be expected, but the decision should be individualized in each case.

INFECTION

Ventilated patients are at high risk for nosocomial respiratory tract infections. Of all ventilator-dependent patients, 10%–70% have been reported to develop nosocomial pneumonias, the risk increasing with ventilation duration. Factors contributing to the increased risk include direct infection from respiratory therapy equipment, increased gram-negative colonization of the oropharynx due to severe illness, increased risk of aspiration due to the endotracheal tube, and altered levels of consciousness caused by the disease or by sedatives, malnutrition, and concurrent antibiotic and corticosteroid therapy. Purulent tracheitis without pneumonia and sinusitis due to nasotracheal intubation are also common problems. Most respiratory tract infections in this setting involve gram-negative bacilli, especially *P. aeruginosa* and anaerobes, or *Staphylococcus*. The most difficult management aspect is distinguishing pneumonia, which requires treatment, from colonization, which does not. Bronchoscopic brushings with quantitative culturing and examination of leukocytes from bronchial secretions for intracellular bacteria may prove helpful in identifying significant infections. Antibiotic prophylaxis has not been shown to be useful in controlling infections among intubated patients.

GASTROINTESTINAL BLEEDING

Upper gastrointestinal (GI) bleeding in ventilated patients is usually due to stress ulceration. The incidence of GI bleeds had been reported at 6%–30% without prophylactic therapy, but more recent studies suggest the true incidence is between 3%–6%. The addition of H2-blockers or antacids to the regimen as standard intensive care therapy has come under question because of the low incidence of significant bleeding and the increased risk of nosocomial pneumonia with antacids. Consideration of ulcer prophylaxis may be appropriate only in mechanically ventilated patients or in individuals with a coagulopathy (46,47). Enteral feeding may be effective in discouraging the development of stress ulceration. Sucralfate may be equally effective in ulcer prevention; it can reduce colonization of the pharynx by intestinal flora by maintaining an acid gastric pH.

VENOUS THROMBOEMBOLISM

Pulmonary thromboembolic disease is difficult to diagnose in the setting of respiratory failure due to obstructive lung disease. The incidence of pulmonary emboli may be as high as 10% in the ICU and 20%–27% of deaths among ventilated patients may result from emboli. Although intermediate probability

$\dot{V}_A/\dot{Q}$ scans are frequent in COPD and require pulmonary angiography for diagnosis, low probability and high probability scans retain their diagnostic validity (48). Venography and other noninvasive evaluations for deep venous thrombosis are further diagnostic choices. Low-dose subcutaneous heparin, 5000–8000 U every 8–12 hours has been shown to be effective in reducing the incidence of embolic events in a medical ICU setting. Unless specifically contraindicated, subcutaneous heparin should be a staple of therapy.

HEART FAILURE

Right-sided heart failure is a common complication of severe COPD, and it may be seen as well in acute severe asthma. Right-sided failure is caused by increased afterload in the pulmonary circuit due either to hypoxic pulmonary vasoconstriction or to loss of alveolar capillaries due to emphysema. The consequences of right-sided heart failure include low cardiac output caused by reduced left-sided filling and systemic edema. The tendency toward fluid retention and edema formation is potentiated by a defect in the renin-angiotensin system. Although digitalis has been shown to produce some improvement in right ventricular performance, in the setting of respiratory failure its use is associated with an increased incidence of arrhythmia due to hypokalemia or hypoxemia. The treatment of fluid retention with diuretics may also pose risks of a low-output state by further reducing left ventricular preload; it may also potentiate hypokalemia. The best therapy of right-sided heart failure in respiratory failure is treatment of the underlying process and correction of hypoxemia. Some evidence suggests that the use of angiotensin-converting enzyme inhibitors may be a safer approach to the problem of edema.

Clinically overt left-sided failure in the absence of intrinsic left ventricular disease is unusual, although abnormalities in left ventricular ejection secondary to stresses caused by right ventricular disease are frequently demonstrable. Pulmonary edema should call for investigation of left ventricular function and exclusion of myocardial ischemia. Weaning may precipitate myocardial ischemia and pulmonary edema by the increase in left ventricular afterload caused by increased inspiratory efforts.

Ventricular and supraventricular tachyarrhythmias, especially multifocal atrial tachycardia, are commonly encountered in respiratory failure. The clinician should be alert to associated precipitants, especially hypoxemia, hypokalemia, toxic levels of theophylline, or combined high-dose theophylline and beta-adrenergic agonists. Every effort should first be expended to correct these abnormalities. If these are normalized, 1–5 mg of intravenous verapamil may succeed in restoring normal sinus rhythm.

Outcome

The in-hospital mortality rate of acute respiratory failure in chronic airflow obstruction is 16%–35%, but approaches 70% over the next 5 years. Pulmonary infiltrates on the chest roentgenogram, low albumin, and $H^+ > 53$ nmol/L identify a poor prognostic group with a fourfold increased risk of death (36,49).

References

1. Williams MH. Increasing severity of asthma from 1960 to 1987. N Engl J Med 329:1015–1016, 1989.
2. CDC. Asthma-United States, 1982–l992. MMWR 43:952–955, 1995.
3. Barrett TE, Strom BL. Inhaled beta-adrenergic receptor agonists in asthma:more harm than good? Am J Resp Crit Care Med 151:574–577,1995.
4. Williams TJ, Tuxen DV, Scheinkestel CD, et al. Risk factors for morbidity in mechanically ventilated patients with acute severe asthma. Am Rev Respir Dis 146:607–615, 1992.
5. Petty TL. Treat status asthmaticus three days before it occurs. J Intensive Care Med 4:135–136, 1989.
6. Bellomo R, McLaughlin P, Tai E, et al. Asthma requiring mechanical ventilation. A low morbidity approach. Chest 105:891–896, 1994.
7. Miller TP, Greenberger PA, Patterson R. The diagnosis of potentially fatal asthma in hospitalized adults. Patient characteristics and increased severity of asthma. Chest 100:515–518, 1992.
8. Rebuck AS, Chapman KR, Abboud R. Nebulized anticholinergic and sympathomimetic treatment of asthma and chronic obstructive airways disease in the emergency room. Am J Med 82: 59–64, 1987.
9. Gluck EH, Onorato DJ, Castriotta R. Helium-oygen mixtures in intubated patients with status asthmaticus and respiratory acidosis. Chest 98:693–98, 1990.
10. Kass JE, Castriotta RJ. Heliox therapy in acute severe asthma. Chest 107:757–760, 1995.
11. Tuxen DV, Lane S. The effects of ventilatory pattern on hyperinflation, airway pressures, and circulation in mechanical ventilation of patients with severe air-flow obstruction. Am Rev Respir Dis 136:872–879, 1987.
12. Smith TC, Marini JJ. Impact of PEEP on lung mechanics and work of breathing in severe airflow obstruction. J Appl Physiol 65:1488–1499, 1988.
13. Gay PC, Rodarte JR, Hubmayr RD. The effects of positive expiratory pressure on isovolume flow and dynamic hyperinflation in patients receiving mechanical ventilation. Am Rev Respir Dis 139:621–626, 1989.
14. Marini JJ. Should PEEP be used in airflow obstruction? Am Rev Respir Dis 140:1–3, 1989.
15. Tuxen DV. Detrimental effects of positive end-expiratory pressure during controlled mechanical ventilation of patients with severe airflow obstruction. Am Rev Respir Dis 140:5–9, 1989.
16. Newhouse MT Fuller HD. Rose is a rose is a rose? Aerosol therapy in ventilated patients:nebulizers versus metered dose inhalers-a continuing controversy. Am Rev Respir Dis 148:1444–1446, 1993.
17. O'Riordan TC, Palmer LB, Smaldone GC. Aerosol deposition in mechanically ventilated patients. Optimizing nebulizer delivery. Am J Respir Crit Care Med 149:214–219, 1994.
18. Fernandez A, Lazaro A, Garcia A, et al. Bronchodilators in patients with chronic obstructive pulmonary disease on mechanical ventilation. Utilization of metered-dose inhalers. Am Rev Respir Dis 141:164–168, 1990.
19. Fuller HD, Dolovich MB, Turpie FH, et al. Efficiency of bronchodilator aerosol delivery to the

lungs from the metered dose inhaler in mechanically ventilated patients. A study comparing four different actuator devices. Chest 105:214–218, 1994.

20. Feihl F, Perret C. Permissive hypercapnia: how permissive should we be? Am J Resp Crit Care Med 150:1722–1737, 1994.

21. Wheeler AP. Sedation, analgesia, and paralysis in the intensive care unit. Chest 104:566–577, 1993.

22. Tuxen DV, Williams TJ, Scheinkestel CD, et al. Use of a measurement of pulmonary hyperinflation to control the level of mechanical ventilation in patients with acute severe asthma. Am Rev Respir Dis 146:1136–1142, 1992.

23. Brochard L, Rauss A, Benito S, et al. Comparison of three methods of gradual withdrawal from ventilatory support during weaning from mechanical ventilation. Am J Respir Crit Care Med 150:896–903, 1994.

24. Esteban A, Frutos F, Tobin MJ, et al. A comparison of four methods of weaning patients from mechanical ventilation. N Engl J Med 332:345–350, 1995.

25. Broseghini C, Brandolese R, Poggi R, et al. Respiratory mechanics during the first day of mechanical ventilation in patients with pulmonary edema and chronic airway obstruction. Am Rev Respir Dis 138:355–361, 1988.

26. Rossi A, Gottfried SB, Higgs BD, et al. Respiratory mechanics in mechanically ventilated patients with respiratory failure. J Appl Physiol 58:1849–1858, 1985.

27. Pepe PE, Marini JJ. Occult positive end-expiratory pressure in mechanically ventilated patients with airflow obstruction. The auto-PEEP effect. Am Rev Respir Dis 126:166–170, 1982.

28. Marcy TW. Barotrauma: detection, recognition, and management. Chest 1104:578–584, 1993.

29. Haake R, Schlichtig R, Ulstad DR, et al. Barotrauma—pathophysiology, risk factors, and prevention. Chest 91:608–613, 1987.

30. Griffin D, Fairman N, Coursin D, et al. Acute myopathy during treatment of status asthmaticus with corticosteroids and steroidal muscle relaxants. Chest 102:510–514, 1992.

31. Douglass JA, Tuxen DV, Horne M, et al. Myopathy in severe asthma. Am Rev Respir Dis 146:517–519, 1992.

32. Albert RK, Martin TR, Lewis SW. Controlled clinical trial of methylprednisolone in patients with chronic bronchitis and acute respiratory insufficiency. Ann Intern Med 92:753–758, 1980.

33. Anthonisen NR, Manfreda J, Warren CPW, et al. Antibiotic therapy in exacerbations of chronic obstructive pulmonary disease. Ann Intern Med 106:196–204, 1987.

34. Aubier M, Murciano D, Fournier M, et al. Central respiratory drive in acute respiratory failure of patients with chronic obstructive pulmonary disease. Am Rev Respir Dis 122:191–199, 1980.

35. Aubier M, Murciano D, Milic-Emili J, et al. Effects of administration of O_2 on ventilation and blood gases in patients with chronic obstructive pulmonary disease during acute respiratory failure. Am Rev Respir Dis 122:747–754, 1980.

36. Jeffrey AA, Warren PM, Flenley DC. Acute hypercapnic respiratory failure in patients with chronic obstructive lung disease: risk factors and use of guidelines for management. Thorax 47:34–40, 1992.

37. Muir JF, Levi-Valensi P. When should patients with COPD be ventilated? Eur J Respir Dis 70:135–139, 1987.

38. Soo Hoo GW, Santiago S, Williams AJ. Nasal mechanical ventilation for hypercapnic respiratory failure in chronic obstructive pulmonary disease: determinants of success and failure. Crit Care Med 22:1253–1261, 1994.

39. Meduri GU, Abou-Shala N, Fox RC, et al. Noninvasive face mask ventilation in patients with acute hypercapnic respiratory failure. Chest 100:445–454, 1991.

40. Meduri GU, Conoscenti CC, Menashe P, et al. Noninvasive face mask ventilation in patients with acute respiratory failure. Chest 95:865–870, 1989.

41. Ravenscraft SA, Burke WC, Nahum A, et al. Tracheal gas insufflation augments CO_2 clearance during mechanical ventilation Am Rev Respir Dis 148:345–351, 1993.
42. Jounieaux V, Duran A, Levi-Valensi P. Synchronized intermittent mandatory ventilation with and without pressure support ventilation in weaning patients with COPD from mechanical ventilation. Chest 105:1204–1210, 1994.
43. Zwillich CW, Pierson DJ, Creagh CE, et al. Complications of assisted ventilation. A prospective study of 354 consecutive episodes. Am J Med 57:161–170, 1974.
44. Baigorri F, deMonte A, Blanch L, et al. Hemodynamic response to external counterbalancing of auto-positive end-expiratory pressure in mechanically ventilated patients with chronic obstructive pulmonary disease. Crit Care Med 22:1782–1791,1994.
45. Stauffer JL, Olson DE, Petty TL. Complications and consequences of endotracheal intubation and tracheostomy. Am J Med 70:65–75, 1981.
46. Ben-Menachem T, Fogel R, Patel RV, et al. Prophylaxis for stress-related gastric hemorrhage in the medical intensive care unit. A randomized, controlled, single-blind study. Ann Intern Med 121:568–575, 1994.
47. Cook DJ, Fuller HD, Guyatt GH, et al. Risk factors for gastrointestinal bleeding in critically ill patients. N Engl J Med 330:377–381, 1994.
48. Lesser BA, Leeper KV, Stein PV, et al. The diagnosis of acute pulmonary embolism in patients with chronic obstructive pulmonary disease. Chest 102:17–22, 1992.
49. Rieves RD, Bass D, Carter RR, Griffith JE, Norman JR. Severe COPD and acute respiratory failure. Correlates for survival at the time of tracheal intubation. Chest 104:854–860, 1993.

Suggested Readings

Corbridge TC, Hall JB. The assessment and management of adults with status asthmaticus. Am J Resp Crit Care Med 151:1296–1316, 1995.
Curtis JR, Hudson LD. Emergent assessment and management of respiratory failure in COPD. Clin Chest Med 15:481–500, 1994.
Derenne J-P, Fleury B, Pariente R. Acute respiratory failure of chronic obstructive pulmonary disease. Am Rev Respir Dis 138:1006–1033, 1988.
Hubmayr RD, Gay PC, Tayyab M. Respiratory system mechanics in ventilated patients: techniques and indications. Mayo Clin Proc 62:358–368, 1987.
Leatherman J. Life-threatening asthma. Clin Chest Med 15:453–479, 1994.
Marini JJ. The physiologic determinants of ventilator dependence. Respir Care 31: 271–282, 1986.
Pingleton SK. Complications of acute respiratory failure. Am Rev Respir Dis 137: 1463–1493, 1988.
Schmidt GA, Hall JB. Acute on chronic respiratory failure, assessment and management of patients with COPD in the emergent setting. JAMA 261:3444–3453, 1989.
Slutsky AS. ACCP consensus conference. Mechanical ventilation. Chest 104:1933–1959, 1993.

21
Ventilatory Support
Following Major Trauma
Robert C. Mackersie

Trauma patients often constitute the single largest group of patients in surgical intensive care units (ICUs), particularly in urban areas. Major injury often involves multiple organ systems and mechanical ventilation, under these circumstances, may have profound effects on central nervous system (CNS), cardiopulmonary, or metabolic functions. This chapter provides an overview of common clinical problems encountered in mechanical ventilation use in trauma patients.

Trauma remains the leading cause of death for persons under the age of 44 years and is responsible for more deaths in persons between the ages of 1 and 34 years than all other diseases combined. Trauma patients are generally young (average age ~33 years), without other significant underlying health problems. Approximately 20%–35% of major trauma victims admitted to a surgical ICU require intubation and mechanical ventilation. These patients frequently have injuries involving the central nervous system (61% of intubated patients), thoracic injuries (32%), and pelvic or abdominal injuries (38%) (1).

The potential need for intubation and mechanical ventilation must be given the highest priority in any critically injured patient. Resuscitation from major trauma should proceed according to the "ABCs" (A = AIRWAY, establishment and maintenance of a secure airway; B = BREATHING, reestablishment and maintenance of oxygenation and ventilation; C = restoration of normal CIRCU-LATION through intravascular volume repletion). Depending on specific injuries, the decision to proceed with tracheal intubation and ventilatory support may be made in the field by appropriately trained paramedic teams, on arrival in the emergency department, or, for a less acute situation, in the operating room or ICU.

The indications for tracheal intubation and mechanical ventilation in the trauma patient are based on principles similar to those used for the general medical or surgical population (Table 21.1). Derangements in oxygenation may be caused by shock or lung injury. Deficits in ventilatory capacity are more commonly caused by direct chest wall trauma or high cervical spine injuries, but may occur also with profound hypotension. Patients with severe head or maxillofacial injuries are generally unable to maintain a secure airway and require tracheal intubation. Injuries associated with peritracheal edema or hemorrhage may also cause airway compromise.

Table 21.1. Indications and Etiology for Intubation and Mechanical Ventilation Following Major Trauma

Compromised airway
  Head injuries
  Maxillofacial injuries
  Neck injuries with hemorrhage and hematoma
  Laryngeotracheal injuries
  Major burns or head/neck burns
  Inhalational injury
Inadequate ventilation
  Major pulmonary contusion
  Profound shock with impending or actual cardiac arrest
  High cervical cord injury
  Pulmonary edema (neurogenic/cardiogenic)
  Head injury: induced hypocapnea
Impaired oxygenation
  Pulmonary contusion
  Pulmonary edema
  Head injury
  Massive aspiration/near drowning

Patients at risk for increased intracranial pressure (Glasgow Coma Score < 8) may benefit from careful mechanical hyperventilation to induce hypocapneic vasoconstriction. These patients typically will require intubation for airway protection also. Hemothorax, pneumothorax, and tension pneumothorax are not indications for mechanical ventilation, per se, and intubation should be undertaken in these patients only where no immediately reversible cause for deficits in oxygenation, ventilation, or airway obstruction exists.

Trauma patients frequently require transport for therapeutic or diagnostic procedures (e.g., computed tomography scan, angiography, operating room). Transport of a critically ill patient always involves some risk and should not be undertaken lightly. Manual ventilation using a bag-valve system (versus controlled ventilation using a transport ventilator) frequently provides inadequate oxygenation and ventilation, particularly in patients with acute lung injury. Similarly, over inflation of injured lungs may occur inadvertently during manual ventilation, producing additional high pressure or volume lung injury. Specifically designed transport ventilators should always be used to transport these patients within the hospital whenever possible.

LUNG MECHANICS AND GAS EXCHANGE: PATHOPHYSIOLOGY IN THE TRAUMA PATIENT

Major changes in lung mechanics and gas exchange occur as a result of major injury. Patients sustaining major injuries who require emergency intubation and mechanical ventilation often have multiple injuries involving the central nervous system, chest, or spinal cord, or they may be in hypovolemic shock.

Shock

Hypotension that follows major injury can be classified into hypovolemic and nonhypovolemic hypotension. Essentially all hypovolemic hypotension occurring in the setting of major trauma is hemorrhagic shock. Healthy trauma victims may lose up to 30%–35% of their circulating blood volume before manifesting hypotension, and they may be in "shock" with a normal blood pressure. Cardiac tamponade, tension pneumothorax, myocardial contusion, or heart failure may produce a hypotensive shock state induced by primary and secondary pump failure. Hypotension that occurs with high spinal cord injuries is usually not a shock (low flow) state.

The principal pulmonary effect of a shock state (inadequate perfusion) relates to changes in diaphragmatic blood flow and dead space ratio. Diaphragmatic blood flow may be preserved with as much as a 35%–40% loss of circulating blood volume. Beyond this point blood flow may decrease, leading to ventilatory fatigue and failure. At the same time, the associated decrease in cardiac output will result in an increased volume of ventilated but nonperfused lung (physiologic dead space), thereby increasing dead space-to-tidal volume ratio (V_D/V_T). This added physiologic dead space will increase minute ventilation requirements for a given $PaCO_2$, thereby increasing the work of breathing and further promoting ventilatory fatigue.

Resuscitation of patients with hemorrhagic shock requires the restoration of circulating blood volume. Resuscitation is usually begun with the rapid administration of 2 L of an isotonic crystalloid solution followed by reassessment. As a rule, roughly two thirds of administered crystalloid eventually extravasates, resulting in increased tissue edema. In large volume resuscitation, the chest wall tissue edema that results, both from crystalloid administration and "third spacing," may add to the work of breathing. In addition to chest wall edema, the resuscitation from major intraabdominal injuries, particularly vascular injuries, is often associated with intraabdominal and retroperitoneal sequestration of edema fluid. In more severe cases, this edema may act secondarily to decrease thoracic compliance through increased diaphragmatic pressure, and further increase the work of breathing.

Head Injury

Patients with severe head injury often present with a number of conditions requiring tracheal intubation and assisted ventilation (see Table 21.1). Gastric aspiration may occur, which compromises both airway and gas exchange. Patients with greatly diminished levels of consciousness may be unable to protect their airways and may require intubation for this reason alone. Occasionally, very combative patients with suspected head injuries may require intubation and paralysis for their own protection.

Gas exchange derangements are common with severe head injuries. The mechanism for this may involve both alterations in ventilation-to-perfusion ratios with increases in physiologic intrapulmonary shunt and accumulation in extra vascular lung water. Clinically evident pulmonary edema, (neurogenic pulmonary edema), occurs less frequently in nonlethal head injuries, but may be associated with significant decreases in lung compliance.

Blunt Chest Trauma

Chest injuries that are most directly associated with changes in gas exchange or lung mechanics include pneumothorax or tension pneumothorax, hemothorax, multiple rib fractures, flail chest with pulmonary contusion, and diaphragmatic rupture. Although direct chest trauma, per se, rarely requires early intubation or mechanical ventilation, it may produce immediate, severe, and prolonged respiratory failure. Simple pneumothorax or hemothorax alone rarely produces acute respiratory failure but, if left untreated, it will result in increased work of breathing and decreased ventilatory capacity. Tension pneumothorax caused by a "ball-valve" effect of the visceral pleura causes progressive trapping of the air within the hemithorax and may create an immediate life-threatening situation. Tension pneumothorax is best treated by simple needle (14-gauge) decompression of the hemothorax followed by tube thoracostomy. Tension pneumothorax by itself should never be treated by intubation and mechanical ventilation. Positive pressure ventilation will reduce venous return to the heart, worsening the associated hypotension, and will exacerbate the high pressures within the airways, causing the further pneumothorax to expand further and compromise circulatory function. The mistaken treatment by intubation and positive pressure ventilation of acute respiratory failure caused by tension pneumothorax may have a lethal outcome if not immediately recognized. Excessive airway pressures, progressive hypotension, asymmetric expansion of the hemithorax, jugular-venous distention, and tracheal deviation all are easily detectable signs.

Multiple rib fractures with or without associated pneumothorax or hemothorax are among the more common thoracic injuries. Rib fractures are often underestimated in terms of their ability to produce ventilatory compromise. They usually produce some degree of chest wall bleeding and edema and cause significant pain-related decreases in ventilatory capacity. The combination of increased work of breathing (secondary to chest wall hemorrhage) and decreased ventilatory capacity can lead to acute ventilatory failure, particularly in elderly patients with underlying lung disease or in those with other major injuries.

Flail chest involves fractures of two or more ribs (or sternum) in two separate places, creating a "free-floating" section of chest wall. The severe gas exchange derangements that may be produced by a flail chest are attributable more to the underlying pulmonary contusion than to either the rib fractures or the paradoxical chest wall motion. Hypoxia that results from pulmonary contusion is a result of direct injury to the pulmonary parenchyma with local edema or frank hemorrhage and, possibly, activation of vasoactive mediators (kinins, prostaglandins) that may exacerbate ventilation-to-perfusion mismatching. In addition to the underlying pulmonary contusion, a large-segment chest wall injury may result in enough impairment in ventilatory capacity to require mechanical ventilation.

Large diaphragmatic tears occasionally present with progressive respiratory distress. With a large defect in the diaphragm, the negative pressure generated in the thoracic cavity will progressively pull abdominal viscera (usually including stomach, spleen, or small bowel) into the left hemithorax. With larger amounts of abdominal visceral displacement, left lung compression may result in diminished ventilatory capacity and increased shunt with resultant hypoxemia. All patients with diaphragmatic rupture require emergent laparotomy to exclude other visceral injuries and to repair the diaphragmatic defect. Repositioning of the abdominal viscera within the peritoneal cavity, with closure of the diaphragmatic laceration and placement of tube thoracostomy, usually corrects most associated physiologic abnormalities.

Spinal Cord Injuries

The muscles of ventilation, in addition to the diaphragm, include the strap muscles of the neck, intercostal muscles, and the thoracoabdominal muscular girdle. Spinal cord motor lesions at the T10 level or above can cause some degree of ventilatory compromise, with higher lesions causing greater compromise. Cord lesions above the C4 level, because of diaphragmatic involvement, are usually incompatible with prolonged spontaneous ventilatory activity. Patients sustaining complete cord lesions of C1 to C3 rarely survive to reach the hospital. Although the chest wall and diaphragmatic muscles' contribution to ventilation are easy to appreciate, the degree of impairment and ventilatory capacity that occurs with abdominal musculature denervation is often underestimated.

In higher cervical spine injuries, with absence of both thoracic wall and abdominal musculature, ventilation occurs entirely by diaphragm contraction and relaxation. This "bellows" activity of the diaphragm requires the downward expansion of both the diaphragm and lungs. For sufficient force to be produced under these circumstances, the diaphragm must be maintained in its normal "dome" configuration position. The abdominal musculature is responsible for preserving this conformation by maintaining a certain amount of intraabdominal pressure. Consequently, a flattened diaphragm results with abdominal muscle denervation.

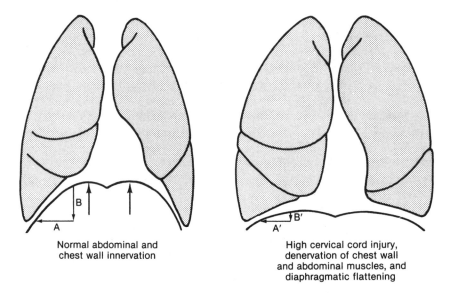

Normal abdominal and
chest wall innervation

High cervical cord injury,
denervation of chest wall
and abdominal muscles, and
diaphragmatic flattening

Figure 21.1. Conformational reduction in the "bellows" component of diaphragmatic force caused by spinal cord injury.

Despite normal contractile strength of the muscle, the efficiency of downward expansion is reduced (Fig. 21.1). This altered mechanical arrangement results in diminished inspiratory force and vital and tussive capacity, particularly for patients in the sitting position. Diminished ventilatory capacity and lack of full lung expansion in patients with spinal cord injuries may lead to decreases in functional residual capacity (FRC) and result in atelectasis and lower respiratory infection. See also Chapter 22, Ventilation of the Neurologically Injured.

SPECIFIC TECHNIQUES IN VENTILATORY MANAGEMENT FOLLOWING MAJOR INJURY

Hypovolemic Shock

Rapid volume resuscitation, not intubation and mechanical ventilation, is generally the most appropriate primary treatment to prevent ventilatory failure in patients with hypovolemic shock. Volume restoration will improve diaphragmatic blood flow and reduce physiologic dead space. Positive pressure ventilation without adequate volume restoration, on the other hand, may exacerbate both hypovolemic and nonhypovolemic shock by increasing mean intrathoracic pressure, thereby decreasing venous return to the heart. Intubation should be reserved for patients with actual or impending cardiopulmonary arrest and those with specific indications (see Table 21.1). For hypotensive patients requiring an emergency operation to control hemorrhage, any anesthetic administration also may have a detrimental effect on blood pressure. Muscle relaxants, which reduce the effect of abdominal muscle wall tone on bleeding tamponade, may also exacerbate hypotension. Under these circumstances, intubation is often best delayed until the patient has been prepared and draped and the operative team is ready to make the incision.

In many regional trauma systems, the military antishock trouser (MAST) suit continues to be used. Hypotensive patients often arrive at the hospital with the suit in place and inflated. Such garments act to improve systolic blood pressure by increasing systemic vascular resistance and causing redistribution of peripheral blood to the central circulation (4). MAST garments may also reduce abdominal and thoracic compliance, increase work of breathing, and precipitate acute ventilatory failure in patients with other major injuries.

Endotracheal intubation, which becomes necessary under certain critical conditions is often associated with some degree of anxiety on the part of the clinician, possibly leading to errors in tube placement. Endotrachael tube positioning must be verified by visualizing its passage through the cords and confirming its placement by auscultation and observation of the chest, ballottement of the tube balloon at the suprasternal notch, and by an end-tidal CO_2 monitor, if available. All patients in shock should be ventilated with 100% oxygen initially at a rate and tidal volume consistent with the maintenance of $PaCO_2$ at a level appropriate to their injuries (head injury patients may require hyperventilation to a $PaCO_2$ level of ~30). Positive end-expiratory pressure (PEEP) and high airway pressures should be avoided until circulating blood volume can be restored and the hemorrhage can be controlled.

Spinal Cord Injury

Paralysis of the diaphragm with cord lesions at or above the C2 level results in rapid asphyxiation. In patients with lower cervical spinal cord injuries, enough diaphragmatic function is usually maintained to allow survival to the hospital. The need for intubation in these patients depends principally on the level of their cord injury and other associated injuries.

Higher spinal cord injuries result in diminished maximal inspiratory force, vital capacity, and FRC and increased risk of atelectasis and pneumonia. Clinical support should be directed toward optimizing ventilatory capacity and preventing infectious complications. Lax abdominal musculature, particularly in the sitting position, reduces diaphragmatic ventilatory efficiency as described (see Fig. 21.1). These effects may be offset somewhat by the application of an abdominal binder. Abdominal binding acts to reestablish the normal domed confirmation of the diaphragm, thus allowing more effective lung expansion. Abdominal binding may also be a useful adjunct to weaning from mechanical ventilation those patients who were intubated primarily because of diminished ventilatory capacity secondary to cord injury.

Mechanical ventilation, except in the unusual circumstance of a C2 to C3 level cord injury, should be regarded as a short-term intervention, during which time the patient recovers from any associated injuries or develops enough diaphragmatic strength and endurance to sustain indefinite spontaneous ventilation. If underlying injuries are not severe, it is reasonable to provide <100% of a patient's ventilatory support. An intermittent mandatory ventilation (IMV) or pressure support (PSV) mode may be used. Because substantial patient anxiety exists with injuries of this type, it is important to allow some flexibility with the ventilatory mode used according to patient comfort. Pressure support ventilation, which allows the patient to set his or her own rate and tidal volume, is often less anxiety provoking in the initial phases than is IMV, assuming no other major injuries are present.

Patients with higher spinal cord injury levels have markedly reduced ventilatory reserve and they produce much less tussive force. They are particularly susceptible to lower respiratory tract infections. The clinical "margin for error" in the development of an often life-threatening pneumonia is low. Careful attention to pulmonary toilet and frequent monitoring with sputum Gram stains and chest radiographs are essential. Nasogastric tubes, which may predispose to reflux of gastric contents and predispose to pneumonia, should be used only as long as any gastric ileus persists. Endotracheal tubes, in addition to nasogastric tubes, are conduits for lower respiratory infections and an aggressive approach should be taken toward weaning and extubation with these patients.

In weaning from mechanical ventilation, bedside pulmonary function tests (maximal inspiratory pressure, vital capacity, maximum voluntary ventilation) should be measured frequently. Because increased diaphragmatic strength and endurance are required to wean successfully, the specific weaning mode is probably not as important as assuring patient cooperation and comfort during the weaning process. It has been our experience that pressure support ventilation produces somewhat less anxiety under these circumstances. See also Chapter 22, Ventilation of the Neurologically Injured.

Maxillofacial Trauma

Patients sustaining major maxillofacial trauma often require intubation for airway maintenance. The swelling or hemorrhage into peritracheal soft tissue that frequently accompanies these injuries may be an indication for emergency cricothyroidotomy in the resuscitation area. No attempt should be made to pass a nasotracheal tube in patients with these types of injuries and even orotracheal intubation may be hazardous. A cricothyroidotomy (an incision in the cricothyroid membrane), not a tracheostomy (an incision usually in the second tracheal ring) should be used to secure an emergency surgical airway. Aspiration of blood, vomitus, or particulate matter, including tissue and teeth, may complicate gas exchange; a diagnostic and therapeutic bronchoscopy following airway placement is indicated with evidence of substantial aspiration of fluid or particulate matter exists.

Isolated maxillofacial injuries are generally not associated with significantly altered ventilatory capacity or ventilatory demands; thus, the amount of mechanical ventilatory support required for these patients is usually limited. For patients intubated solely for control of the airway, spontaneous ventilation with a low level of continuous positive airway pressure (CPAP) may be used to optimize FRC and overcome the airway resistance inherent in the endotracheal tube. When edema, hemorrhage, and other factors causing airway obstruction have resolved (for patients without surgical airways), extubation can usually be accomplished without the need for prolonged ventilator weaning. Determining at what point sufficient resolution of airway edema has occurred occasionally requires bronchoscopic inspection. Cuff leaks with minimal pressure (<10 cmH$_2$O) and an ability to breathe around the endotracheal tube with the balloon deflated also suggest an adequate airway.

Head Injury

Early therapeutic intervention in patients with severe head injury is directed toward airway control, avoiding hypercapnia, maintaining cerebral oxygenation, and controlling intracranial pressure (ICP). The indications for intubation and mechanical hyperventilation following head injury may be based on the Glasgow Coma Score (GCS, Table 21.2) (3). These more profound decreases in the level of consciousness are often associated with increases in ICP and are indications for control of ventilation. It has been our routine practice to intubate patients with a Glasgow Coma Score <8.

Hyperventilation may be an effective, rapid means of reducing ICP in selected patients. CO_2 is a potent vasoconstrictor and acute reductions in arterial PCO$_2$ produce cerebral vasoconstriction, a reduction in cerebral blood volume, and a resultant decrease in intracranial pressure (2). Because of more recent concerns about over ventilation and cerebral ischemia, more emphasis has been place on the maintenance of cerebral perfusion pressure, (CPP = mean arterial pressure − intracranial pressure), than on simple ICP manipulations.

Ventilator settings that act to increase mean airway pressure may exacerbate ICP by impeding venous return to the chest. The application of expiratory pressure (PEEP, CPAP) may cause increases in ICP. Similarly, elevations in mean airway pressure caused by change in rate or tidal volume may also be associated with increases in ICP. In patients with normal chest compliance, the use of larger tidal volumes (15–18 ml/kg) with corresponding reductions in ventilatory rate may be useful in reducing mean airway pressures. This technique should not be used,

Table 21.2. The Glasgow Coma Score[a]

Verbal response
   1 = None
   2 = Incomprehensible sounds
   3 = Inappropriate words
   4 = Confused
   5 = Oriented
Eye opening
   1 = None
   2 = To pain
   3 = To speech
   4 = Spontaneously
Motor response
   1 = None
   2 = Abnormal extension to pain
   3 = Abnormal flexion to pain
   4 = Withdraws to pain
   5 = Localizes to pain
   6 = Follows commands

[a] *The GCS ranges from 3 to 15 and evaluates the best patient response in three areas: verbal response, eye opening, and motor response.*

however, in patients with decreased chest and lung compliance because of the associated increases in peak airway pressures and the potential for producing high volume-high pressure lung injury.

Recent outcome data from patients with major head injury suggest that two factors, hypotension and hypoxia, may exacerbate preexisting cerebral injury and worsen the outcome (10). It is crucial, therefore, that head injured patients be kept well oxygentated. Although the addition of end-expiratory pressure, by impeding venous return, may cause increases in ICP in some patients, the effect is by no means universal. Mild increases in ICP may be compensated for by corresponding increases in mean arterial pressure to maintain cerebral perfusion pressure in patients requiring the addition of PEEP for oxygenation.

The control of intracranial pressure may work at cross purposes with efforts to clear secretions and maintain adequate gas exchange. Methods used to control intracranial pressure usually involve bed elevation, adjusted hyperventilation, mannitol administration, ventriculostomy drainage, and paralytic agents. In more severe cases, high-dose barbiturates may be necessary. Patients with elevated ICP frequently are positioned with the head of bed elevated; they are immobilized for prolonged periods. The combined effects of the absence of cough, endotracheal intubation, and the supine position may act to decrease both FRC and a predisposition to respiratory infection. Unfortunately, methods used to help clear secretions (e.g., postural drainage or tracheal suctioning) may produce marked increases in ICP and are often inadvisable.

Many head-injured patients are intubated via the nasal route because of ease and convenience as well as the concern for cervical spine injury. The prolonged use of nasotracheal intubation, however, has been associated with an increased incidence of purulent sinus infection. Bacterial reservoirs in the sinuses may also contribute to the high incidence of pulmonary infections seen in patients. For this reason, our practice is to change nasotracheal tubes to the orotracheal route in patients without cervical spine injury whenever this can be done without adverse effects on ICP.

Patients sustaining severe head injuries often receive paralytic agents or barbiturates and require controlled hyperventilation. Control or assist-control mechanical ventilation modes are appropriate for these patients. End-expiratory pressure should be limited to ≤ 5 unless required for oxygen exchange. Ventilator weaning in patients recovering from severe head injuries ultimately involves the following steps: (*a*) reversal of paralytic agents and discontinuation of any barbiturates; (*b*) normalization of $PaCO_2$ by reductions in ventilatory rate or tidal volume; (*c*) stepwise reductions in ventilatory support; (*d*) complete spontaneous ventilation (CPAP or T-piece); and (*e*) careful assessment of airway reflexes prior to extubation. Weaning ultimately depends on the extent and rapidity of neurologic recovery. Patients without underlying lung disease or injury generally wean without much difficulty. Patients in vegetative states require permanent tracheostomy. The weaning method of choice depends on the severity of underlying lung and neurologic injury, the duration of intubation, and the patient's age.

Chest Trauma

There is a wide spectrum of chest injuries, from minor insignificant chest wall contusions to more severe crushing injuries involving the lung, heart, and even contents of the abdominal cavity. Indications for ventilatory support in patients following blunt chest trauma should follow conventional guidelines in terms of requirements for oxygenation and ventilation and maintenance of a secure airway. With the exception of the physiologic derangements in specific injuries previously discussed, no absolute mandatory indications exist for intubation following blunt chest trauma, including flail chest and pulmonary contusion.

Historically, the management of flail chest has consisted of external stabilization of the chest wall, often with crude arrangements consisting of external clips and pulleys. Further experience in the 1960s and 1970s suggested that many of these patients could be stabilized internally by the mandatory use of mechanical ventilation. With the recognition that much of the acute impairment in oxygenation occurs as a result of pulmonary contusion and not due to flail chest, per se, Richardson et al. (6) demonstrated that many patients with these injuries may be managed without either external stabilization or mechanical ventilation but with close attention to pulmonary toilet, alleviation of pain, and avoidance of infectious complications.

Chest wall injuries requiring ventilatory support usually consist of major pulmonary contusions with or without flail chest, combined pulmonary and myocardial contusions, or less severe injuries in elderly patients with underlying cardiopulmonary disease. Patients with multiple rib fractures frequently have an associated hemo- or pneumothorax secondary to muscular or intercostal rib bleeding or lung laceration. The presentation of hemo- or pneumothorax may be delayed and all patients should have a repeat chest radiographic study within 4–6 hours following admission.

Multiple rib fractures are virtually always associated with significant pain. Failure to alleviate pain may result in reduced ventilatory capacity, atelectasis, and pneumonia. It has been shown that alleviation of pain with these types of injuries acts to restore ventilatory function. Specific techniques for pain relief include continuous intravenous administration of opiates, patient-controlled analgesia, intercostal nerve blocks using local anesthetics, intrapleural local anesthetics, or epidural opiates with or without local anesthetics added. We prefer the use of epidural opiate analgesia, which provides good restoration of ventilatory function, without the problems of hypotension and motor or sensory symptoms associated with the addition of local anesthetics (7). Daily ventilatory function tests should be monitored to assess the adequacy of analgesia and the degree of ventilatory impairment.

The required duration of mechanical ventilation for isolated chest wall injuries in younger patients is usually short. The edema associated with pulmonary contusion resolves relatively quickly over the first 2–3 days, with associated improvements in gas exchange and reduced work of breathing. With the exception of elderly patients and patients with very severe chest contusions or rib fractures, most patients wean quickly once their oxygenation has improved and their pain is well controlled. A rapid weaning program using either IMV or pressure support ventilation is appropriate for these patients. Patients with more severe lung injury and more severe decreases in ventilatory capacity or increases in ventilatory requirements usually benefit from a weaning program consisting of periods of high ventilatory demand interspersed with periods of complete ventilatory rest. In patients with blunt trauma, large flail segments may produce major instability of the chest wall and impede ventilator weaning. On rare occasions, surgical stabilization of the ribs, either with K-wires or fixation using external plates, may be indicated. Rib stabilization can be performed concomitantly in patients who have major chest wall disruption and require a thoracotomy to control bleeding.

Bronchopleural fistulae often occur following chest trauma and usually consist of only a transient air leak from a tube thoracostomy in patients on positive pressure ventilation. Most leaks are small and do not compromise ventilation.

With more severe lung parenchymal injury, larger leaks may occur, particularly in patients with noncompliant lungs and high peak airway pressures. Ventilatory adjustments should be made that will reduce peak airway pressure and thereby reduce the amount of air leakage. These include reduced peak inspiratory flow rate, adjustment of inspiratory-to-expiratory (I/E) ratios, reduced PEEP/CPAP, smaller tidal volumes, and a change in the inspiratory flow pattern. In extreme circumstances with very large air leaks, high-frequency ventilation may be useful. All postinjury patients with very large air leaks or with pneumothorax unresponsive to tube thoracostomy should undergo bronchoscopy to exclude a bronchial tear as the source of an air leak.

Other ventilatory techniques of potential benefit in the face of massive chest trauma with large bronchopleural fistulae include independent lung ventilation (differential lung ventilation) and high-frequency ventilation. The need for these specialized ventilatory techniques is extremely rare in our experience. Bronchopleural fistulae large enough to require independent lung or high-frequency ventilation should prompt a bronchoscopic examination for tracheal injury. Occasionally, patients with penetrating chest injury and subsequent infection (empyema, lung abscess) who develop large bronchopleural fistulae are not surgical candidates and may benefit from local reductions in peak airway pressures afforded by differential or high-frequency ventilation.

An air embolism is a rare but often a lethal complication of pulmonary injury that usually occurs shortly after injury. More often associated with penetrating lung injury, an air embolism is the result of positive pressure ventilation forcing air into open pulmonary veins at the site of injury. Air embolism usually presents as a sudden cardiac arrest or hypotension at the time of endotracheal intubation, often associated with vigorous positive pressure ventilation by hand. Air aspirated from an arterial line is a universally fatal sign. Treatment consists of immediate decompression of the involved hemithorax, positioning (head down, left side up), and thoracotomy with open cardiac massage and left ventricular venting. High airway pressures should always be avoided in patients with penetrating chest injuries, and ambu bags are best equipped with "pop-off" valves to prevent the generation of excessive airway pressures.

Orthopedic Injuries

Major orthopedic injuries have important implications for the potential development of acute respiratory failure. The two principal clinical scenarios are (*a*) adult respiratory distress syndrome occurring acutely following long bone or pelvic fractures; (*b*) progressive respiratory failure or pneumonia associated with delayed fixation and prolonged immobilization. Adult respiratory distress syndrome (ARDS) developing soon after long bone fractures has typically been referred to as *fat embolism syndrome,* but it is probably more appropriately called *marrow embolism syndrome.* The syndrome has also been observed following intramedullary reaming and femur fixation. In its milder form, gas exchange derangements generally do not require intubation and mechanical ventilation. In the more severe form, pulmonary edema, severe gas exchange impairment, pulmonary fibrosis, and death may occur. Sepsis is generally not implicated in this form of ARDS and the precise sequence of lung inflammatory events that occurs is still not well understood.

The optimal timing of operative fixation for long bone fractures has yet to be determined. It appears as though a long delay (>7 days), may be associated with a high incidence of pulmonary dysfunction and longer hospitalization (8). The precise mechanism by which unstabilized orthopedic injuries result in pulmonary dysfunction is unclear, but it is likely related in some degree to the enforced bed rest that these injuries require. More recently, the immediate (<24 hours) fixation of long bone fractures was associated with a higher incidence of ARDS in patients with combined thoracic injuries (12). Clearly, the ventilatory management of these patients requires careful consideration with respect to the relative risks and benefits of immediate, early, and delayed fixation of these injuries, particularly with preexisting chest injury or acute lung injury.

References

1. Mackersie, RC. University of California, San Diego Trauma Registry; Unpublished data 1987–1988.
2. Lundberg N, Kjallquist A, Bien C. Reduction of increased intracranial pressure by hyperventilation. Acta Psychiatr Scand 34:4–64, 1959.
3. Teasdale G, Jennett B. Assessment of coma and impaired consciousness: a practical scale. Lancet 2:81, 1974.
4. McSwain NE. Pneumatic Anti-Shock Garment: state of the art 1988. Ann Emerg Med. 17:506–525, 1988.
5. Carlon GC, Ray C Jr, Miodownik S, Kopec I, et al. Capnography in mechanically ventilated patients. Crit Care Med 16(5):550–556, 1988.
6. Richardson JD, Adams L, Flint LM. Selective management of flail chest and pulmonary contusion. Ann Surg 196:481–487, 1982.
7. Mackersie RC, Shackford SR, Hoyt DB, Karagianes TG. Continuous epidural fentanyl analgesia: ventilatory function improvement with routine use in the treatment of blunt chest injury. J Trauma 27(11):1207–1212, 1987.
8. Seibel R, LaDuca J, Hassett JM, Babikian G, Mills B, Border DO, Border JR. Blunt multiple trauma (ISS 36), femur traction, and the pulmonary failure-septic state. Ann Surg 202:283–295, 1985.
9. Mackersie RC, Christensen JM, Pitts LH, Lewis FR. Pulmonary extravascular fluid accumulation following intracranial injury. J Trauma 23:968, 1983.
10. Chesnut RM, Marshall LF, Klauber MR et al. The role of secondary brain injury in determining outcome from severe head injury. J Trauma 34(2):216–222, 1993.
11. Reynolds MA, Richardson JD, Spain DA et al. Is the timing of fracture fixation important for the patient with multiple trauma? Ann Surg 222:470–481, 1995.
12. Pape HC, Auf'm'Kolk M, Paffrath T et al. Primary intramedullary femur fixation in multiple trauma patients with associated lung contusion—a cause of posttraumatic ARDS? J Trauma 34:540–548, 1993.

22
Ventilation of the Neurologically Injured

William T. Peruzzi

James A. Colombo

Ventilation of the patient with neurologic impairment requires well-defined goals based on several factors. These include the location of the injury in the nervous system, the ability to correct the underlying problem, and projected needs for ongoing ventilatory support. After careful consideration of these factors, the goals for mechanical ventilation of the neurologically injured patient can be specifically addressed.

This chapter addresses the more common neurologic disease processes that lead to respiratory difficulties and require mechanical ventilatory support. A brief discussion of the pathophysiology of each neurologic aberration, and its appropriate treatment, is provided so the reader may understand the various functional derangements that occur and the appropriate steps that must be taken to correct them. Topics covered include brain and spinal cord injury, neuromuscular diseases, and the brain dead patient. The discussion of these neurologic process focuses on decisions pertaining to airway management, the initiation of mechanical ventilation, and the management of short- and long-term mechanical ventilatory support.

GENERAL CONSIDERATIONS

The most common respiratory complications in neurologically injured patients are related to the loss of respiratory muscle activity, which is imperative for deep breathing, cough, and airway protection. The degree of respiratory impairment associated with neurologic injury varies depending on both the etiology and severity of the underlying process. Often, the etiology of respiratory complications in a neurologically impaired patient is multifactorial and may require more than one intervention to address current and future problems.

There are three major factors requisite for normal mechanical respiratory function: (*a*) central ventilatory drive, (*b*) ventilatory muscle function, and (*c*) normal lung parenchyma (Fig. 22. 1). Neurologic insults may affect any or all of these factors. For example, central ventilatory drive might be affected by brain injury or drug overdose; ventilatory muscle function might be compromised by spinal

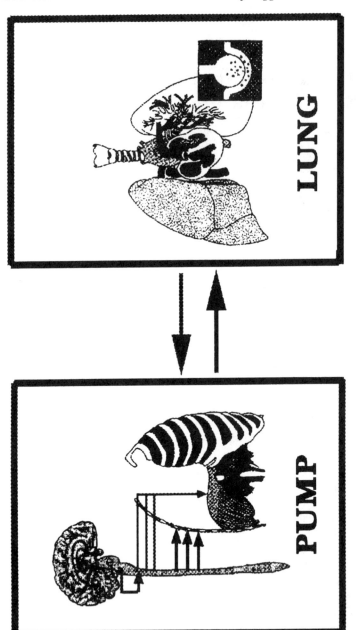

Figure 22.1. Normal ventilatory function requires the interaction of three system components: 1) the central nervous system, 2) the musculoskeletal system, and 3) the pulmonary system. The respiratory centers of the brainstem send signals to the phrenic nuclei in the spinal cord which, in turn, send nerve impulses to the diaphragm which stimulate contraction. Intercostal muscles are stimulated via the thoracic nerves which are also regulated by signals from the brainstem. This neuromuscular activity will result in tidal ventilation if the lungs are appropriately functioning. (Modified with permission from Shapiro BA, Kacmarek RM, Cane RD, Peruzzi WT, Hauptman D. Clinical application of respiratory care, 4th ed. Chicago, Mosby–Year Book, 1991.)

cord injury or neuromuscular disease; and lung parenchymal function can be impaired by neurogenic pulmonary edema.

The combination of objective clinical findings and subjective information generally guides medical decision making. In the setting of neurologic injury, objective data are particularly helpful because the patient's ability to formulate or verbalize feelings or symptoms is often compromised or eliminated completely. Bedside spirometry (i.e., tidal volume, vital capacity, or negative inspiratory force), arterial blood gas analysis, and vital signs are the most useful objective measures in neurologically injured patients. Such measurements are easily obtained, easily repeated and, if obtained sequentially, can provide trend information on which to base clinical decisions. Clinical observations (i.e., the volume and consistency of pulmonary secretions or the overall clinical work of breathing) are important subjective data to be considered when making decisions regarding airway management and mechanical ventilatory support in the neurologically impaired patient.

ARTIFICIAL AIRWAYS AND MECHANICAL VENTILATION

Artificial airways (endotracheal tube or tracheostomy) are indicated in the presence of four clinical situations: (*a*) upper airway obstruction; (*b*) loss or impairment of airway protective reflexes; (*c*) the inability to maintain adequate clearance of bronchial secretions; and (*d*) the need for mechanical ventilatory support. Some would include hypoxemia as an indication for an artificial airway; however, this is not necessarily the case because there are many ways to establish adequate arterial oxygenation without intubation or tracheostomy.

Airway Obstruction

Several pathophysiologic processes can produce acute airway compromise necessitating the urgent or emergent establishment of an artificial airway, including trauma, central nervous system disease, drug overdose, and others. Direct trauma to the larynx or trachea can result in partial or complete airway obstruction. Foreign bodies, oral secretions, or vomitus in patients with impaired mental status can present serious problems. Inflammation or rapidly expanding lesions (e.g., hematomas, abscesses, diffuse infections) in the supraglottic region can result in airway compromise.

Obstructive sleep apnea is a less obvious problem that is associated with obesity, day time somnolence, frequent headaches, snoring, intermittent night time airway obstruction with apnea, hypercapnia, and hypoxemia. This situation can often be alleviated with continuous positive airway pressure (CPAP) applied by nasal mask at bedtime, tracheostomy placement, or surgical alteration of the soft palate. These patients do not usually require urgent or emergent intubation unless their condition is related to other pathologic states.

Airway Protection

Airway protective reflexes can be impaired by processes similar to those outlined for airway obstruction. However, loss of airway protection may be more insidious and not as obvious as airway obstruction. Patients may maintain their airway patency, but when a foreign substance (e.g., food, vomitus) is introduced into the mouth or posterior pharynx, it may readily be aspirated into the trachea. Airway protection is primarily dependent on the swallow reflex, although gag reflex assessment provides some indication of the patient's overall neurologic status. Assessment of these reflexes is critical in the examination of anyone with an altered mental status. The absence of these reflexes mandates an artificial airway be established unless a decision has been made to forego supportive care.

Bronchial Hygiene

The ability to clear respiratory secretions is paramount in maintaining both oxygenation and spontaneous ventilation. Retained secretions can result in segmental and lobar lung collapse, hypoxemia, and increased work of breathing. The ability to clear secretions is based on the patient's capability to generate an effective cough. The three basic prerequisites to an effective cough are (*a*) the ability to take a deep breath, (*b*) an intact glottic mechanism, and (*c*) the muscular ability to generate positive intrathoracic pressure. The ability to take a deep breath is quantified by measuring the vital capacity (VC) or the peak maximal negative inspiratory pressure (PImax). A vital capacity of ≥ 15 ml/kg is generally associated with the ability to breathe sufficiently deep to clear secretions in the presence of the other prerequisites listed above (1). A PImax of -20 cmH$_2$O usually corresponds to a VC of ≥ 15 ml/kg (2).

The VC is measured by having the patient take in the deepest inspiration possible and then exhale completely through a spirometer. When measured properly in a cooperative patient, vital capacity is a good indicator of respiratory reserves. It is also a simple measurement that can be performed at the bedside and repeated frequently. Unfortunately, the VC is a very effort-dependent maneuver that is subject to large and inconsistent errors if the patient does not cooperate fully. For this reason, the PImax is often used in place of the VC measurement in patients who are unwilling or unable to cooperate. The PImax is measured by placing a manometer on the artificial airway followed by airway occlusion for ~20 seconds. At the end of this time, patients capable of breathing, will attempt to make a maximal inspiratory effort regardless of willingness or ability to cooperate. This maneuver can also be performed by applying a face mask to the patient;

however, the tight face mask seal required to make an accurate measurement is often difficult, and frequently impossible, to obtain. Care must be taken when making this measurement in the neurologically impaired patient because it may result in autonomic imbalance and precipitate cardiac arrhythmias.

It is unusual for a patient to have glottic dysfunction so severe as to prevent the generation of an effective cough on the basis of neurologic impairment alone. However, if necessary, glottic function can be evaluated by direct or indirect larynx examination.

Generating positive intrathoracic pressure requires active expiratory muscle activity. Such expiratory muscles include the intercostal and abdominal muscles. The function of these muscles is not easily measured or quantified. However, the degree of impairment can be predicted if a dermatomal level of motor impairment, as is associated with spinal cord injury, can be identified. Although spinal cord injury patients can often breathe deeply, their inability to generate a sufficiently high intrathoracic pressure renders their cough ineffective and often necessitates establishing an artificial airway despite what appear to be adequate ventilatory parameters. Many patients with neurologic injuries have no awareness of the need to cough. The degree of impairment that this imposes cannot be prospectively quantified.

Tracheostomy

Tracheostomy is often necessary in the neurologically injured patient. As with mechanical ventilatory support, the approach to tracheostomy requires a clear definition of needs and goals. A tracheostomy is a way to provide stable, comfortable, long-term airway management that will not cause laryngeal injury.

The first step in the decision-making process regarding tracheostomy is to define the clinical indication. As discussed, there are four indications for an artificial airway such as a tracheostomy: (*a*) airway obstruction, (*b*) airway protection, (*c*) bronchial hygiene, and (*d*) mechanical ventilation. Frequently, patients with brain injury do not have intact airway protective reflexes and will aspirate. Tracheostomy placement does not prevent microaspiration around the tracheostomy cuff because of capillary action; however, in the presence of an appropriately functioning cuff, a tracheostomy tube generally prevents massive aspiration of food particles or gastric and oral secretions. Thus, the problems of aspiration pneumonitis associated with aspiration of large amounts of acid-containing gastric secretions and airways obstruction due to aspiration of particulate food material will be eliminated.

Patients with brain or spinal cord injury are frequently unable to make effective cough efforts and require an artificial airway for safe and effective suctioning of bronchial secretions. Upper airway obstruction may be a problem in patients with head and neck trauma or malignancies, patients who have undergone cervical spine surgery via the anterior approach, or those who have neuromuscular disorders that preclude maintenance of appropriate head positioning. In these circumstances the upper airway (glottis) must be bypassed to maintain appropriate air movement into and out of the lungs.

Patients who require mechanical ventilatory support for a prolonged period must have a tracheostomy to allow positive pressure ventilation administration. Even patients who benefit from alternative modes of ventilatory support (i.e., negative pressures ventilation) almost always require a tracheostomy to facilitate bronchial hygiene and to provide positive pressure ventilation outside of the acute care setting as a "backup" to the alternative mode of ventilation.

Tracheostomy timing can be a rather controversial subject; however, if a consistent and straightforward approach is used, such decisions become much simpler. The most useful approach is to determine if the neurologic injury that necessitates an artificial airway is reversible. If it is not, then there is little sense in waiting a predetermined interval with an oral or nasal endotracheal tube in place, which allows for greater risk of laryngeal injury and the potential for accidental loss of the airway. In this circumstance, it is best to proceed to tracheostomy immediately to avoid these complications.

If the pathology necessitating an artificial airway is reversible, it is often prudent to wait and observe the patient for clinical improvements that would permit extubation. Based on the general recommendations of the Consensus Conference on Artificial Airways, if the pathology has persisted for 7–10 days and is not predicted to resolve within the next 3 days, it is best to proceed with tracheostomy (3). Early tracheostomy seems to be effective in reducing both days on the ventilator and days in the intensive care unit (ICU) (4). Although such data are not available specifically for the neurologically injured patient population, common sense suggests that these guidelines should be applicable to the patient with neurologic injury.

Tracheostomy procedures are traditionally performed in the sterile environment of the operating suite. Although this practice offers both real and perceived benefits, it is of questionable necessity in the critical care patient population. Bedside procedures in the ICU are becoming more routine because interhospital transport of potentially unstable patients carries risks of both morbidity and mortality. Additionally, the cost associated with such procedures is higher, and the time is constrained when working in the operating suite. The standard ICU milieu, however, is more flexible in terms of time constraints and adds little cost beyond the basic ICU costs. It has been shown that tracheostomies can be performed in the ICU without difficulty or additional complications with the availability of appropriate personnel and equipment (5).

Mechanical Ventilation

There are four basic clinical indications for mechanical ventilatory support: (*a*) apnea, (*b*) acute ventilatory failure, (*c*) impending ventilatory failure, and (*d*) hyperventilation for intracranial pressure (ICP) control. *Apnea* is a circumstance that can occur in a variety of clinical situations. It is often related to prescribed or illicit drug administration, such as neuromuscular blocking agents or narcotics. It can also occur with certain types of central nervous system (CNS) injury or profound cardiovascular instability. *Acute ventilatory failure* is a diagnosis based on arterial blood gas (ABG) analysis demonstrating an acute rise in $PaCO_2$ and an acute fall in pH. Such circumstances indicate that, for whatever reason, the patient is incapable of spontaneously maintaining normal carbon dioxide homeostasis. If the situation is not corrected and the patient is not appropriately supported, the process can lead eventually to death. *Impending ventilatory failure* is a clinical diagnosis made independent of ABG analysis. In this circumstance, the clinician is making the assessment that the patient's clinical presentation is consistent with significantly increased work of breathing that exceeds cardiopulmonary reserves and is *detrimental* to physiologic homeostasis. Therefore, if left unabated, this condition will eventually progress to respiratory muscle fatigue and acute ventilatory failure. Clinical signs of detrimental work of breathing include tachypnea, dyspnea, intercostal retractions, use of accessory muscles of ventilation, tachycardia, hypertension, diaphoresis, and so forth. *Hyperventilation for ICP control* is included here because, although many patients with CNS injuries will hyperventilate spontaneously, mechanical ventilation is the only way to assure the consistent maintenance of a desired $PaCO_2$.

BRAIN INJURY

Brain pathology requiring mechanical ventilatory support covers a wide range of neurologic insults, including trauma, tumors (primary brain or metastatic), and cerebral edema from various causes. Depending on the type of brain injury and its sequelae, the need for mechanical ventilatory support may be short term or chronic. Among the most common reasons for mechanical ventilatory support in this patient population is hyperventilation for ICP control, which should be considered a short-term proposition with clearly defined endpoints. It is usually recommended that this procedure be accomplished with tidal volumes of 12–15 ml/kg and ventilator rates of ~10 cycles/minute. The target $PaCO_2$ should be in the range of 28–32 mmHg (Fig. 22.2) (6). This hyperventilation level is usually sufficient to cause intracranial blood vessel consriction, decrease intracranial volume, and improve intracranial pressure.

Caution must be taken to avoid excessive hyperventilation. It has been demonstrated that acute hyperventilation to a $PaCO_2$ <20 mmHg results in brain tissue ischemia (7). This ischemia results in localized tissue acidosis, which causes a compensatory vasodilation; thus, brain perfusion is maintained by the mechanism for which hyperventilation is applied to prevent. Good evidence exists that even

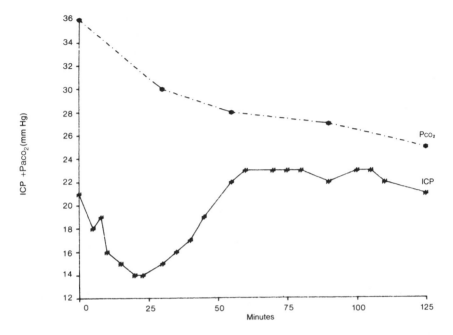

Figure 22.2. Typical temporal profile of intracranial pressure change after acute and sustained mechanical hyperventilation. Minute ventilation is increased at time = 0. (Reproduced with permission from Ropper AH. Neurological and neurosurgical intensive care, 3rd ed. New York, Raven Press, 1993.)

clinically acceptable levels of hyperventilation, although improving intracranial pressure, impair cerebral blood flow and oxygen delivery (8). Jugular venous bulb oxyhemoglobin saturation ($S_{jv}O_2$) can be used in conjunction with hyperventilation to guide therapy. The normal $S_{jv}O_2$ is ~75%; hyperventilation may be safely carried out to the point that the $S_{jv}O_2$ falls to ~50%. At this juncture, further hyperventilation-induced vasoconstriction will result in cerebral ischemia due to excessive reduction in cerebral blood flow.

Hyperventilation should be used primarily as a temporizing means by which to acutely control intracranial pressure. Hyperventilation alone is not sufficient to accomplish sustained control of intracranial hypertension (see Fig. 22.2). Other means of controlling intracranial pressure (e.g., osmolar diuresis, pharmacologic therapy) should be instituted as quickly as possible.

The need for aggressive pharmacologic interventions for intracranial pressure or seizure control can also make mechanical ventilatory support a necessity. For instance, although they lower cerebral oxygen utilization, provide cerebral protection, and raise the seizure threshold, barbiturates and benzodiazepines also can severely suppress the central medullary ventilatory centers to a point requiring mechanical ventilation to avoid serious hypercapnia or apnea. Neuromuscular blockade, which is frequently required as adjunctive therapy for intracranial pressure control, always results in apnea due to inactivation of the neuromuscular junction. Again, conventional volume-preset ventilatory modes are usually the most efficacious because they are consistent, they do not carry any significant detrimental effects when applied to the normal lung, and they help to prevent atelectasis and hypoxemia.

These indications for mechanical ventilation are acute and generally short term. However, chronic ventilatory support may be necessary when the injury affects the respiratory centers of the brain or when the combination of underlying cardiopulmonary disease and brain injury renders the patient unable to maintain current work of breathing. In this circumstance, it is important to simplify the mechanical ventilatory regimen as much as possible. Frequently, patients with neurologic injury who require mechanical ventilation are cared for in extended care facilities or at home where staffing or family members have minimal technical training related to medical devices. Therefore, the less complex the device and ventilator settings, the easier and more cost-effective is patient care. For example, unless positive end expiratory pressure (PEEP) is required to maintain oxygenation, it should be eliminated so that additional PEEP settings or valves do not need to be included in the system and periodically checked. Oxygen therapy should be minimized or eliminated, if possible. Other ventilatory maneuvers (i.e., inspiratory pause, expiratory retard, pressure support) should be discontinued and ventilatory modes chosen that are consistent with what is available on the commonly used portable ventilators.

Patients with brain injuries frequently have abnormal ventilatory patterns and varying degrees of autonomic instability (9). The clinical presentation then appears to be that of detrimental work of breathing and impending ventilatory failure, which results in the institution of mechanical ventilatory support. Although an abnormal ventilatory pattern and clinical presentation may represent increased work of breathing, they do not necessarily represent detrimental work of breathing. Therefore, mechanical ventilatory support may not be necessary. A useful approach to this situation is to evaluate the patient carefully for any underlying disease processes, such as infections (pulmonary and otherwise), cardiac failure, and so forth, which would account for the detrimental work of breathing, and to be certain to reverse any such processes. If the abnormal pattern of ventilation remains, mechanical ventilation should be withdrawn in a carefully monitored setting (i.e., neurologic ICU). The patient should be observed closely for evidence of clinical deterioration, and blood gases should be frequently monitored for evidence of acute ventilatory failure ($\uparrow$ $PaCO_2$, $\downarrow$ pH). If this does not occur after a reasonable time frame (24–48 hours), then the abnormal ventilatory pattern is central in origin and mechanical ventilatory support is not necessary. In such a circumstance, the ventilatory pattern frequently returns to normal several months following the brain injury.

SPINAL CORD INJURY

In the United States, traumatic injury of the spinal cord occurs ~10,000 times each year and primarily affects previously healthy young men 16–35 years of age. Mortality approaches 50% and is due to both the spinal cord injury and to concurrent traumatic injuries. Although this mortality is of great concern, the morbidity associated with spinal cord injury is equally significant, both in terms of lifestyle and in societal costs. Despite a great deal of research and improvements in the treatment of complications associated with spinal cord injury, the degree of neurologic recovery following serious spinal cord injuries remains dismal.

Spinal cord injuries are classified by neurologic impairment type and injury level, both dermatomal and vertebral. A commonly used neurologic injury classification system is the Frankel Classification (Table 22.1) (10). Classifying the level of injury is usually intuitive; however, there are instances where the level of vertebral injury differs from that of the neurologic injury. This discrepancy may be due to incomplete neurologic injuries or secondary factors (e.g., spinal cord edema, hemorrhage, infarction) that cause neurologic impairment above or below the level of vertebral column disruption.

Spinal cord injuries affect respiratory function in various ways that result in the need for mechanical ventilation. The degree to which respiratory function is impaired relates directly to the level and type of spinal cord injury. The higher into the thoracic and cervical region the injury extends and the more complete the neurologic injury, the greater the degree of respiratory embarrassment. This is demonstrated by the data in Table 22.2 relating the level of complete neurologic injuries to respiratory complication rates and mortality (11).

The neurologic pathways controlling the respiratory musculature descend from the brainstem through the spinal cord to the levels of the phrenic nuclei (C3–5)

Table 22.1. Frankel Classification of Neurologic Injury

Class	Neurologic Injury
A	Complete lesion, loss of sensory and motor function below the level of injury.
B	Incomplete lesion, sensory function present below level of injury.
C	Incomplete lesion, nonfunctional motor activity present below level of injury.
D	Incomplete lesion, functional motor activity present below level of injury.
E	Neurologically intact, no motor or sensory deficits associated with spine fracture.

Table 22.2. Relationship Between Pulmonary Complications, Mortality, and Level of Neurologic Injury[a]

| | Level of Neurologic Injury (% of Patients) | | | | | | | Total |
Pathology	C1–C2	C3–C5	C6–C8	T1–T6	T7–T12	L1–L5	S1–S5	(N = 1698)
Pneumonia	37.5	16.7	8.9	13.2	7.1	4.2	0.0	8.2
Acute ventilatory failure	25.0	15.1	7.3	5.5	1.9	1.6	0.0	5.9
Death	37.5	7.1	4.7	7.1	2.6	1.6	0.0	4.4

[a] *Data pertain to 1698 patients admitted to Midwest Regional Spinal Cord Injury Center.*

in the spinal cord (see Fig. 22.1). Disruption of these pathways at or above the level of C2 results in apnea and death if resuscitative efforts are not undertaken immediately; chronic ventilatory support is then required if life is to be sustained. Injuries below the C5 level seldom require mechanical ventilatory support, at least not on a long-term basis, unless there are other mitigating circumstances (e.g., head injury, underlying severe cardiopulmonary disease). Injuries at C3–C4 occasionally require some level of chronic mechanical ventilatory support, depending on the patient's underlying cardiopulmonary reserves and associated chest injuries.

Methods by which clinicians provide ventilatory support for patients with such neurologic injuries range from conventional positive pressure ventilation techniques to phrenic nerve or diaphragmatic pacing systems (negative pressure ventilation). Other negative pressure ventilation techniques, such as "iron lungs," are primarily of historical interest. The choice of artificial ventilatory method depends on the injury type and any underlying clinical conditions. Conventional positive pressure ventilation is always the simplest and most available option under most clinical conditions. However, select patients may be given a great deal more mobility with alternative ventilatory methods.

Conventional positive pressure ventilation using standard tidal volumes (12–15 ml/kg) and ventilator rates (8–10 cycles/minute for full ventilatory support; ≤6 cycles/minute for partial ventilatory support) usually suffice for mechanical ventilatory support in the acute phase of spinal cord injury. Once the patient demonstrates the need for mechanical ventilation on a chronic basis, several modifications of standard ventilatory techniques are frequently necessary to maintain patient comfort and restore the ability to vocalize. Frequently patients with spinal cord injury express subjective feelings of breathlessness despite adequate ventilation or even hyperventilation. The reason for this may be related to the loss of somatic and visceral sensory function, but the mechanism of this phenomenon is complex and poorly understood. This subjective breathlessness often can be alleviated by using larger than normal tidal volumes (>15 ml/kg) and lower ventilator rates.

When adjusting ventilator tidal volumes for this reason, it is important to assess the effects on $PaCO_2$ to avoid severe hypocapnia and respiratory alkalemia. A $PaCO_2$ <30 mmHg is also considered acceptable if the pH is <7.55. Tidal volumes producing airway plateau pressures <35 cmH_2O are generally considered within the safe range. Excessively large tidal volumes that might induce pulmonary volutrauma should also be avoided.

Restorating vocalization is an important aspect in the rehabilitation of patients with spinal cord injury. This sometimes can be accomplished with specially de-signed tracheostomy tubes that permit airflow past the vocal cords; however, the failure rate of such devices is high. Therefore, special airway and ventilator manipu-lations are often necessary to accomplish this goal. The most useful and straightfor-ward method to reestablish vocalization is to deflate the tracheostomy cuff until there is a sufficient air leak past the vocal cords to permit speech. This requires that the patient learn to speak during inspiration rather than exhalation, but this is not usually a significant problem in the motivated patient. Again, the tidal volume, air flow patterns, and ventilator rate must be adjusted to compensate for the air leak and to maintain adequate alveolar ventilation. Generally this requires larger tidal volumes and higher ventilator rates. In this circumstance, the more frequent the ventilator breaths, the more frequently the patient is able to vocalize. It is not possible to predict what ventilator settings is required to optimize vocaliza-tion; therefore, it is a "trial-and-error" process that requires close monitoring of the patient's respiratory and hemodynamic status. One-way valves can be used in the ventilator circuit to force all exhaled gases to pass through the vocal cords and enhance vocalization (12). However, appropriate monitoring is especially impor-tant in this situation because severe air-trapping may occur, which can result in significantly increased intrathoracic pressure with subsequent hemodynamic instability.

Noninvasive methods of assessing $PaCO_2$, such as capnography or transcutane-ous PCO_2, may be used during the abovementioned ventilator adjustments; how-ever, the limitations of these monitoring methods must be understood and the information obtained from them should be confirmed with appropriate blood gas analysis.

Phrenic nerve or diaphragmatic pacing devices have been available for many years (13). These devices function in a fashion similar to cardiac pacemakers; however, because the muscular structure and neurologic innervation of the dia-phragm is very different from that of the heart, the pacing electrodes are most effectively placed around the phrenic nerve rather than in the muscle itself. Because of this requirement, intact phrenic nerves are needed for use of this technology. Candidates for phrenic nerve or diaphragm pacer implantation are those with spinal cord lesions at the C1–C2 level or those with abnormalities of the medullary respiratory centers (i.e., central hypoventilation syndrome). The C1–C2 lesion must be "clean" in that the spinal cord below that level, primarily the area of

C3–C5 (which contains the phrenic nerve nuclei) must be intact. If the C1–C2 lesion occurs because the original spinal cord lesion began at a lower level and ascended through secondary processes (i.e., edema or hemorrhage), the phrenic nerve nuclei will be damaged, the phrenic nerve will undergo Wallerian degeneration, and pacing will be rendered impossible. There are intercostal-to-phrenic-nerve grafting procedures that may permit phrenic nerve pacing in such individuals; however, these techniques are still early in development (14).

Phrenic nerve pacing systems include several components: (*a*) implanted electrodes, (*b*) implanted receiver system, (*c*) external antennas, and (*d*) an external transmitter system (Fig. 22.3). Some phrenic nerve pacing systems use one stimulating electrode that consistently stimulates one region of the phrenic nerve, whereas other phrenic nerve pacing systems use a quadripolar electrode system that stimulates different areas of the phrenic nerve sequentially with each breath. The quadripolar electrode system is not currently commercially available. Research centers working with it, however, have found that it has several advantages over the unipolar systems in terms of more rapid conditioning and improved endurance (15).

The electrodes are implanted around the phrenic nerve in a noncircumferential fashion to avoid nerve constriction and subsequent damage (see Fig. 22.3, *inset*). Electrode implantation can occur around the phrenic nerve as it courses through the neck or the chest. Neck implantation is preferred in adults because the procedure is less invasive than a thoracotomy and the nerve is larger and more easily located. In children, thoracic implantation is often preferred because the thoracic phrenic nerve is larger and more easily identified.

The transmitter generates a radio signal that is picked up by the receivers and converted into a series of electrical impulses which, in turn, stimulate the phrenic nerves and cause diaphragmatic contraction. The stimuli amplitude and frequency are adjusted to provide adequate tidal volumes and carbon dioxide excretion with minimal stimulus amplitude to avoid nerve damage. Following implantation and recovery from the surgery (~2 weeks), pacing and phrenic nerve-diaphragm conditioning can begin. This is accomplished by pacing until the phrenic nerve-diaphragm unit fatigues. Fatigue is monitored by sequentially or continuously measuring tidal volumes, which decrease progressively as fatigue develops. After an adequate period of rest, pacing is again instituted and progressively prolonged as tolerated. The pacing pattern with the unipolar electrode system often requires alternating unilateral pacing. This allows rest of the phrenic nerve-diaphragm unit on one side while the alternate side is being paced. It may take several weeks before 24-hour pacing can be done with this process and with the unipolar system.

Phrenic nerve pacing process appears to be much more rapid with the quadripolar electrode system in that simultaneous bilateral pacing can often be accomplished within 24–48 hours of initiation of conditioning (unpublished results). Such systems allow much greater patient mobility because it is not necessary to

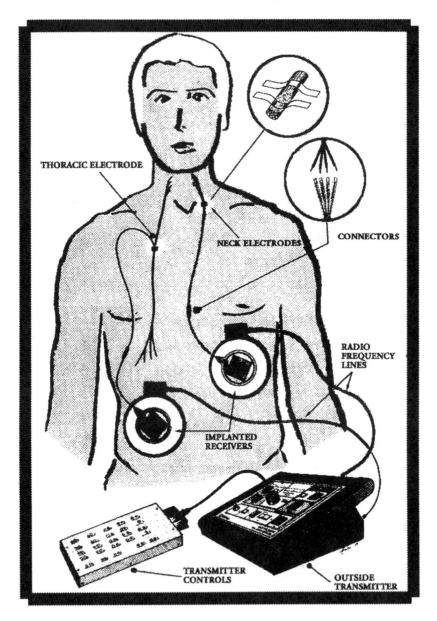

Figure 22.3. The receiver components are implanted subcutaneously on the chest or abdominal wall and connected to the electrodes with wires that are burrowed under the skin and through the chest wall, if necessary. The antennas lie outside the chest wall, over the implanted receiver components. (Modified with permission from Atrotech CO., Tampere, Finland.)

carry along a heavy and cumbersome ventilator during routine trips. Although these systems eliminate the need for a mechanical ventilator in the home, a self-inflating manual resuscitation bag is necessary in case of a pacing system malfunction or pathophysiologic problems encountered with the patient.

NEUROMUSCULAR DISEASES

Several neuromuscular disease groups alter respiratory muscle function either in a periodic or progressive fashion. Myasthenia gravis is a disease that is typically insidious in onset and presents as fluctuating voluntary muscle weakness. It is a relatively rare disease that occurs predominately in women (two thirds of patients) with an incidence of ~1 in 30,000. Women usually present with the disease as young adults; whereas, men rarely develop symptoms before the age of 40. Approximately 10% of all cases occur in the pediatric age group. The disease is felt to be due to destruction or inactivation of the postsynaptic neuromuscular junction by antibodies that recognize the neuromuscular junction as foreign. Between 70% and 80% of functional acetylcholine receptors are lost by the time the patient is symptomatic. The origin of this autoantibody is not known, but the thymus gland has been implicated in that (*a*) thymic hyperplasia is present in >70% of patients with myasthenia gravis and (*b*) ~75% of patients who undergo thymectomy undergo remission. Nonsurgical therapeutic modalities include anticholinesterase drugs, corticosteroids, direct immunosuppressant agents, and plasmapheresis. Excessive anticholinesterase therapy can result in cholinergic crisis, which also manifests as skeletal muscle weakness. This situation can be differentiated from worsening of the underlying disease by the administration of an additional dose of intravenous anticholinesterase (i.e., 1 to 2 mg of edrophonium). Worsening of symptoms, plus muscarinic side effects (e.g., miosis, salivation, bradycardia) confirms the diagnosis of cholinergic crisis. The disease is exacerbated by exercise and improves after a periods of rest.

Respiratory muscle weakness rarely is a presenting symptom of myasthenia gravis; however, it is seen later in the course of the progressive form of the disease. Ventilator support is usually necessary only for short periods of time during acute exacerbations of the disease process. Ventilatory failure is secondary to neurotransmission failure at the neuromuscular junction. When ventilation must be initiated, full ventilatory support should be started with a conventional volume preset ventilatory mode that delivers a consistent tidal volume and minute ventilation (i.e., synchronized intermittent mandatory ventilation). In addition to providing for CO_2 excretion, this mechanical ventilatory support system also prevents widespread atelectasis. As the acute exacerbation abates or control is gained with a new medication regimen, mechanical ventilatory support usually can be withdrawn rapidly by any of several techniques.

Assistance with bronchial hygiene usually precedes the need for mechanical ventilation because the vital capacity falls to a level where an adequate cough cannot be generated (<15 ml/kg). This frequently requires the establishment of an artificial airway which may be necessary on a chronic basis (tracheostomy) if uncontrolled exacerbations occur with any frequency. Proceeding to tracheostomy must be predicated on the ongoing needs of the patient rather than a single disease exacerbation episode.

Guillain-Barré syndrome typically presents as a rapidly progressive, ascending peripheral neuropathy. Neurologic defects are usually limited to motor paralysis and autonomic dysfunction, both of which can be severe and prolonged if untreated. Sensory symptoms may be present, but objective sensory loss is rare. The etiology of the Guillain-Barré syndrome is not clear, but it has been linked to viral infections, vaccinations, and immunosuppressive therapy. About one half of the patients suffering from this syndrome report a recent history of respiratory or gastrointestinal tract infections prior to onset of symptoms. Treatment is mainly supportive and symptomatic; however, plasmapheresis appears to quicken recovery. Mortality is <5%, but autonomic nervous system instability is the primary cause of death due to this syndrome. Recovery is not always complete and axonal degeneration may leave some patients with permanent weakness in affected muscle groups.

When ventilatory support is required, it is usually for a limited time because the disease often responds well to appropriate therapy. However, ventilatory support becomes a major part of the patient's care as neurologic dysfunction begins to affect the nerves innervating the respiratory musculature. The gradual progression usually permits ventilatory assistance to be initiated in a planned rather than an emergent fashion. Serial measurements of vital capacity and blood gases best assist in deciding when to establish an artificial airway and institute mechanical ventilatory support. Any patient with questionable ventilatory function who is required to leave the ICU, either for diagnostic studies or for transfer to another institution, should be intubated and ventilated prior to leaving the critical care setting. When mechanical ventilatory support is necessary, conventional modes and ventilatory techniques are usually adequate. With appropriate therapy, recovery is often within weeks and tracheostomy is currently often unnecessary.

Amyotrophic lateral sclerosis is a progressive demyelinating disease that ultimately results in the paralysis of all skeletal muscles. The need for mechanical ventilation usually occurs late in the disease process and is very gradual in onset. Patients may be provided ventilatory support initially with noninvasive mechanical ventilatory techniques (e.g., bi-level positive airway pressure therapy), constant airflow generators or negative pressure ventilatory techniques (e.g., chest cuirass) (Fig. 22.4). The goal of such therapy is not to provide complete ventilatory support; rather, it is to eliminate only that work of breathing that is detrimental to the

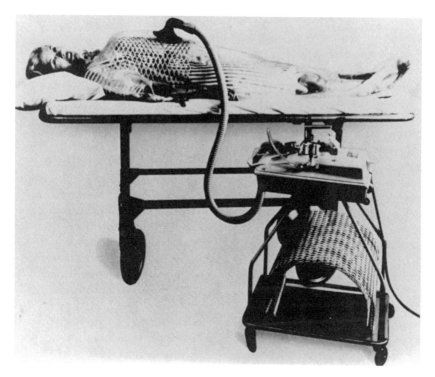

Figure 22.4. Emerson cuirass. (Courtesy of J. H. Emerson Co., Cambridge, Massachusetts.)

patient and which might lead to acute ventilatory failure. The degree of difficulty initiating ventilation varies depending on the technique chosen.

Continuous air flow generators basically function like vacuum cleaners in reverse. Air is blown out through a tube, into the patient's mouth, through the glottis and, ultimately, into the lungs. Such a device requires that patients are able to manipulate a circular object into their mouths, form a seal with their lips, and open and close their glottis. Patients can perform this maneuver as frequently or infrequently as they choose, thus, titrating the ventilatory support level to their subjective symptoms of breathlessness or fatigue. These devices are relatively portable and inexpensive, but not commonly used. The utility of these devices is limited because the patient's clinical condition is progressive and the necessary motor skills required for their use eventually become inadequate.

The chest cuirass requires that a "turtle shell" type of device be applied to the anterior chest and abdomen (see Fig. 22.4) with a good seal around the edges. A vacuum is then generated between the shell and the patient, which results in chest expansion, anterior abdominal wall motion with subsequent descent of the diaphragm and tidal ventilation. The problem with this technique is that the fit and seal are not always adequate and it is frequently necessary to have a custom chest piece manufactured. Additionally, changes in body size and shape, as occurs with degenerative diseases, periodically necessitate refitting of the chest piece.

Bi-level positive airway pressure entails the application of an expiratory airway pressure and an inspiratory airway pressure to the patient's airway via a face mask. This face mask is usually an appropriately fitting nasal mask. Air flow is directed into the mask to maintain the chosen expiratory positive airway pressure (EPAP); additional airflow is applied with inspiration to maintain the desired inspiratory positive airway pressure (IPAP). In this patient population, it is the gradient between the EPAP and IPAP levels that is most important because this gradient determines the degree of tidal volume augmentation that will occur. The EPAP level is set and usually maintained constant. The IPAP level is titrated upward to whatever level is tolerated by the patient. An IPAP level that is too high can become uncomfortable, whereas a low IPAP level will not produce adequate augmentation of tidal volume. Correct initiate and adjustment of the various ventilatory parameters associated with bi-level positive airway pressure require close clinical monitoring and the constant attention of various medical personnel (i.e., physician, respiratory therapist, nurse).

Unfortunately, these "noninvasive" methods become progressively less effective as the disease advances. Eventually the patient's ability to clear bronchial secretions and maintain CO_2 excretion becomes so severely compromised to require a tracheostomy and chronic mechanical ventilatory support. It is important to discuss the clinical situation thoroughly with the patient and define the desired goals while the patient can communicate effectively. Some patients do not desire to initiate or to continue mechanical ventilatory support beyond a certain point of disability. The patient's wishes must be completely clear to all concerned so that the desired care is provided and inappropriate interventions are not made.

BRAIN-DEAD PATIENT

The diagnosis of brain death requires that there be a complete lack of brain activity at all levels. This means that all basic reflexes must be absent, including corneal, occulovestibular, gag, and carinal (cough) reflexes. After confirmation that these reflexes are absent, the final step in the clinical diagnosis of brain death requires the demonstration of apnea. This demonstration must be accomplished in the absence of any drugs that might interfere with the central or peripheral neuromuscular function. Also, the patient must not be hypothermic when the diagnosis of brain death is made.

To document apnea there must be complete absence of ventilatory activity in the face of a maximal stimulus to breathe. Such a stimulus requires that a $PaCO_2$

>60 mmHg and an arterial pH <7.3 be attained; however, it is critical that oxygenation be maintained while minute ventilation is decreased to allow the $PaCO_2$ to rise. Apnea can confirmed in different ways depending on the subsequent clinical plan. If organ donation is planned, then the aforementioned parameters (pH, $PaCO_2$, PaO_2 ventilatory efforts) must be clearly measured and documented in an organized and defined fashion, which has been termed the *ventilatory challenge*. If organ donation is not part of the plan following the diagnosis of brain death, then an *apneic challenge*, which accomplishes the same goal with fewer blood tests, may be performed.

The ventilatory challenge requires that a trained professional (i.e., physician, nurse, respiratory care practitioner) provide appropriate bedside monitoring and support during the procedure. During the ventilatory challenge, the patient should be given one breath with an oxygen-enriched atmosphere ($F_IO_2 = 0.5$–1.0) every 30 seconds. This should permit a gradual rise in $PaCO_2$ while ensuring that adequate arterial oxygenation is maintained. The patient should be closely observed for evidence of spontaneous ventilatory efforts and cardiopulmonary instability. Arterial blood gases should be obtained at 5-minute intervals until the appropriate endpoints (pH <7.3, $PaCO_2$ >60 mmHg) are documented. Once these endpoints are reached and there is no evidence of spontaneous ventilatory efforts, the declaration of brain death is made and the patient is again placed on full ventilatory support until organs can be harvested.

If organ donation is not an option, then establishing brain death and withdrawing ventilatory support can be done simultaneously. In this procedure, the apneic challenge, the patient is preoxygenated with 100% oxygen for 5–10 minutes, and is then removed from the ventilator and placed on a T-piece delivering 100% oxygen. In this manner, oxygenation will be maintained while the $PaCO_2$ rises to the appropriate level. If the patient is indeed brain dead, cardiac function eventually ceases due to hypercapnia and acidosis. Oxygenation will be maintained because of the preoxygenation and because of ongoing entrainment of oxygen through the endotracheal tube as it is used at the alveolar level (apneic oxygenation). If extubation is desired, oxygen can be delivered via a face mask if the airway remains patent; however, it is probably best to document apnea with the ventilatory challenge first and then extubate the patient without concern for maintaining a patent airway or oxygenation.

In both the ventilatory challenge and the apneic challenge, it is important that the patient be permitted the opportunity to develop spontaneous ventilatory efforts without being allowed to succumb to hypoxia. Only in this way can one be certain that the brainstem is nonfunctional and that all the criteria for the declaration of brain death have been met.

On rare occasions it is necessary to support a patient who is known or suspected to be brain dead for an extended period of time. The reasons for this include maintaining a pregnant patient until fetal maturity is achieved, allowing metabolism of drugs known to confuse the clinical picture, or permitting the appropriate timing of transplantation. The primary goals in such supportive ventilatory care are to minimize ventilator-induced lung injury, maintain physiologic homeostasis, and compromise hemodynamics as little as possible. Most individuals who are selected for organ donation have a premorbid level of health that is near normal; therefore, preexisting lung pathology is not usually a complicating issue when maintaining ventilatory support. However, the lungs are the most frequently refused organs offered for transplantation. This is partly due to the propensity of the lungs to mount nonspecific inflammatory responses to a variety of systemic insults, but this can also be attributed to unnecessary ventilator-induced lung injury. Although it is not currently possible to avoid all inflammatory responses, eliminating ventilator injury is an attainable goal. Factors responsible for ventilator-induced lung injury include oxygen toxicity and alveolar overdistension (16). Maintaining the F_IO_2 <0.5 helps to preserve normal function in lungs being considered for transplantation. Alveolar trauma caused by excessive tidal ventilation is another avoidable causative mechanism in ventilator-induced lung injury. These patients often require hyperventilation prior to being declared brain dead. This hyperventilation can be done using tidal volumes that maintain alveolar pressures believed to be in the nontraumatic range (30–40 cmH$_2$O) and higher respiratory rates if necessary.

By following the relatively simple guidelines outlined herein, ventilator-induced lung injury can be minimized. Often conflicting therapeutic goals arise in bridging the gap from declaration of brain death to organ harvesting in the brain dead patient. These conflicts are best resolved by the regional organ bank overseeing and directing the patient's preharvest care. Organ banks and procurement agencies are most familiar with local organ needs and can help to prioritize management issues in individual patients.

CONCLUSIONS

The neurologically injured patient often has very little preexisting pulmonary disease and responds to positive pressure ventilation well. Although sophisticated ventilatory support techniques may be necessary in certain clinical situations, successful ventilation of the neurologically injured is usually accomplished with conventional ventilatory techniques and minor modifications. Although the artificial airways and mechanical ventilation that these patients often require can add to their disability and to the complexity of their care, when appropriately managed the impact of these needs can be reduced.

References

1. Shapiro BA, Kacmarek RM, Cane RD, Peruzzi WT, Hauptman D. Retained secretions. In: Clinical application of respiratory care, 4th ed. Chicago, Mosby-Year Book, Inc., 1991, pp 49–56.

2. Shapiro BA, Kacmarek RM, Cane RD, Peruzzi WT, Hauptman D. Clinical evaluation of the pulmonary system. In: Clinical application of respiratory care, 4th ed. Chicago, Mosby-Year Book, Inc., 1991, pp 29–45.

3. Consensus Conference on Artificial Airways in Patients Receiving Mechanical Ventilation (Consensus Conference). Chest 96:178–180, 1989.

4. Lesnik I, Rappaport W, Fulginiti J, Witzke D. The role of early tracheostomy in blunt, multiple organ trauma. Am Surg 58:346–349, 1992.

5. Stock MC, Woodward CG, Shapiro BA, Cane RD, et al. Perioperative complications of elective tracheostomy in critically ill patients. Crit Care Med 14:861–863, 1986.

6. Ropper AH. Treatment of intracranial hypertension. In: Ropper AH (ed.). Neurological and neurosurgical intensive care, 3rd ed. New York, Raven Press, 1993, pp 29–52.

7. Plum F, Posner JB. Blood and cerebrospinal fluid lactate during hyperventilation. Am J Physiol 212:864–870, 1967.

8. Fortune JB, Feustel PJ, Graca L, Hasselbarth J, Kuehler DH. Effect of hyperventilation, Mannitol, and ventriculostomy drainage on cerebral blood flow after head injury. Journal of Trauma: Injury, Infection, and Critical Care 39:1091–1099, 1995.

9. Plum F, Posner JB. The pathologic physiology of signs and symptoms of coma. In: The diagnosis of stupor and coma, 3rd ed. Philadelphia, FA Davis, 1984, pp 1–73.

10. Frankle HL, Hancock DO, Hyslop G, et al. The value of postural reduction in the initial management of closed injuries of the spine with paraplegia and tetraplegia: Part I. Paraplegia 7: 179–192, 1969.

11. Meyer PR. Pulmonary effects of acute spinal cord injury: assessment and management. In: Surgery of spine trauma. New York, Churchill Livingstone, 1989, pp 173–183.

12. Manzano JL, Lubillo S, Henriquez D, Martin JC, Perez MC, Wilson DJ. Verbal communication of ventilator-dependent patients. Crit Care Med 21:512–517, 1993.

13. Glenn WWL, Brouillette RT, Dentz B, Fodstad H, Hunt CE, Keens TG, Marsh HM, Pande S, Piepgras DG, Vanderlinden RG. Fundamental considerations in pacing of the diaphragm for chronic ventilatory insufficiency: a multi-center study. PACE Pacing Clin Electrophysiol 11: 2121–2127, 1988.

14. Krieger AJ, Mitchell RG, Adler RJ. Electrophrenic respiration after intercostal to phrenic nerve anastomosis in a patient with anterior spinal artery syndrome: technical case report. Neurosurgery 35:760–764, 1994.

15. Baer GA, Talonen PP, Hakkinen V, Exner G, Yrjola H. Phrenic nerve stimulation in tetraplegia. Scand J Rehabil Med 22:107–111, 1990.

16. Shapiro BA, Peruzzi WT. Changing practices in ventilator management: a review of the literature and suggested clinical correlations. Surgery 117:121–133, 1995.

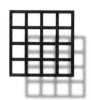

23
Weaning from Mechanical Ventilation

Ashvini H. Gursahaney • *Stewart B. Gottfried*

When ventilatory support is no longer required, the process of transferring the task of breathing from the ventilator to the patient has been referred to as *weaning.* In the broadest sense, weaning refers to all methods of discontinuing mechanical ventilation. In most patients, especially those requiring short-term ventilatory support for an acute and rapidly reversible condition, discontinuing ventilatory support is not difficult. In patients requiring more prolonged ventilatory assistance, however, the ability to resume spontaneous breathing is often fraught with difficulty and can represent a more gradual and time-consuming process. In particular, weaning may be problematic in patients with severe preexisting lung disease or in those with significant residual respiratory dysfunction related to an acute illness. To predict which patients are capable of breathing spontaneously, it is important to understand the balance between the amount of work required for breathing and the capability of the ventilatory pump to perform that work. Management of the patient who experiences difficulty during weaning requires recognition of the imbalance between these factors and prompt institution of appropriate measures to return this relationship back toward normal.

DETERMINANTS OF WEANING OUTCOME

The ability to tolerate the discontinuation of mechanical ventilation depends on the integrity of both the mechanical components of the respiratory system and its gas exchanging capacity. In this regard, it is conceptually helpful to classify respiratory failure into two major categories: Type I hypoxemic respiratory failure (i.e., lung failure) and type II hypercapnic respiratory failure (i.e., pump failure). Although abnormalities in oxygenation may lead to failure to wean, most cases requiring prolonged mechanical ventilation can be attributed to ventilatory pump failure. This may be related to neuromuscular dysfunction, increased ventilatory loads, or a combination of the two. To understand why an individual patient fails to wean, it is important to identify which of these physiologic variables are altered,

Table 23.1. Determinants of Weaning Outcome

Oxygenation
Decreased respiratory capacity
  Decreased respiratory center output
  Phrenic nerve dysfunction
  Peripheral nerve dysfunction
  Disorders of neuromuscular junction
  Muscular disorders
Increased ventilatory demand
  Abnormal respiratory mechanics
  Dynamic hyperinflation
  Ventilator circuit load
  Increased dead space ventilation
  Increased central drive and minute ventilation

keeping in mind that one or potentially even several factors may be responsible (Table 23.1).

Oxygenation (Type I Hypoxemic Respiratory Failure)

Hypoxemia can occur for many different reasons. These include severe hypoventilation, ventilation-perfusion ($\dot{V}_A/\dot{Q}$) mismatch, true shunt, diffusion impairment, or reduced oxygen delivery (which by reduces the oxygen content of venous blood and worsens existing hypoxemia). Intubation and mechanical ventilation may improve hypoxemia by affecting one or more of these variables. Endotracheal tube placement ensures a specific and increased inspired oxygen concentration. Positive pressure ventilation itself can improve oxygenation owing to a better $\dot{V}_A/\dot{Q}$ matching or a reduction in shunt, particularly in the case of retained secretions or atelectasis. In addition, positive pressure ventilation may be beneficial because of its effects on cardiac function or the oxygen cost of breathing. Although mechanical ventilation provides supportive care in patients with hypoxemia, it is still necessary to identify and treat the underlying cause of lung failure. Typically, this includes parenchymal lung disease characterized by distal airspace filling with fluid (cardiogenic or noncardiogenic pulmonary edema), inflammatory exudate (infection, alveolitis), or blood (pulmonary hemorrhage).

Ventilatory Pump Failure
(Type II Hypercapnic Respiratory Failure)

Neuromuscular dysfunction, excessive ventilatory load, or a combination of both can lead to ventilatory pump failure. Neuromuscular impairment may be due to abnormalities anywhere along the neuraxis from the central nervous system

| RESPIRATORY CAPACITY | | VENTILATORY LOAD |

DEPRESSED DRIVE
    Narcotics, Sedatives
    Metabolic Alkalosis
    Hypothyroidism

IMPAIRED TRANSMISSION

    SPINAL CORD DISEASE
    - Multiple Sclerosis
    - Amyotrophic Lateral Sclerosis
    - Trauma

    PHRENIC NERVE INJURY
    - Cardiac Surgery
    - Central Venous Catheterization
    - Other Trauma
    - Post Viral Illness

    PERIPHERAL NEUROPATHY
    - Guillain-Barre
    - ICU Polyneuropathy

    NEUROMUSCULAR JUNCTION
    - Myasthenia Gravis

MUSCLE WEAKNESS
    Malnutrition
    Electrolyte Imbalance
    Endocrinopathies

INCREASED CENTRAL DRIVE
    Sepsis
    Fever
    Pain, Anxiety
    Agitation

INCREASED DEAD SPACE VENTILATION
    Pulmonary Embolism
    ARDS
    COPD

RESISTIVE LOADS
    Bronchospasm
    Secretions
    Endotracheal Tube
    Ventilator Circuit

LUNG ELASTIC LOADS
    Pulmonary Edema
    Pneumonia
    Atelectasis

CHEST WALL ELASTIC LOADS
    Pleural Fluid
    Abdominal Distension
    Ascites
    Obesity

THRESHOLD LOADS
    Ventilator Trigger
    Intrinsic PEEP

Figure 23.1. Failure to wean from mechanical ventilation. The balance between respiratory capacity and ventilatory load.

to the respiratory muscles themselves (Fig. 23.1). These abnormalities include decreased central drive, impaired neural transmission along the spinal cord or peripheral nerves, or primary muscle weakness. If isolated, these abnormalities are generally associated with a normal or only mild reduction in arterial PO_2.

Although a proportion of hypercapnic respiratory failure is due to some form of neuromuscular dysfunction, mechanical derangement of the respiratory system (e.g., pulmonary edema, pneumonia, status asthmaticus, chronic obstructive pulmonary disease [COPD]) is perhaps more common. In considering weaning a patient from mechanical ventilation, it is useful to review the general factors that may be responsible for success or failure.

DECREASED RESPIRATORY CENTER OUTPUT

Central respiratory drive impairment may be a cause of weaning failure that may be an obvious consideration in patients recovering from a recent cerebrovascular accident, neurosurgical procedure, or head trauma. A reduction in central drive for other reasons may not be readily apparent, however, but nevertheless can contribute to ventilatory failure. This notion is particularly true if superimposed on significant acute or chronic respiratory disease, which may render the balance between respiratory capacity and ventilatory demand tenuous. For example, occult hypothyroidism may reduce central drive while impairing respiratory muscle strength. The most common reasons for central respiratory drive depression are iatrogenic factors such as the effects of sedative and opiod medications.

NEURAL CONDUCTION

Although there may be adequate output from the respiratory center, the signal must be successfully transmitted to the various muscles of respiration. A defect in neural transmission may occur at the level of the spinal cord, phrenic nerve, other peripheral nerves, or at the neuromuscular junction (see also Chapter 22, Ventilation of the Neurologically Injured). Abnormalities within the spinal cord are most commonly posttraumatic. Other common nontraumatic disorders include ischemia, malignancies (e.g, direct compression or paraneoplastic syndrome), demyelinating or degenerative diseases (e.g., multiple sclerosis, amyotrophic lateral sclerosis). Spinal cord lesions below the C5 level rarely result in ventilator dependence, except when accompanied by other abnormalities in respiratory function or ventilatory load. For example, the development of pneumonia in a low cervical quadriplegic may precipitate acute respiratory failure.

Because the diaphragm is the primary muscle of respiration, phrenic nerve dysfunction is associated with significant reduction in the ability to generate inspiratory force. Although phrenic nerve injury may be postinfectious or idiopathic, it is much more commonly seen in the postoperative setting. Patients undergoing coronary artery bypass surgery are particularly susceptible, where direct thermal injury to the phrenic nerve is associated with the use of cold cardioplegia. Phrenic nerve injury has also been reported as a complication of central venous catheterization. Lastly, routine upper abdominal surgery has been associated with transient reduction in diaphragmatic pressure generation, which improves progressively over the first postoperative week. This defect has been thought to be neurally mediated because external electrical stimulation of the phrenic nerve has been shown to produce normal transdiaphragmatic pressure. This problem has been ascribed to reflex inhibition from abdominal visceral afferents. Because of the physiologic reserve present in a previously healthy individual, however, isolated phrenic nerve injury should not result in respiratory failure unless other significant coexistent pulmonary function abnormalities are also present.

A polyneuropathy with conduction abnormalities diffusely involving the muscles of respiration may also result in respiratory failure. A typical example is the Guillain-Barré-Strohl syndrome, an acute inflammatory polyneuropathy, where mechanical ventilation is necessary in 15%–20% of patients. Critical illness itself has been associated with the development of a sensory-motor polyneuropathy referred to as *critical care polyneuropathy* or *(intensive care unit ICU) neuropathy.* In general, there tends to be a gradual recovery as the underlying illness improves. This may be prolonged, however, and patients may be left with significant residual dysfunction.

Disorders of the neuromuscular junction (e.g., myasthenia gravis or Eaton-Lambert syndrome) may impair weaning owing to decreased respiratory muscle strength or endurance. Although the diagnosis is generally apparent prior to the onset of respiratory symptoms, these disorders may first present with unexplained ventilatory failure.

MUSCULAR DISORDERS

A variety of primary pathologic conditions affecting skeletal muscle may adversely affect respiratory muscle function. This diagnosis could include, for example, relatively unusual disorders such as muscular dystrophy as well as mitochondrial or enzyme abnormalities. However, undernutrition is a much more common cause of respiratory muscle weakness in the mechanically ventilated patient. Because respiratory muscle mass correlates well with total body mass, reduced respiratory muscle strength occurs quickly in the critically ill, mechanically ventilated patient because of an imbalance between nutritional support and metabolic demands. In addition, metabolic abnormalities frequently are found in patients in the ICU, and they easily can be overlooked. Disorders of potassium and, particularly, magnesium, calcium, and phosphate metabolism have all been shown to adversely affect respiratory muscle strength. Mechanically ventilated patients are prone to develop electrolyte imbalances owing to inadequate oral intake, excess loss (e.g., diuretic use, vomiting, diarrhea), or inadequate replacement (e.g., total parenteral nutrition). Endocrinologic abnormalities (e.g., hypothyroidism) may also go unrecognized clinically unless one has a high index of suspicion and the appropriate tests are performed. A number of medications have been reported to cause neuromuscular dysfunction. Specifically, persistent paralysis due to decreased metabolism of non-depolarizing neuromuscular blockers (e.g., pancuronium, vecuronium) should be considered in the appropriate setting. Such paralysis is likely to occur with impaired liver or renal function, use of continuous infusion, and failure to monitor the level of neuromuscular blockade. In addition, a myopathic disorder has been well documented with corticosteroid administration. It is suspected that this may occur more commonly when administered in patients who have also received neuromuscular blocking agents.

INCREASED RESPIRATORY SYSTEM LOAD

Respiratory Mechanics

Standard tests of pulmonary function are not feasible in intubated, mechanically ventilated patients because of the patient effort and cooperation required as well as other considerations. However, measurements of the passive mechanical properties of the respiratory system can be used to determine the loads contributing to increased respiratory effort and work of breathing performed in the difficult to wean patient. For example, end-inspiratory occlusions performed during constant flow inflation and end-expiratory occlusions may be used to assess respiratory system resistance, compliance, and intrinsic positive end-expiratory pressure (PEEP) (discussed below).

Common factors contributing to an increase in respiratory resistance in the mechanically ventilated patient include a small or narrowed endotracheal tube (see below), bronchospasm, or excessive tracheobronchial secretions. Diseases associated with reduced compliance of the respiratory system will increase the elastic load imposed on the respiratory muscles.

This change in lung mechanics may be due to lung or chest wall abnormalities. For example, reduced lung compliance is commonly seen with cardiogenic or noncardiogenic pulmonary edema, pneumonia, or atelectasis. A reduction in chest wall compliance has a comparable effect and may be due to the presence of pleural fluid (effusion, chylothorax, hemothorax), pneumothorax, or abdominal distension (ileus, ascites). Abnormal respiratory mechanics due to preexisting pulmonary disorders (COPD, pulmonary fibrosis) also add to the resistive and elastic loads placed on the respiratory muscles.

Some of the current generation of mechanical ventilators and commercially available free-standing devices can provide automated measurements of respiratory resistance and compliance using one of several approaches. However, to date, the results obtained from these monitoring packages have not been extensively validated in patients with ventilatory failure. Based on previous experience, there are a number of situations in which one might expect these automated calculations to be in error. For example, many of these devices do not account for intrinsic PEEP (see below), which leads to an underestimation of respiratory system compliance. Incomplete relaxation of the respiratory muscles adversely affects measurements of respiratory system resistance as well as compliance. Therefore, caution must be exercised when using automated measurements of respiratory mechanics to aid in clinical decision making.

Dynamic Hyperinflation and Intrinsic PEEP

The work of breathing is generally increased in patients with acute hypercapnic respiratory failure due to underlying obstructive airways disease. In patients with severe COPD, for example, the rate of lung emptying is unduly prolonged relative to the available expiratory duration. As a result, expiratory flow is interrupted by the subsequent breath before a complete exhalation has had adequate time to occur, such that end-expiratory lung volume is dynamically increased. This phenomenon has been aptly termed *dynamic hyperinflation*. A physiologic conse-

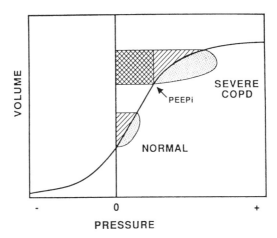

Figure 23.2. Schematic respresentation of the volume-pressure relationship of the respiratory system demonstrating the manner in which the mechanical work of breathing is increased in a patient with severe COPD and acute respiratory failure. Compared with a normal subject, the inspiratory resistive work of breathing (*stippled area*) is significantly increased. In addition, the extensive degree of hyperinflation forces the COPD patient to breathe on the relatively flattened portion of the volume-pressure relationship, considerably increasing the elastic work of breathing (*diagonally striped area*) as well. Inspiratory effort is also required to overcome the positive recoil pressure present at end expiration, or intrinsic PEEP (PEEP$_I$), further adding to the increased elastic (*cross-hatched area*) and total work of breathing that must be performed.

quence of dynamic hyperinflation is that alveolar pressure remains positive throughout expiration, in contrast with the normal circumstance. The positive pressure present at end expiration is referred to as *auto* or *intrinsic* PEEP.

The impact of intrinsic PEEP and dynamic hyperinflation on the inspiratory effort and work of breathing can perhaps be best understood by reviewing the dynamic volume-pressure relationship of a patient with COPD illustrated in Figure 23.2. The area contained within the volume-pressure loop is a quantitative reflection of the physical work that the respiratory muscles must perform. As can be seen, the total work is markedly increased in the COPD patient compared with normal. This change is due to a considerable elevation in the resistive work of breathing as would be expected. However, the elastic work of breathing is also excessive, because the extensive degree of hyperinflation forces the COPD patient to breathe along the relatively flattened portion of the volume-pressure relationship, where the respiratory system appears stiffer or less compliant. Additional effort is required to overcome the opposing positive recoil pressure offered by intrinsic PEEP. In this respect, intrinsic PEEP acts as an inspiratory threshold load. In addition to increasing the work of breathing, dynamic hyperinflation impairs the mechanical efficiency of the respiratory muscles owing to length-tension considerations, abnormal thoracic geometry, and various other factors.

Ventilator and Equipment Load

Intubation and mechanical ventilation, per se, impose a load owing to the inspiratory and expiratory components of the ventilator and tubing system. Breathing through the ventilator requires opening of a demand valve to achieve gas flow with each breath. Specifically, a large decrease in airway pressure to trigger the machine, an excessive time delay before the onset of inspiratory flow, and insufficient flow relative to patient demand during the positive pressure breath all contribute to increasing the work of breathing. More sensitive or modified demand valve systems, including the use of a flow trigger, may serve to reduce this inspiratory load.

The flow resistance of an artificial airway generally exceeds that of the native upper airway. This increase may be worsened as a result of tube deformation, airway secretions, and other factors. As a result, endotracheal tube resistance represents a significant portion of the total resistance measured in intubated patients mechanically ventilated for the treatment of acute respiratory failure. Differentiating between increases in endotracheal tube and intrinsic patient resistance may be clinically difficult. Monitoring endotracheal tube resistance using recently described techniques is feasible, however, and may help identify patients in whom excessive tube resistance contributes to weaning failure.

Minute Ventilation Load

Minute ventilation is a major determinant of the amount of pressure work that must be performed per unit of time. Assuming respiratory system mechanics to be constant, the work of breathing rises as ventilatory requirements increase. This may be an important factor contributing to weaning failure in patients in whom the balance between respiratory capacity and demand is marginal.

Increased minute ventilation may be due to elevated respiratory drive, increased CO_2 production ($\dot{V}CO_2$), or increased dead space-to-tidal volume ratio (V_D/V_T). Respiratory drive may be inordinately elevated because of anxiety, agitation, or pain. It may also be increased owing to disorders involving the lung parenchyma, which enhance afferent sensory information from chemoreceptors and mechanoreceptors. Even if the work of breathing for each breath remains constant, the rise in breathing frequency needed to increase minute ventilation will also increase energy requirements. The rapid respiratory rate can also further increase the work of breathing owing to a number of other factors, including increased respiratory resistance, the development of intrinsic PEEP, and a reduction in intrinsic efficiency of the contracting respiratory muscles.

$\dot{V}CO_2$ often is elevated in critically ill patients, most commonly owing to fever, sepsis, agitation, or muscular exertion. Rarely, unrecognized hyperthyroidism may markedly increase CO_2 production. The amount of CO_2 produced is also integrally related to the amount of O_2 consumed. This relationship is known as the *respiratory quotient* (RQ), where $RQ = \dot{V}CO_2/\dot{V}O_2$. The RQ depends in part on the substrate for metabolism. Overfeeding, particularly with carbohydrates, may impede weaning owing to the high respiratory quotient associated with the metabolism of an overabundance of carbohydrates. Specifically, conversion of carbohydrates to fat (lipogenesis) results in a marked increase in CO_2 production.

Minute ventilation also may be increased to maintain a stable level of alveolar ventilation. This change suggests that the anatomic or physiologic dead space (areas characterized by a high ventilation-to-perfusion ratio) has increased. The anatomic deadspace may be increased by excessive length or compliance of tubing within the ventilator circuit. Elevated physiologic dead space may be due to preexisting respiratory disease, particularly severe emphysema. Increased dead space may also be the result of pulmonary embolism, hypovolemia, or advanced adult respiratory distress syndrome (ARDS). Application of PEEP may further increase dead space through a variety of physiologic mechanisms. For a given level of minute ventilation, the smaller tidal volume seen with a rapid, shallow breathing pattern will lead to an increase in the dead space fraction (V_D/V_T).

PREDICTING WEANING OUTCOME

Successful weaning from the ventilator requires that the imbalance between respiratory capacity and ventilatory load be returned toward normal. However, prior to extubating a patient recovering from acute respiratory failure, some basic criteria must be fulfilled. These include that the patient be clinically and hemodynamically stable and that the cause of respiratory failure has decreased significantly, if not resolved. In addition, the patient must have an adequate level of consciousness and upper airway function, both to protect the airway and to clear secretions.

Although clinical experience is of importance in predicting weaning outcome, a variety of parameters have been used to aid in assessing an individual patient's ability to discontinue mechanical ventilation. The capacity to reliably predict weaning success has been generally disappointing. As noted, failure to wean from mechanical ventilation may be attributed to inadequate oxygenation, reduced respiratory capacity, or increased ventilatory demand. In Table 23.2, commonly used predictors of weaning success are provided. In addition, other indices that are more complex to obtain or less well accepted are also listed. These indices may provide an objective assessment of physiologic variables that may account for failure to wean and may guide the weaning process.

Table 23.2. Weaning Indices/Predictors of Success

Oxygenation
  $PO_2 \geq 60$ mmHg on $F_IO_2 \leq 35\%$
  $PO_2/F_IO_2 \geq 200$ mmHg
  PEEP ≤ 5 cmH$_2$O
Breathing pattern
  $f \leq 30$ breaths/minute
  $V_T \geq 5$ ml/kg
  $\dot{V}_E \leq 10$ l/min
  $V_C \geq 10$ ml/kg
  $V_T/V_C \leq 0.4$
  MVV $\geq 2 \cdot \dot{V}_E$
Neuromuscular capacity/drive
  $PI_{MAX} \leq -20$ cmH$_2$O
  $P_{0.1} < 5.5$ cmH$_2$O
Integrative indices
  $f/V_T \leq 105$
  $PI/PI_{MAX} \leq 0.3$
  $P_{0.1}/PI_{MAX} \leq 0.15$
  $P_{0.1} \times f/V_T \leq 450$
  Cdyn*PI_{MAX}*(PaO_2/P_AO_2)/Rate ≥ 13 ml/min

PO_2, oxygen tension (or partial pressure); F_IO_2, fraction of inspired oxygen; PEEP, positive end-expiratory pressure; V_T, tidal volume; $\dot{V}_E$, expired minute ventilation; V_C, vital capacity; MVV, mandatory minute ventilation; P_{IMAX}, maximal inspiratory pressure, P_I, peak negative airway pressure generated during the first attempt at a sustained airway occluded maneuver; Cdyn*P_{I-MAX}, total respiratory system compliance in dynes and maximal inspiratory pressure; $P_{0.1}$ = airway occlusion pressure, the pressure generated during the first 100 msec of an occluded inspiratory effort.

Oxygenation

Different criteria exist to predict weaning success in relation to arterial oxygen content relative to inspired F_IO_2. These include an arterial $PO_2 \geq 60$ mmHg on an $F_IO_2 \leq 35\%$, or a PO_2 to F_IO_2 ratio >200. However, no index of oxygenation is universally accepted as being prohibitive to weaning. Nonetheless, it is difficult to ensure inspired O_2 concentrations $>50\%$ without tight-fitting, high flow mask systems or intubation. In general, it should be noted that inadequate oxygenation is usually associated with other abnormalities of respiratory capacity and ventilatory load that preclude weaning success.

Breathing Pattern

Several studies have shown that patients failing to wean from mechanical ventilation generally have a rapid shallow breathing pattern. This pattern is not surprising because it is often a consequence of severe respiratory dysfunction, whether it be due to increased respiratory load or to decreased respiratory capacity. A respiratory frequency of <30 breaths/minute and a tidal volume of >5 ml/kg have been associated with a favorable weaning outcome. In addition, a vital capacity of >10 ml/kg and a tidal volume to vital capacity ratio of <0.4 have also, traditionally, been used to predict weaning success. However, these indices have high sensitivities but poor specificity and, as a result, the positive predictive value tends to be low.

Despite its simplicity, Yang and Tobin demonstrated that the ratio of breathing frequency to tidal volume ($f/V_T \leq 105$) was more accurate in predicting weaning outcome than other conventional weaning criteria. Specifically, the sensitivity and specificity were 0.97 and 0.64, respectively, whereas the positive and negative predictive values were 0.78 and 0.95, respectively. Subsequent studies generally support the utility of this index, although some controversy remains as to the precise utility in specific patient populations.

Minute Ventilation

As stated, work of breathing rises as ventilatory requirements increase. Minute ventilation in normal subjects is ~6 L/minute and weaning success has been associated with a minute ventilation requirement of <10 L/minute. However, a number of studies have reported positive and negative predictive values of only 40% to 50% when using this variable alone. The ability to double minute ventilation voluntarily has also been associated with weaning success. Patients who can double minute ventilation may have adequate ventilatory reserve and, therefore, will tolerate weaning. It is, therefore, important to treat causes of excessive CO_2 production and, when possible, to minimize dead space related to the ventilator circuit. Frequently, it is difficult to reduce the high ventilatory requirement associated with the underlying disease process, such as in patients with severe COPD or advanced ARDS.

Maximal Inspiratory Pressure

Respiratory muscle strength is an important determinant of weaning success. Maximal inspiratory pressure (PI_{MAX}) has been used as a global assessment of respiratory muscle capacity. It had been felt that a value less negative than -20 cmH_2O was useful in predicting weaning failure. However, a number of investigators have found that this value also has poor positive and negative predictive values, especially in patients requiring prolonged ventilatory support. This result is not at all surprising given that the value takes into account ventilatory muscle strength but does not reflect the ventilatory load imposed, the fraction of available capacity required to maintain spontaneous breathing, or a more direct measure of respiratory muscle endurance. As will be discussed, derived indices attempt to combine variables to account for the multifactorial nature of weaning failure.

Airway Occlusion Pressure

Airway occlusion pressure (i.e., the pressure generated during the first 100 msec of an occluded inspiratory effort, or $P_{0.1}$), has been used to assess neuromuscular output from the medullary respiratory center in a variety of research settings, including mechanically ventilated patients. For example, Murciano et al. examined the relationship between $P_{0.1}$ and clinical outcome in patients with COPD in acute respiratory failure. $P_{0.1}$ was markedly elevated but fell significantly in patients who were successfully weaned, in contrast with those individuals requiring continued ventilatory support. Fernandez et al. demonstrated that sensitivity and specificity in differentiating between patients who needed full, partial, or no further ventilatory support were improved by using the ratio of $P_{0.1}$ to PI_{MAX} rather than $P_{0.1}$ alone.

Currently, however, $P_{0.1}$ is not measured routinely in mechanically ventilated patients, primarily because of technical considerations and the need for additional specialized equipment. However, some of the newer generation ventilators and free-standing monitoring units now provide automated measurements of $P_{0.1}$. Based on studies such as those cited above, bedside measurements of $P_{0.1}$ may be routinely performed. However, further work is still required to validate the reliability of such measurements and the ability of $P_{0.1}$ to aid clinical decision making in the patient who is difficult to wean.

Derived Indices

Several investigators have attempted to improve on the above indices by combining them with other parameters. For example, Sassoon and Mahutte hypothesized that the shallow breathing pattern characteristic of the imbalance between ventilatory capacity and demand in difficult to wean patients is associated with increased respiratory drive. To test this hypothesis, airway occlusion pressure ($P_{0.1}$) and f/V_T were prospectively measured in 45 patients with acute respiratory failure. The product of $P_{0.1}$ and an f/V_T was found to be as sensitive but more specific in comparison with other weaning indices, including the f/V_T ratio alone. Both positive and negative predictive values were also slightly higher. Similarly, Yang reasoned that the relationship between ventilatory demand and capacity could be represented by the ratio of the peak negative airway pressure generated on the first (PI) and last (PI_{MAX}) inspiratory effort during a sustained 20- to 30-second airway occlusion. This approach assumes that the ratio of PI to PI_{MAX} obtained in this manner represents the fraction of maximal inspiratory force generating capacity used during tidal breathing. In this study, a ratio of PI to PI_{MAX} of 0.3 was retrospectively found to provide the best separation between weaning success and failure. Although this ratio was not as discriminatory as f/V_T in predicting weaning outcome, the combination of f/V_T and PI/PI_{MAX} had the highest positive predictive value. Both of these studies confirmed the relative utility of f/V_T and demonstrated the potential to improve its accuracy by taking into account other parameters. More complicated derived indices, which attempt to incorporate these parameters, are shown in Table 23.2.

Spontaneous Breathing Trial

Irrespective of which method of discontinuing mechanical ventilation is used (see below), a potential criterion for extubation would be the ability to breathe spontaneously without any form of assistance for a prescribed period of time (e.g., 0.5–2.0 h). This is often done using a simple T-piece system, where the patient breathes from an oxygen source with gas flowing past the open end of the endotracheal tube. With many of the newer generation ventilators, an alternative approach is to have the patient breathe spontaneously through the ventilator circuit. The latter offers the potential advantages of convenience, ease of application, access to the ventilator's monitoring systems and alarms, and avoidance of additional equipment. However, spontaneous breathing through the ventilator circuit may further add to the ventilatory load owing to factors such as circuit dead space, inspiratory and expiratory circuit resistance, and demand valve operation.

During spontaneous breathing trials using either system, it should be recognized that endotracheal tube resistance is significant, and it often greatly exceeds that of the native upper airway. In fact, patients may do better without the endotracheal tube in place owing to an improved ability to cough and spontaneously clear secretions. Conversely, upper airway dysfunction postextubation may require reintubation and be the principal factor contributing to weaning failure in a patient who otherwise could breathe spontaneously without positive pressure assistance from the ventilator.

METHODS OF DISCONTINUING MECHANICAL VENTILATION

Most patients who require short periods of ventilatory support resume spontaneous breathing without difficulty. In particular, patients who are mechanically ventilated for surgical procedures can often resume spontaneous breathing when the effects of anesthesia and sedation have dissipated. However, such is often not the case in patients who have required prolonged mechanical ventilatory support or in those with significant preexisting lung disease. In these situations, attempts may be made to discontinue mechanical ventilation with intermittent trials of T-piece breathing, or with a progressive graded reduction in the ventilatory support level provided in either the volume-cycled or pressure-regulated mechanical ventilation mode. It should be noted that multicenter trials comparing the efficacy of various weaning modalities have provided conflicting results. In fact, it has been suggested that weaning outcome is likely related to how the mode is employed rather than the specific advantages or disadvantages associated with the mode itself.

Intermittent T-Piece Breathing

Weaning may be attempted by using spontaneous breathing trials of increasing duration mixed with periods of "rest" using positive pressure ventilation. The progressively increasing frequency and duration of these trials may eventually enable the patient to resume spontaneous breathing without any form of ventilatory support. The optimal duration and interval between spontaneous breathing trials needed to maximize the "training effect" is unknown. Although this method theoretically may allow recovery from fatigue, it has not been shown to be superior to other methods of weaning. Whether a subgroup of patients recovering from respiratory failure would benefit from this approach remains unclear.

Synchronized Intermittent Mandatory Ventilation

During synchronized intermittent mandatory ventilation (SIMV), the patient receives a fixed number of positive pressure volume-cycled breaths per minute. In addition, the patient is able to breathe spontaneously between these breaths. During weaning from mechanical ventilation, the number of SIMV breaths provided is progressively reduced until the patient is breathing spontaneously through the ventilatory circuit for all (or nearly all) breaths. During this gradual reduction of support, patients are monitored in terms of respiratory rate, minute ventilation, gas exchange, and ventilation adequacy. By reducing the SIMV rate, it is possible to produce a graded increase in inspiratory effort performed by the patient.

A number of potential advantages of SIMV exist. The presence of a backup rate and preset tidal volume ensure a minimal mandatory minute ventilation. However, some limitations of increased load of the ventilator circuit discussed above for spontaneous breathing apply on both supported and nonsupported breaths during SIMV. Since its introduction in the early 1970s, it has been assumed that the positive pressure volume-cycled breaths during IMV require minimal work of breathing by the patient. However, the workload required to open the ventilator demand valve as well as the fixed inspiratory flow may actually require a relatively high level of work during both assisted and spontaneous breaths. In particular, the large drop in airway pressure required to trigger the ventilator, the excessive time delay from the onset of breathing effort to the onset of flow delivery, and the potential for insufficient flow delivery may all significantly increase the work of breathing. Owing to the limitations discussed, it is perhaps not surprising that SIMV use has not been proven to be superior to T-piece trials or pressure support. At this time, SIMV remains a commonly employed weaning method in many ICUs.

Pressure Support Ventilation

Pressure support is a unique mode of partial ventilatory support. It offers several possible advantages over other conventional modes of assisted ventilation. It allows the patient to vary the level of inspiratory flow as well as tidal volume and respiratory rate, while machine assistance is provided with each spontaneous effort. In addition, minute ventilation generally increases with the amount of pressure support applied, while providing a graded reduction in the work and oxygen cost of breathing. Therefore, pressure support seems well suited to a gradual transition from assisted ventilation to spontaneous breathing. In fact, it has been suggested that pressure support can simulate spontaneous breathing in the extubated subject by adjusting the level to a point that just overcomes the flow resistance of the endotracheal tube and ventilator circuit. In principle, this requires precise knowledge of the resistive pressure drop across the endotracheal tube, which may be quite different in vivo from the value measured in vitro.

A relative disadvantage of pressure support, not unlike other modes of assisted ventilation, is the potential added work required to initiate and maintain airflow through the ventilator's demand valve system. In a multicenter, randomized prospective study, pressure support was compared with SIMV and T-piece weaning. In this study, patients were weaned more quickly with pressure support than with the other two modalities. A subsequent trial, however, could not corroborate these findings. Therefore, the superiority of pressure support compared with other weaning modalities remains to be determined.

PEEP or CPAP During Weaning from Mechanical Ventilation

PEEP traditionally has been used to improve oxygenation in mechanically ventilated patients by the reexpansion of flooded or atelectatic alveoli. This use is generally associated with an increase in functional residual capacity and an improvement in lung compliance. In contrast, in the mechanically ventilated patient with severe COPD, PEEP may be of therapeutic benefit not because of its effects on gas exchange but rather its ability to reduce inspiratory effort. In the presence of dynamic hyperinflation, PEEP acts by offsetting the positive recoil pressure present at end-expiration. In effect, PEEP replaces PEEPi and in this manner, eliminates the inspiratory threshold load imposed. This notion has been shown to be the case when applying PEEP in spontaneously breathing COPD patients (i.e., continuous positive airway pressure [CPAP]) during weaning as well as during assisted ventilator modes (e.g., assist mode ventilation [AMV], SIMV, and pressure support [PS]) and is, perhaps, unique to COPD patients, where the presence of expiratory flow limitation enables PEEP to counterbalance intrinsic PEEP without further increasing lung volume.

Proportional Assist Ventilation

Although not yet clinically available, proportional assist ventilation is a new mode of assisted ventilation where pressure can be applied by the ventilator in proportion to the volume and flow generated. By adjusting the proportionality between applied pressure and volume as well as applied pressure and flow, it should therefore be possible to control separately the decrease in magnitude of the elastic and resistive work of breathing performed.

In principle, unloading the respiratory muscles in this fashion acts to restore the relationship between patient effort and its ventilatory output toward normal. In comparison with other forms of assisted ventilation, proportional assist ventilation therefore offers a unique ability to regulate the amount of ventilatory support in proportion to the identified abnormalities in respiratory function. Although preliminary results in patients with acute respiratory failure are encouraging, no information is as yet available with regard to the efficacy of weaning patients with this ventilation mode.

Mask Ventilation

Although it would be ideal to predict reliably the weaning and extubation success in all patients, options other than reintubation exist for the patient who has failed extubation, namely noninvasive mask ventilation. This is particularly true for the individual in whom a new and rapidly reversible problem has been identified. Volume-cycled and pressure-regulated mechanical ventilation modes as well as CPAP can be provided in this manner. Technological improvements in ventilator design in addition to an increasing number of comfortable patient-ventilator interfaces have broadened the use and potential success of noninvasive ventilatory support in this and other settings.

APPROACH TO WEANING FROM MECHANICAL VENTILATION

Prior to weaning and extubation, certain basic criteria must be fulfilled. Patients must have an adequate level of consciousness to protect the upper airway and be able to eliminate tracheal secretions. Mental status may be improved by optimizing sleep-wake cycles with appropriate sedation with special attention paid to avoiding oversedation. Optimizing body position during weaning as well as the time of day which weaning trials are performed may be of further assistance.

Table 23.3. Approach to Weaning from Mechanical Ventilation

Goal	Assessment/Intervention
Ensure adequate level of consciousness	
Assess ability to protect airway/clear secretions	
Ensure adequate body position	
Assess oxygenation	Arterial blood gas/SaO$_2$
Assess respiratory capacity	
Ensure adequate respiratory drive	Minimize sedation
	Optimize time of weaning trials
	Improve sleep/wake cycles
	Arterial blood gas (PaO$_2$, PaCO$_2$)
Assess neuromuscular capacity	Breathing pattern assessment (f, V_T, $\dot{V}_E$)
	Measure maximal inspiratory pressure (PI$_{MAX}$)
Correct fluid and electrolyte imbalance (pH, K$^+$, Mg^{++}, PO$_4^{-2}$, Ca^{++})	
Ensure adequate O$_2$ delivery	
Ensure adequate nutrition	
Rule out endocrinopathies (thyroid function tests)	
Assess ventilatory load	
Measure respiratory system mechanics	
Resistive load	Bronchodilators
	Clearance of secretions
	Consider endotracheal tube resistance
Elastic load	Treat underlying disorder (pulmonary edema, abdominal distension)
Dynamic hyperinflation	Adjust ventilator settings (decrease $\dot{V}_E$, increase V, increase T$_E$)
	Bronchodilators
	Change endotracheal tube
Measure ventilatory dead space	V$_D$/V$_T$ 0.65
Tract causes of increased respiratory drive	Fever, pain, anxiety

As stated, most patients requiring short-term mechanical ventilation are weaned successfully and extubated without difficulty. However, an ordered and systematic approach is necessary in the patients in whom weaning is unsuccessful (Table 23.3). In these patients, it is important to assess each determinant of weaning outcome, including oxygenation, respiratory capacity adequacy, and ventilatory demand level. As each of these areas is assessed, efforts should be made to correct or optimize each abnormality identified, because the inability to resume spontaneous breathing is often multifactorial. Despite an organized approach, a small percentage of patients, particularly those with preexisting severe respiratory disease or those with significant residual disease, may remain chronically ventilator dependent.

Oxygenation adequacy can readily be assessed noninvasively using a pulse oximeter. Continuous monitoring of oxygen saturation in this manner should eliminate unrecognized or prolonged periods of hypoxemia and also help identify hypoxemia as a contributing factor in weaning failure.

Respiratory capacity also should be evaluated carefully. This includes ensuring adequate central respiratory drive by minimizing use of sedative drugs and correcting any metabolic alkalosis. Respiratory muscle strength should be monitored routinely; it can be maximized by improving nutritional status, as well as correcting abnormalities in fluid-electrolyte status. Other less obvious conditions (e.g., hypothyroidism, ICU polyneuropathy) should be sought in patients with otherwise unexplained neuromuscular weakness.

Lastly, special attention must be paid to the potential importance of increased ventilatory demand. Assessment of spontaneous breathing parameters, particularly respiratory rate, tidal volume, and minute ventilation, may alert the physician to problems of both decreased respiratory capacity and increased ventilatory load. These changes may be due to mechanical abnormalities of the respiratory system (including dynamic hyperinflation), ventilator circuit impedance, or excessive minute ventilation. Serial measurements of resistance and compliance of the respiratory system as well as intrinsic PEEP may be useful in identifying specific problems and in providing objective improvement criteria over time. In addition, minimizing the load imposed by the endotracheal tube and ventilator circuit may aid in the weaning process. Finally, methods to minimize dynamic hyperinflation serve both to decrease the inspiratory threshold load imposed by intrinsic PEEP and to improve on the mechanical disadvantage placed on the respiratory muscles.

In general ICU populations, the vast majority of patients are rapidly and successfully weaned from mechanical ventilation. However, the small fraction of patients who are difficult to wean use a disproportionate amount of physical and monetary resources. Therefore, it is important to address this problem in a systematic fashion and promptly to identify and correct those factors contributing to the disturbed relationship between ventilatory demand and respiratory capacity.

Suggested Readings

1. Aubier M, Murciano D, Fournier M, et al. Central respiratory drive in acute respiratory failure of patients with chronic obstructive pulmonary disease. Am Rev Respir Dis 122:191–199, 1980.
2. Aubier M, Murciano D, Lecocguic Y, et al. Effect of hypophosphatemia on diaphragmatic contractility in patients with acute respiratory failure. N Engl J Med 313: 420–424, 1985.
3. Aubier M, Trippenbach T, Roussos C. Respiratory muscle fatigue during cardiogenic shock. J Appl Physiol 51:499–508, 1981.

4. Brochard L, Harf A, Lorino H, Lemaire F. Inspiratory pressure support prevents diaphragmatic fatigue during weaning from mechanical ventilation. Am Rev Respir Dis 139:513–521, 1989.

5. Brochard L, Rauss A, Benito S, et al. Comparison of three methods of gradual withdrawal from ventilatory support during weaning from mechanical ventilation. Am J Respir Crit Care Med 150:896–903, 1994.

6. Brochard L, Rua F, Lorini H, et al. Inspiratory pressure support compensates for the additional work of breathing caused by the endotracheal tube. Anesthesiology 75: 739–745, 1991.

7. Calderini E, Petrof B, Gottfried SB. Continuous positive airway pressure improves efficacy of pressure support ventilation in severe COPD. Am Rev Respir Dis 139: A155, 1989.

8. Covelli HD, Black JW, Olsen MS, et al. Respiratory failure precipitated by high carbohydrate loads. Ann Intern Med 95:579–581, 1981.

9. Dureuil B, Vires N, Cantineau JP, et al. Diaphragmatic contractility after upper abdominal surgery. J Appl Physiol 61:1775–1780, 1986.

10. Esteban A, Frutos F, Tobin MJ, et al. A comparison of four methods of weaning patients from mechanical ventilation. N Engl J Med 332:345–350, 1995.

11. Fernandez R, Cabrera J, Calaf N, Benito S. P100/PIMax: an index for assessing respiratory capacity in acute respiratory failure. Intensive Care Med 16:175–179, 1990.

12. Ford GT, Whitelaw WA, Rosenal TW, et al. Diaphragm function after upper abdominal surgery in humans. Am Rev Respir Dis 127:431–436, 1983.

13. Gottfried SB, Rossi A, Higgs BD, et al. Non-invasive determination of respiratory system mechanics during mechanical ventilation for acute respiratory failure. Am Rev Respir Dis 131:414–420, 1985.

14. Gottfried SB. The Role of PEEP or CPAP in the mechanically ventilated COPD patient. The Thorax, Part C 85:2471–2500, 1995.

15. Grassino A, Macklem PT. Respiratory muscle fatigue and ventilatory failure. Ann Rev Med 35:625–647, 1984.

16. Gursahaney AH, Gottfried SB. Monitoring respiratory mechanics in the intensive care unit. Current Opinion in Critical Care 1:32–42, 1995.

17. Hansen-Flaschen J, Cowen J, Raps EC. Neuromuscular blockade in the intensive care unit: more than we bargained for. Am Rev Respir Dis 147:234–236, 1993.

18. Hill N.S. Noninvasive ventilation. Am Rev Respir Dis 147:1050–1055, 1993.

19. Hussain SNS, Simkus G, Roussos C. Respiratory muscle fatigue: a cause of ventilatory failure in septic shock. J Appl Physiol 58:2033–2040, 1985.

20. Laub GW, Muralidharan S, Chen C, Perritt A, Adkins M, Pollick S, Bailey B, McGrath LB. Phrenic nerve injury: a prospective study. Chest 100:376–379, 1991.

21. Lopez Messa JB, Garcia A. Acute polyneuropathy in critically ill patients. Intensive Care Med 16:159–162, 1990.

22. MacIntyre NR. Respiratory function during pressure support ventilation. Chest 89: 677–683, 1986.

23. Marini JJ. Should PEEP be used in airflow obstruction? Am Rev Respir Dis 140:1–3, 1989.

24. Marini J, Rodriguez M, Lamb V. The inspiratory workload of patient-initiated mechanical ventilation. Am Rev Respir Dis 134:902–909, 1986.

25. Marini JJ, Smith TC, Lamb VJ. External work output and force generation during synchronized intermittent mechanical ventilation: effect of machine assistance on breathing effort. Am Rev Respir Dis 138:1169–1179, 1988.
26. Murciano D, Boczkowski J, Lecocguic Y, Milic-Emili J, Pariente R, Aubier M. Tracheal occlusion pressure: a simple index to monitor respiratory muscle fatigue during acute respiratory failure in patients with chronic obstructive pulmonary disease. Ann Int Med 108:800–805, 1988.
27. Navalesi P, Hernandez P, Laporta D, Landry J, Maltais F, Navajas D, Gottfried SB. Influence of site of tracheal pressure measurement on in situ estimation of endotracheal tube resistance: J Appl Physiol 77:2899–2906, 1994.
28. Navalesi P, Hernandez P, Wongsa A, LaPorta D, Goldberg P, Gottfried SB. Proportional assist ventilation in acute respiratory failure: effects on breathing pattern and inspiratory effort. Am J Respir Crit Care Med 153:,1996; in press.
29. Olopade CO, Staats BA. Time course of recovery from frostbitten phrenics after coronary artery bypass graft surgery. Chest 99:1112–1115, 1991.
30. Pepe PE, Marini JJ. Occult positive end-expiratory pressure in mechanically ventilated patients with airflow obstruction. Am Rev Respir Dis 126:166–170, 1982.
31. Petrof B, Légaré M, Goldberg P, Milic-Emili J, Gottfried SB. Continuous positive airway pressure reduces work of breathing and dyspnea during weaning from mechanical ventilation in severe chronic obstructive pulmonary disease. Am Rev Respir Dis 141:281–289, 1990.
32. Ranieri M, Calderini E, Eissa T, Petrof B, Gottfried SB. PEEP reduces inspiratory effort during synchronized intermittent mandatory ventilation (SIMV) in COPD. Am Rev Respir Dis 141:A572, 1990.
33. Rossi A, Gottfried SB, Zocchi L, Higgs B, Lennox S, Calvery P, Begin P, Grassino A, Milic-Emili J. Respiratory mechanics in mechanically ventilated patients with respiratory failure. J Appl Physiol 58:1849–1858, 1985.
34. Sassoon CSH, Mahutte CK. Airway occlusion pressure and breathing pattern as predictors of weaning outcome. Am Rev Respir Dis 148:860–866, 1993.
35. Tobin MJ, Perez W, Guenther SM, et al. The pattern of breathing during successful and unsuccessful trials of weaning from mechanical ventilation. Am Rev Respir Dis 134:1111–1118, 1986.
36. Whitelaw WA, Derenne J-P. Airway occlusion pressure. J Appl Physiol 74:1475–1483, 1993.
37. Wright PE, Marini JJ, Bernard GR. In vitro vs. in vivo comparison of endotracheal airflow resistance. Am Rev Respir Dis 140:10–16, 1989.
38. Yang KL. Inspiratory pressure/maximal inspiratory pressure ratio: a predictive index of weaning outcome. Intensive Care Med 19:204–208, 1993.
39. Yang K, Tobin M. A prospective study of indexes predicting the outcome of trials of weaning from mechanical ventilation. New Eng J Med 324:1445–1450, 1991.
40. Younes M. Proportional assist ventilation, a new approach to ventilatory support. Am Rev Respir Dis 145:114–120, 1992.

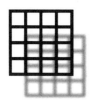

24
Ventilatory Support: Temptations and Pitfalls
Azriel Perel • M. Christine Stock

This final chapter summarizes the basic principles of ventilatory support. A fairly comprehensive variety of ventilatory modes were described in the preceding chapters. We limited the following discussion to practical remarks, pointing out common pitfalls encountered during the administration of ventilatory care.

As ventilatory options increase and as ventilators become more sophisticated, enabling the control of more complex parameters, there is more room for error in the ventilatory management of critically ill patients. In addition, new concepts in ventilatory care of patients with respiratory failure are being introduced constantly. Among these concepts are noninvasive ventilation, pressure-limited ventilation, permissive hypercapnia, and patient-ventilator interfaces, to name a few. Although these developments are effective and useful in some cases, they may be misused in others. We cannot, therefore, recommend a best overall ventilatory mode; such a panacea does not exist. Moreover, even though various modes are recommended highly by some authors, in general, there is inconclusive evidence to support the superiority of one single ventilatory mode. This lack is due to the scarcity of prospective well-controlled studies comparing ventilatory options, the inhomogeneity of the population in need of ventilatory support, the large interpatient differences in measurable respiratory variables, and the subtle differences in ventilator technology and exact mode of its operation. These problems result in sufficiently large standard deviations so that prohibitively large numbers of patients must be studied.

Optimal ventilatory support requires the clinician to recognize the diversity of respiratory failure. Identifying and understanding each patient's pathophysiology, combined with thorough knowledge of the available ventilatory options, are often the most vital elements in the treatment of critically ill patients. Therapeutic efforts should be aimed at understanding and correcting the pathogenesis of ventilatory failure or acute lung injury and improving total patient care. Technology by itself is unlikely to solve these patients' complex pathophysiology because in most cases, mechanical ventilation is *only* supportive, not therapeutic. However, in the more severely affected patients the choice of ventilatory mode and its correct application can make a critical difference. Several questions should be considered when ventilatory assistance may be necessary.

IS THE PATIENT IN NEED OF VENTILATORY SUPPORT?

There are five distinct major categories for instituting ventilatory support:

1. Neuromuscular inability to breathe (lung parenchyma usually normal).
2. Depressed ventilatory drive (drugs, brain stem injury).
3. Acute lung disease:
   a. Those with previously normal lungs (e.g., acute respiratory distress syndrome [ARDS] following trauma or aspiration).
   b. Those with chronic lung disease (e.g., the chronic obstructive pulmonary disease [COPD] patient who gets pneumonia).
4. Heart disease (both ischemic and heart failure).
5. Other severe systemic disease (e.g., burns, head injury, sepsis).

The requirement for ventilatory support is obvious in the case of complete central nervous system depression or profound neuromuscular failure. However, when ventilatory drive or the neuromuscular ability to breathe is partial, the decision to institute ventilatory support requires critical timing. The critical nature of this decision-making process is especially true in patients suffering from progressive degenerative muscle diseases, who can be supported for a considerable period of time by noninvasive ventilatory modes through a mask, mouthpiece, or perithoracic cuirass-type instrument. Much progress has been made in recent years, both conceptually and technologically, and the options to support patients with chronic partial ventilatory failure due to muscle weakness have developed considerably.

Drug-induced ventilatory depression should be assessed only when the patient is not stimulated in any manner because breathing may result from stimulation of higher cortical areas in response to command or pain. For example, large doses of opioids may result in a patient who is arousable and follows commands, but who is apneic unless instructed to breathe. Tests that reflect neuromuscular ability (e.g., forced vital capacity or maximal inspiratory pressure) can be fatally misleading. These patients are typically "strong" and normal vital capacity can be measured; however, once left unstimulated, these patients become apneic. These considerations are also important when contemplating the withdrawal of mechanical ventilatory support in an overly sedated patient.

Another reason for instituting ventilatory support is the patient's inability to meet the demands of increased breathing work. Increased resistive breathing work is due to increased resistance to the flow of gas. It may precipitate ventilatory failure either by acute CO_2 retention or by ventilatory muscle fatigue. Ventilatory failure due to increased elastic breathing work (increased *inspiratory* work that is required to expand stiff lungs) is less common because the human respiratory system is handle increases in elastic work better than increased resistive work. It is important to watch for the development of ventilatory failure because intervention aimed at the primary pathologic process may prevent progress to overt ventilatory failure. Further, close observation of such patients may allow the timely institution of continuous positive airway pressure, noninvasive ventilatory support, or tracheal intubation before the patient becomes moribund.

Organ system failure, other than the central nervous system, the neuromuscular systems, and the lungs, may precipitate ventilatory failure. Patients with severe hemorrhagic; cardiogenic or septic shock states; and those with extensive burns or head injury should receive mechanical ventilatory support before sudden, severe, respiratory failure occurs. In addition to the complications of positive airway pressure, complications due to intubation, pulmonary toilet, sedation, and equipment failure are associated with ventilatory support. Thus, the decision to ventilate a patient's lungs deserves critical assessment and mature clinical judgment.

When the patient no longer needs ventilation, ventilatory support should be discontinued. Although this advice sounds rather elementary, plans for discontinuation of ventilatory support should begin when the support is instituted. If the reason ventilation was instituted resolves, but the patient appears to continue to require mechanical ventilation, other and possibly new pathology must be sought (e.g., muscle paralysis after prolonged use of muscle relaxants). Further, if the patient's course varies significantly from what one would anticipate as the natural course of disease, other previously unrecognized disease should be sought (e.g., the development of sepsis in a chronic obstructive pulmonary disease [COPD] patient).

WHAT IS THE NATURE OF THE RESPIRATORY FAILURE?

In the first years of positive-pressure ventilatory support outside the operating room, from the 1950s to the early 1970s, all patients in need of ventilatory support received controlled mechanical ventilation (CMV), which enabled the titration of tidal volume, respiratory rate, and later on, F_IO_2. Because many more options are currently available, ventilatory support can be better tailored to the patient's needs. Thus, it is mandatory to clarify the nature of the disease process that makes ventilatory support necessary and to choose the right ventilatory mode accordingly.

Straightforward CMV can be used safely in patients who have no ventilatory activity at all and no respiratory failure. These include patients with inadequate ventilatory drive, neuromuscular disability, or drug-induced paralysis (such as during general anesthesia). When the patient has spontaneous ventilatory activity, a ventilatory mode that allows some form of patient-ventilator interaction should be employed. The most common modes include assist/control (A/C), intermittent mandatory ventilation (IMV), or pressure support (PS). When the mechanical support depends solely on patient triggering, it is important to ensure adequate minute ventilation in case apnea occurs. This safety net can be accomplished by setting a minimal number of mechanical breaths per minute as a backup rate or the use of apnea ventilation parameters available in some ventilators. It is important to stress that PS ventilation should not be used alone for patients with depressed ventilatory drive because it only augments spontaneous ventilatory efforts. If the patient makes no attempt to breathe, PS ventilation will deliver no ventilatory support. Hence, the necessity for the careful setting of apnea ventilation parameters in those ventilators that are equipped with this option, and the extra vigilance that is mandatory when using pressure support as a sole ventilation mode with ventilators that do not have this option.

When ventilatory failure is due to reduced functional residual capacity (FRC) and increased extravascular lung water (e.g., in ARDS), minute ventilation usually is elevated and does not need further augmentation. When such patients retain airway reflexes and are awake and cooperative, the hypoxemia and increased elastic work of breathing can be corrected with a continuous positive airway pressure (CPAP) mask, thus obviating the need for intubation and positive pressure ventilation. CPAP mask is also valuable to support hypoxemia and the increased elastic work of breathing in patients with flail chest or pulmonary contusion, and in those with hypoxemia induced by *Pneumocystis carinii.* Tracheal intubation may predispose patients, especially those who are immunosupressed, to secondary nosocomial, life-threatening infection, and can be avoided for some patients treated with a CPAP mask. CPAP also can be the sole supportive mode in tracheally intubated patients whose spontaneous minute ventilation is adequate or whose lung mechanics have improved greatly after CPAP institution. In addition, supportive therapy with CPAP alone is useful for patients with cardiogenic pulmonary edema and acute intravascular volume overload. Noninvasive ventilation modes, such as pressure support and bi-level positive airway pressure (BiPAP), can delay or prevent intubation even in patients with inadequate spontaneous minute ventilation.

Between CMV (full ventilatory support) and spontaneous ventilation with CPAP (no *ventilatory* support) lies partial ventilatory support with its infinite possibilities. Partial ventilatory support allows patients to perform whatever part of their work of breathing they are capable, with the ventilator performing the remainder of the work. It is useful for those patients who suffer from an imbalance between the required work of breathing and their ability to perform such work. Patients with COPD, asthma, severe adult respiratory distress syndrome (ARDS), severe lung infection or injury, or multiple organ failure may demonstrate such an imbalance, although this list is not exhaustive. Administering partial ventilatory support is more complex owing to the delicate interaction between ventilator and patient.

Understanding the pathophysiology that precipitated ventilatory failure (identifying the adequacy of chest mechanics, derangements of resistance and compliance, the nature of parenchymal injury, the presence of air-trapping, the influence of nonpulmonary organ failure on lung function, and principles of airway management) may help the clinician implement mechanical ventilation, choose the appropriate mode, and set up correctly the available multitude of ventilatory parameters.

THE EFFECTS OF VENTILATORY SUPPORT ON OTHER ORGAN SYSTEMS

Mechanical ventilation is used to augment CO_2 elimination and to promote adequate oxygen delivery to all organs. Augmenting oxygen delivery by optimizing arterial oxygen content is a major component in the treatment of low flow or low perfusion states. It may improve the function of organs that have inadequate oxygen supply (e.g., the brain, liver, kidneys, and gut). Occasionally, mechanical ventilation is used to improve the function of a specific organ system; for example, employing deliberate hyperventilation for patients with increased intracranial pressure. Another example is to supply mechanical normoventilation to reduce diaphragmatic and intercostal muscle oxygen consumption, which can be quite considerable during respiratory failure. This support allows a limited cardiac output to reestablish blood flow to other organs or to decrease myocardial oxygen consumption.

Positive intrathoracic pressure may influence cardiac function beneficially or detrimentally, depending on the patient's volume status and cardiac function. The normal preload-dependent heart will decrease its output when the increase in intrathoracic pressure depresses venous return during mechanical ventilation. This common detrimental effect of positive pressure ventilation is seen most dramatically in hypovolemic patients, especially when associated with the simultaneous administration of anesthetic agents, which abolish the intense contraction of the vascular system. The increased intrathoracic pressure further decreases an already inadequate venous return, thus further compromising cardiac output. One must carefully evaluate improved arterial oxygenation after institution of positive pressure maneuvers to ensure that PaO_2 has not been improved at the expense of cardiac output and oxygen delivery.

Therefore, when hypovolemia is present or suspected, appropriate intravenous fluids must be administered and a ventilatory mode is used that offers low mean airway pressure until euvolemia is achieved. These patients typically fare better with as much spontaneous ventilation as possible to preserve the thoracic venous pump, a slow rate of mechanical ventilation, and ambient expiratory airway pressure. Almost all ventilatory parameters alter mean airway pressure; thus, changes in tidal volume, rate of controlled or assisted mechanical breaths, inspiratory-to-expiratory time (I/E) ratio, positive end-expiratory pressure (PEEP)/CPAP level, and pressure control level, may influence the patient's cardiovascular system, intra-cranial pressure, as well as renal and hepatic perfusion. Switching from one ventila-tory mode to another (e.g., from CMV to A/C or from IMV to PS) may cause inadvertent increases in mean airway pressure.

Alternatively, patients with abnormally increased preload due to heart failure or excessive intravascular volume, will experience improved cardiac function as raised airway pressure decreases both cardiac preload and afterload. The afterload reducing effect of positive pressure ventilation is due to the portion of the positive pressure being transmitted to the left ventricle and intrathoracic aorta, thus de-creasing the force that the left ventricle has to develop to eject blood. Observing the effects of positive pressure ventilation on the arterial wave form can be helpful in determining its effects on the cardiovascular system (see Chapter 5, Cardiac Effects of Mechanical Ventilation).

CHOOSING VENTILATORY VARIABLES

Tidal Volume

During ventilatory support of patients with normal lungs (e.g., during anesthe-sia), the administration of low tidal volumes (5–7 ml/kg) may lead to a progressive decrease in FRC, increase in venous admixture, and possible atelectasis. However, larger tidal volumes (12–15 ml/kg) may cause parenchymal injury at the alveolar level—even in healthy lungs. Therefore, modest tidal volumes (8–10 ml/kg) with a low level of CPAP to prevent atelectasis is desirable for *most* patients receiving conventional mechanical ventilation. Because the tidal volume is one of the impor-tant determinants of mean airway pressure, it should be restricted in hypovolemic patients, as well as in those who are prone to develop barotrauma. Periodic breaths of 15–18 ml/kg (a "sigh" breath) to prevent microatelectasis are used rarely and the "sigh" mechanism has disappeared from most newer ventilators. To prevent possible decrease in FRC in intubated patients with normal lungs, it is common to apply "physiologic" PEEP/CPAP of 4–5 cmH$_2$O.

The choice of tidal volume in patients who are in severe respiratory failure is a subject of much recent debate. Many studies have convincingly shown that large tidal volumes can cause lung damage by a combination of overdistension and large traction forces on lung units. Moreover, the damage is considered to be a direct result of the tidal volume (volutrauma) rather than to an increased airway pressure (barotrauma). These observations have led to frequent restriction of the set tidal volume (6–8 ml/kg) or to the use of pressure controlled ventilation. Using low tidal volumes use during respiratory failure usually is associated with PEEP levels that are above the "inflection point" of the pressure-volume curve. Such ventilation strategies are often associated with high PaCO$_2$ levels ("permissive hypercapnia"). Periodic inflations with larger tidal volumes may prove valuable in this setting and their effect should be examined empirically.

When using ventilatory modes, such as pressure support or pressure-limited ventilation, the tidal volume is no longer a preset parameter. However, it is important to monitor tidal volume because it may reflect the progress or decline of lung mechanics and inspiratory effort. In ventilators that do not contain microprocessors the tidal volume should be quantitatively assessed by measuring *expired tidal volume* at the proximal port of the endotracheal tube.

Respiratory Rate

During full ventilatory support with tidal volumes of ~10 ml/kg, a mechanical ventilatory rate of 8–10 breaths per minute will result, approximately, in normocarbia. Mechanical ventilatory rate may have to be increased when using small tidal volumes or for patients with increased dead space or increased CO_2 levels (e.g., during laparoscopic surgery). Higher rates allow less time for expiration, increase mean airway pressure, and may cause air-trapping, especially in the presence of increased airway resistance. It is important to realize that reducing the respiratory rate in time-cycled ventilators should be usually accompanied with readjustment of the I/E ratio to prevent long inspiration times. Using permissive hypercapnia is usually achieved by reducing the tidal volume rather than the respiratory rate.

Supplemental Oxygen Therapy

To minimize the problem of cellular oxygen toxicity and absorption atelectasis, the lowest F_IO_2 level that produces satisfactory arterial oxygenation should be used. There is no evidence that the prolonged use of an $F_IO_2 \leq 0.40$ damages critically ill patients and, therefore, no excessive effort to reduce the F_IO_2 usually is indicated in this range, for fear of oxygen toxicity. An $F_IO_2 = 0.40$ may result in a false sense of well-being for the patient, because, at $F_IO_2 = 0.40$, venous admixture measurements are at their nadir with respect to F_IO_2.

Diagnostically, the response of PaO_2 to an F_IO_2 increase can help differentiate between hypoxemia due to low $\dot{V}_A/\dot{Q}$ relationships; for example, COPD (relatively good response) and hypoxemia due to true intrapulmonary shunt; for example, ARDS (minimal response). For a single patient, F_IO_2 does influence the calculated intrapulmonary shunt. Physiologic shunt fraction varies with F_IO_2 and will be lowest at $F_IO_2 = 0.4$–0.6.

Airway Pressure

Peak airway pressure is determined by the compliance, resistance, and inspiratory flow pattern and rate. However, the change in the airway pressure during the mechanical breath may reveal changes in lung mechanics. High peak airway pressure that is associated with a much lower plateau (end-inspiratory) airway pressure reflects abnormally increased resistance which may be due to a narrow tracheal tube or bronchospasm. A small difference between a high peak airway pressure and plateau pressure reflects low lung compliance. Ideally, one would measure airway pressure near the carina, thus eliminating the influence of the tracheal tube. Airway pressure should be measured no farther from the patient than the tracheal tube. The disconnect alarm on most ventilators is based on airway pressure. Setting the *low* pressure alarm at ~10–15 cmH$_2$O below peak inspiratory pressure not only will detect ventilator disconnection, but also will detect a leak or improved resistance or compliance. Similarly, setting the *high* pressure alarm 5–10 cmH$_2$O above peak airway pressure will give early warning of increased resistance, decreased compliance, or the patient coughing or "fighting" the ventilator.

Following the degree of the negative airway pressure swing at the beginning of inspiration may give a clue to possible increases in ventilator resistance and increased work of breathing. Such increased inspiratory effort can be managed by increasing the ventilator's sensitivity, switching to a decelerating flow pattern to minimize the pressure rise-time, and ruling out sources of increased inspiratory resistance (e.g., an occluded tracheal tube).

When using pressure-limited ventilation to reduce lung damage in patients with acute lung injury, one should limit the end-inspiratory (plateau) pressure to 35–45 cmH$_2$O, although lower pressures may be used if gas exchange is favorable.

Inspiratory/Expiratory Ratio

Conventional ventilatory techniques employ I/E ratios of $<1:1$ and more typically $<1:2$. The interval during which gas actually enters the lung normally should not be <1.5 seconds or an unacceptably high peak airway pressure may result. Increasing the I/E ratio will increase mean airway pressure and may cause air-trapping and generate intrinsic PEEP. Pressure-controlled inverse ratio ventilation is a ventilatory mode that specifically uses this feature to achieve better alveolar recruitment during ventilation, but its efficiency has not been demonstrated unequivocally, and cardiovascular side effects are significant. Following the flow wave form in ventilators with a graphics screen may be the easiest way to identify air-trapping, which can be identified when new inspiration starts before expiratory flow is completed.

In systems that include a continuous fresh gas flow (e.g., anesthesia machines and some IMV systems) and when combining high-frequency jet ventilation (HFJV) with a conventional ventilator, increasing inspiratory time may increase tidal volume.

TEMPTATIONS AND PITFALLS OF VARIOUS VENTILATORY MODES

In addition to the nature of the patient's primary pathology, choice of ventilatory mode is influenced by (*a*) the equipment available, (*b*) reading the literature, and (*c*) previous experience. After making an initial choice, it is necessary to verify that it continues to answer the patient's needs, both in theory and in practice.

Control Mode Ventilation

Control mode ventilation is the ventilatory method of choice when the patient has no spontaneous breathing effort, as during central respiratory depression, neuromuscular failure, or extreme fatigue of the ventilatory muscles. CMV is used also when the respiratory efforts are so inefficient that they may be harmful to the patient. Thus, although never the first choice, CMV use during muscle paralysis may be effective for patients with severe status asthmaticus or for those with severe respiratory or multiorgan failure.

Intermittent Mandatory Ventilation

Intermittent mandatory ventilation gained widespread popularity because it was the first ventilatory mode available for adults that allowed spontaneous breathing and titration of mechanical ventilation according to the patient's needs (i.e., partial ventilatory support). The fear of simultaneously delivering a ventilator breath concomitant with the patient's spontaneous breath ("stacking") prompted the introduction of synchronized IMV (SIMV). No benefit has ever been demonstrated when comparing SIMV and IMV. Further, such synchronization requires a demand valve for spontaneous ventilation, which, at least in older ventilators, increased the work of breathing detrimentally. Even with newer demand valves, the work of breathing can be significant due to a clinically imperceptible delay in the available gas flow and in the pressure "rise time."

A general rule in choosing an appropriate mechanical ventilatory rate during IMV is to reduce the mandatory rate as long as the arterial pH exceeds 7.35 in patients with adequate ventilatory drive and no clinical signs of ventilatory muscle fatigue, particularly no increase in respiratory rate. When a demand valve is used, care must be exercised to ensure that the ventilator's demand valve is sensitive enough and has low enough inertia so as not to increase the work of breathing. Transient airway pressure swings below expiratory pressure at the outset of spontaneous inspiration should not be >2 cmH$_2$O below expiratory pressure. The pressure changes in the trachea are greater and are best measured near the carina rather than in the distal respiratory circuitry.

When using a homemade continuous-flow spontaneous ventilation system with an inspiratory reservoir bag, the continuous flow of gas must be controlled attentively. When flow is too low, inspiratory effort will increase and thereby increase the patient's work of breathing. When the flow is too high, it may increase the mechanically delivered tidal volume owing to late closure of the valve.

The most common mistake in weaning patients with IMV is that the weaning process is too gradual, reducing ventilatory frequency only one breath at a time, and analyzing an excessive number of arterial blood samples for gas analysis. Such gradual weaning is justified only for patients with severe respiratory failure or for those demonstrating ventilatory muscle fatigue. In most patients, and especially in those who receive mechanical ventilation postoperatively, adapting a set schedule for weaning frequently results in unnecessarily prolonged ventilation. A much faster weaning rate can be achieved by individually assessing the patient's ability to breathe spontaneously and reducing the mechanical ventilatory rate accordingly.

Pressure Support Ventilation

Pressure support ventilation is now used widely and has replaced IMV in many places as the choice method for partial ventilatory support and weaning. Its popularity stems from the elegance with which it reduces the work of breathing on a breath-by-breath basis and the ease with which it is used as a weaning method. PSV breaths are pressure-limited; thus, using PSV in patients with low lung compliance may decrease peak airway pressure and may increase mean airway pressure, especially in tachypneic patients. Increased mean airway pressure, in turn, may decrease venous return. Despite many patients' apparent comfort, avoid perceiving the patient as breathing spontaneously, especially when high pressure levels are employed. When determining the PSV level, take into account the underlying pathophysiology, gases, and the desirable level of patient effort. Tidal volume should be monitored closely, as with any pressure-limited mode of ventilation. PSV should be used as a stand-alone method of ventilation only in patients with reliable respiratory drive, preferably with ventilators that have the capacity to recognize and supply "backup" positive pressure breaths.

Inverse Ratio Ventilation

Inverse ratio ventilation requires sedation and paralysis and does not allow spontaneous ventilation. Its safe use requires pressure-limited mechanical inspiration. IRV usually results in high mean airway pressure and gas-trapping intrinsic PEEP. The high mean airway pressure may reduce severely cardiac output; therefore, intensive hemodynamic monitoring, as well as close monitoring for the development of barotrauma, is imperative.

High-Frequency Ventilation

High-frequency ventilation can be delivered as high-frequency positive pressure ventilation (using a conventional ventilator with noncompliant tubings that minimize the compressible volume), high-frequency jet ventilation (HFJV), or high-frequency oscillatory ventilation (currently limited to pediatric patients). The classic (and FDA-approved) indication for HFJV is the presence of significant bronchopleural fistula.

The main problems in the clinical use of HFJV are the difficulties with accurately measuring airway pressures and volumes and with adequate inspired gas humidification. Estimation of tidal volume is difficult because it is composed of both the jet volume and entrained gas. The entrained volume is influenced by the site of the jet (when proximal it creates more entrainment and, hence, larger tidal volume), by changes in the patient's pulmonary compliance and resistance, gas velocity, and by the gas available for entrainment. Airway pressure should be measured in the distal trachea, well below the jet port. When measuring airway pressure proximal to the jet, airway pressure will show a negative deflection during inspiration and mean airway pressure will be underestimated grossly. When measured immediately below the jet, an artifactual increase in airway pressure may result. Another common phenomenon that escapes simple observation is the increase in FRC due to air-trapping, which may improve gas exchange. Mean airway pressure should be monitored continuously, as should the hemodynamic consequences of raised mean airway pressure.

Airway Pressure Release Ventilation

Airway pressure release ventilation (APRV) is not available in most ventilators, although the use of two expiratory pressure levels in the form of BiPAP is gaining popularity especially as a noninvasive ventilatory mode through a face mask. Choosing the appropriate CPAP and release pressure levels is not as yet a standardized procedure and should be determined by the level of CPAP necessary for oxygenation, the patient's compliance, and the required tidal volume. APRV is useful for patients who have no increase in airway resistance. Although designed for those with decreased lung compliance, APRV can be used for any patient with normal airway resistance.

PEEP/CPAP

Low-level PEEP/CPAP of 4–6 cmH_2O are kept to prevent microatelectasis during mechanical ventilation, especially when lower tidal volumes are used. Further, extubation of the trachea from these low PEEP/CPAP levels rather than from ambient pressure may improve postextubation pulmonary function. Using

PEEP/CPAP prophylactically for patients who are at high risk for developing respiratory failure is probably not effective. However, early aggressive use of PEEP/CPAP in those with early evidence of lung injury may decrease the duration of therapy. PEEP/CPAP does not reduce extravascular lung water and, in fact, may cause it to increase. Nevertheless, in patients with pulmonary edema, PEEP/CPAP effectively increases FRC, flattens the alveolar edema fluid on the wall of the tracheobronchial tree, improves compliance, reduces work of breathing, and causes coarse rales to disappear. Its use for patients with cardiogenic pulmonary edema in the emergency room, therefore, has increased widely.

Not all hypoxemic patients are responsive to PEEP/CPAP (e.g., those with emphysema). In patients with ARDS, the response to CPAP is also indicative of disease severity because lower PEEP/CPAP levels fail to recruit truly consolidated lungs. The demonstrated inhomogeneity of pulmonary injury in ARDS, as well as the growing evidence that pulmonary damage can occur as a result of high airway pressure use, has tempered enthusiasm for high PEEP/CPAP level use. Thus, PEEP/CPAP should be used so that it either allows F_IO_2 reductions to nontoxic concentrations (<0.50), or so that it demonstrably improves lung mechanics.

When using PEEP/CPAP, one must be familiar with the system's mechanical characteristics and choose either a high-flow system or a system with a sensitive demand valve, thereby minimizing inspiratory effort. Further, the expiratory valve must be a true threshold resistor to prevent significant increases in airway pressure during coughing or increases in the circuit's gas flow.

Respiratory advantages of PEEP/CPAP use always should be weighed against its potential cardiovascular side effects—both good and bad. At higher levels, PaO_2 should be used in conjunction with other variables reflecting the effects of PEEP/CPAP on cardiac function and, ultimately, on total oxygen delivery.

SUMMARY

The goal of mechanical ventilatory support is to allow the patient to survive past a critical illness and, it is hoped, to return to a fairly normal life. Because of the variety of mechanical ventilatory modes, the large interpatient variation, a wide spectrum of disease, and limited financial resources, it is unlikely that large prospective multi-institutional studies will be performed to examine the efficacy and outcome of various ventilatory modes. As a result, mechanical ventilatory support must be based on sound knowledge of physiology and physical principles. Rational care of the critically ill patient who needs ventilatory support requires knowledge of both normal and pathologic respiratory physiology. Further, intimate knowledge of how the machines work and how they interface with the patient's physiology is also imperative. This book imparts only fundamental knowledge and information concerning mechanical ventilatory support, respiratory physiology, and related science. It is meant to guide the novice and refresh the experienced clinician. We encourage the reader to seek more detailed texts and the original literature to gain a more intimate knowledge of the field.

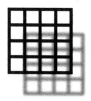

Index

Note: Page numbers in *italics* denote figures; those followed by a t denote tables.

Absorption atelectasis, 91
Acidosis, for asthma, 283
A/CMV. *See* Assist/controlled mechanical
    ventilation (A/CMV)
Acute lung injury (ALI). *See also* Adult
    respiratory distress syndrome
    (ARDS)
  definition of, 249
  mechanisms of, 251–254
    cellular elements and, 252
    humoral elements and, 252–254
ADH (antidiuretic hormone), positive-pressure
    ventilation and, 78
Adult respiratory distress syndrome (ARDS),
    249–269
  clinical management of, 254–268
    inspiratory muscle load reduction and,
      258–260
    mechanical ventilatory techniques for,
      263–265
    minimal excursionary ventilation in,
      265–268
    oxygenation in, 254–256
    positive airway pressure in, 261, 263
    respiratory system compliance reduction
      and work of breathing and,
      256–257, *257–262*
  definition of, 249–250
  extracorporeal respiratory support in, 243t,
    243–244
    logistic and personnel problems with,
      244
    rationale for, 243
  mechanisms of acute lung injury and,
    251–254
    cellular elements and, 252

    humoral elements and, 252–254
  outcome of, 268–269
  pathogenesis of, 250–251
  prevalence of, 249
  pulmonary vascular resistance and, 268
  risk factors for, 251
  tachypnea and agitation in, 107–108
Afterload, effects of mechanical ventilation on,
    61, 63
Agitation, in adult respiratory distress
    syndrome, 107–108
Air embolism, ventilatory management
    techniques for, 315
Airway(s), artificial. *See* Endotracheal
    intubation; Neurologic injuries,
    artificial airways with
Airway obstruction, auto-PEEP in, 105–107,
    106
Airway pressure(s), 365–366
  end inspiratory lung volume versus, in acute
    lung injury, 264–265
  with intermittent mandatory ventilation and
    synchronized intermittent
    mandatory ventilation, 130, *131,*
    132
  measurement of, 37–39
    approaches for, 16
    site of, 13, *14,* 15–16
  monitoring of, with high frequency
    ventilation, 226–228, *227–229*
  occlusion, weaning outcome and, prediction
    of, 350
  transmission to cardiovascular system,
    57–59, *59, 60*

Airway pressure release ventilation (APRV), 183–191
  in acute lung injury, 266–267
  advantages and disadvantages of, 369
  clinical application of, 188–190
    for patients with moderately to severely decreased lung compliance, 189–190, 190t
    for patients with relatively normal lung compliance, 188–189, 189t
  clinical efficacy of, 184–186
  effects on cardiovascular system, 68
  equipment for, 183–184, *184, 185*
  ventilatory parameters for, 186–188
  weaning from, 190–191
Alarms, initial ventilator settings and, 99, 101
Albuterol, for asthma, 275, 275t, 282
Aldosterone, positive-pressure ventilation and, 78–79
Algorithms, operating, for microprocessor-controlled generators, 29, *30*
ALI. *See* Acute lung injury (ALI)
Alkalemia, assist/controlled mechanical ventilation and, 105
Alveolar collapse, 144–146, *145, 146*
Alveolar hyperoxia, in acute lung injury, 255
Amyotrophic lateral sclerosis, 332–334, *333*
Anesthesia
  high frequency ventilation in, 229–230
  inhalation, for asthma, 278–279
Aneurysms, resection of, high frequency ventilation in, 230
Angiotensin, positive-pressure ventilation and, 78–79
Antibiotics, for asthma, 277
Anticholinergics, for asthma, 275t, 275–276
Anticoagulation
  for extracorporeal CO_2 removal, 240
  for extracorporeal membrane oxygenation, 235
Antidiuretic hormone (ADH), positive-pressure ventilation and, 78
Apneic challenge, in brain dead patients, 335
Apneic diffusion oxygenation, 205–209, *206, 207*
  low flow extracorporeal removal of carbon dioxide and, 209–215
    clinical investigation of, 211–215, *212, 213*, 214t
    experimental work on, 209–211, *210*

Apneic ventilation, constant flow, 209–215
  clinical investigation of, 211–215, *212, 213,* 214t
  experimental work on, 209–211, *210*
APRV. *See* Airway pressure release ventilation (APRV)
Arachidonic acid metabolites, in acute lung injury, 253
ARDS. *See* Adult respiratory distress syndrome (ARDS)
Arrhythmias, in chronic obstructive pulmonary disease, 298
Arterial blood gas analysis, 42
Arterial pressure wave form, as reflection of effects of mechanical ventilation on cardiovascular function, *68–71, 68–72*
Artificial airways. *See* Endotracheal intubation; Neurologic injuries, artificial airways with
Artificial lungs, extracorporeal CO_2 removal and, 239
Assist/controlled mechanical ventilation (A/CMV), 101–108
  effects on cardiovascular system, 65
  limitations of, 123
  pressure targeted (preset), 103–104
    volume targeted ventilation versus, 104–108
Asthma, 273–290
  antibiotics for, 277
  anticholinergics for, 275t, 275–276
  bronchodilators for, 274–275
  bronchoscopy for, 279
  helium for, 278
  incidence of, 273–274
  inhalation anesthetics for, 278–279
  magnesium sulfate for, 278
  outcome of, 290
  oxygen therapy for, 278
  steroids for, 276–277, 277t
  theophylline for, 276
  ventilation in, 279–290
    adjunctive measures with, 283–285
    bronchodilator delivery and, 281–282
    complications of, 288–290
    controlled hypoventilation and, 282–283
    fluids and, 282
    indications for, 279
    monitoring during, 285–286, *287*

Asthma (*Continued*)
  ventilator settings and, 280–281, *281*
  weaning from, 286, 288
Atelectasis, absorption, 91
Atrial natriuretic factor, positive-pressure
      ventilation and, 79–80
Autonomic innervation, positive-pressure
      ventilation and, 77–78
Auto-PEEP
  in airway obstruction, 105–107, *106*
  in asthma, 288–289
  in chronic obstructive pulmonary disease,
      295–296, *296*
Ayre's T-piece, *124,* 124–125, *125*

Bag-valve ventilation, during patient transport,
      304
Barotrauma, 50–51
  assist/controlled mechanical ventilation and,
      104–105
  in asthma, 289
  continuous positive airway pressure and
      positive end-expiratory pressure
      and, 151
Beta agonists, for asthma, 274–275, 275t
Bile duct pressure, increase with positive-
      pressure ventilation, 82
Bi-level positive airway pressure, in
      neuromuscular diseases, 334
Bleeding
  extracorporeal CO_2 removal and, 241t,
      241–242
  gastrointestinal, in ventilator-dependent
      patients, 297–298, *297*
Blood flow, renal, redistribution with positive-
      pressure ventilation, 77
Brain death, 334–336
Brain injury, 323–326, *324*
  lung mechanics and gas exchange and,
      305–306
  ventilatory management techniques for,
      311–313, 312t
Breathing, work of. *See* Work of breathing
Breathing circuits, 116, *117–121,* 118–121
  continuous flow, 116, *117–119,* 118
  for continuous positive airway pressure, 111
  demand regulators and, 118–119
  for extracorporeal membrane oxygenation,
      234–235
  for high frequency jet ventilation, *222,*
      223–224
  pressure valves and, 119–121, *120, 121*

Breathing pattern, weaning outcome and,
      prediction of, 348–349
Bronchial hygiene, with artificial airways,
      320–321
Bronchodilators
  for asthma, 274–275
    delivery of, 281–282
  for chronic obstructive pulmonary disease,
      291
Bronchopleural fistulae
  with large air leak flows, high frequency
      ventilation for, 231
  ventilatory management techniques for,
      314–315
Bronchoscopy, for asthma, 279

Cannulas, injector, for high frequency
      ventilation, 225
Cannulation
  for extracorporeal CO_2 removal, 237–238
  for extracorporeal membrane oxygenation,
      234–235
Capnography, 40, 328
Carbon dioxide
  elimination during high frequency
      ventilation, mechanisms of,
      227–228
  end-tidal, monitoring of, 40–41
  extracorporeal removal of. *See* Extracorporeal
      CO_2 removal ($ECCO_2R$)
  retention of, with intermittent mandatory
      ventilation and synchronized
      intermittent mandatory
      ventilation, 134–135
  transcutaneous, monitoring of, 41
Cardiac contractility, effects of mechanical
      ventilation on, 60
Cardiac decompensation, with intermittent
      mandatory ventilation and
      synchronized intermittent
      mandatory ventilation
    avoidance of, 134
    increased likelihood of, 136
Cardiac disease, 46
Cardiac output
  decrease with positive-pressure ventilation
    hepatic function and, 81
    renal function and, 76–77
  effects of mechanical ventilation on, 59–61,
      62, 63–64

Cardiopulmonary bypass, separation from, systolic pressure and, 71
Cardiovascular function
  continuous positive airway pressure and positive end-expiratory pressure and, 147–151, *148*
  effects of mechanical ventilation on, 57–72, 363–364
    airway pressure release ventilation and, 68
    airway pressure transmission and, 57–59, *59, 60*
    arterial pressure wave form as reflection of, *68–71,* 68–72
    assist/controlled mechanical ventilation and, 65
    cardiac output and, 59–61, *62,* 63–64
    controlled mechanical ventilation and, 65
    high frequency ventilation and, 67
    intermittent mandatory ventilation/ synchronized intermittent mandatory ventilation and, 65–66
    inverse-ratio ventilation and, 67–68
    positive end-expiratory pressure/ continuous positive airway pressure and, 66–67
    pressure support ventilation and, 67
    spontaneous ventilation and, 64–65
Central processing units (CPUs), for microprocessor-controlled generators, 26–27
CFAV (constant flow apneic ventilation), 209–215
  clinical investigation of, 211–215, *212, 213,* 214t
  experimental work on, 209–211, *210*
CFI (constant flow insufflation), 215–216
CFV (constant flow ventilation), 209–215
  clinical investigation of, 211–215, *212, 213,* 214t
  experimental work on, 209–211, *210*
Chest cuirasses, in neuromuscular diseases, *333,* 333–334
Chest trauma
  lung mechanics and gas exchange and, 306–307
  ventilatory management techniques for, 313–315
Chest wall injuries, ventilatory management techniques for, 314
Chronic obstructive pulmonary disease (COPD), 290–299

medical management of, 290–292
outcome of, 299
precipitants for, 290
ventilation in, 292–298
  complications of, 295–298
  home, chronic, 294
  indications for, 292–293
  noninvasive, 293–294
  perithoracic, 194
  positive pressure, 195
  tracheal gas insufflation, 294
  weaning from, 294–295
Circuit(s). *See* Breathing circuits
Circuit modification techniques, for differential lung ventilation, 178–179
Circulation, monitoring of, 45–47
Circulatory shock, respiratory failure with, high frequency ventilation for, 230
Closed reservoir systems, for intermittent mandatory ventilation, 126, *127*
Closed-loop control systems, for microprocessor-controlled generators, 28–29
CMV. *See* Controlled mechanical ventilation (CMV)
Complement, in acute lung injury, 253
Congestive heart failure, end-expiratory pressure in, 149–150
Constant flow apneic ventilation (CFAV), 209–215
  clinical investigation of, 211–215, *212, 213,* 214t
  experimental work on, 209–211, *210*
Constant flow insufflation (CFI), 215–216
Constant flow ventilation (CFV), 209–215
  clinical investigation of, 211–215, *212, 213,* 214t
  experimental work on, 209–211, *210*
Continuous gas flow systems, 116, *117–119,* 118
  in neuromuscular diseases, 333
Continuous positive airway pressure (CPAP), 3, 12–13, *13,* 195, 362
  advantages and disadvantages of, 369–370
  breathing circuits for, 111
  differential, for differential lung ventilation, 178
  effects on cardiovascular system, 66–67
  hemodynamic effects of, 63–64

Continuous positive airway pressure (*Continued*)
  physiologic, 152
  physiologic considerations with, 142–151
    respiratory gas exchange, 142
    respiratory system mechanics, *143,* 143–151, *145, 146*
  release of, 187–188
  technical considerations with, 139–142, *140, 141*
  titration of, 152–153
  during weaning, 353–354
Continuous positive-pressure ventilation (CPPV), 8
Controlled mechanical ventilation (CMV), 8, *9,* 101–108, 361. *See also* Assist/controlled mechanical ventilation (A/CMV)
  advantages and disadvantages of, 367
  for asthma, 280
  effects on cardiovascular system, 63, 65
  limitations of, 123
  pressure targeted (preset), 103–104
    volume targeted ventilation versus, 104–108
COPD. *See* Chronic obstructive pulmonary disease (COPD)
Corticosteroids
  for asthma, 276–277, 277t
  for chronic obstructive pulmonary disease, 291
CPAP. *See* Continuous positive airway pressure (CPAP)
CPPV (continuous positive-pressure ventilation), 8
CPUs (central processing units), for microprocessor-controlled generators, 26–27
Critically ill patients, transport of, 304
Cuirasses, in neuromuscular diseases, *333,* 333–334
Cycling mechanisms, 18–24, 19t
  flow-cycled mechanical inhalation and, 23–24
  pressure-cycled mechanical inhalation and, 22–23, 24t
  time-cycled mechanical inhalation and, 18–19, *20,* 20t
    pressure-limited, 19, 21, *21*

volume-cycled mechanical inhalation and, 21–22, 22t, *23*
Cycling synchrony, 159
Cytokines, in acute lung injury, 252–253

Dead space, elimination of, in acute lung injury, 266
Demand regulators, 118–119
  for intermittent mandatory ventilation, 127, *128*
Diaphragmatic pacing, 328–329
Diaphragmatic tears, lung mechanics and gas exchange and, 307
Differential lung ventilation (DLV), 173–181, *174, 175*
  discontinuation of, 180
  endobronchial intubation for, 175–178, *177*
  indications for, 173–174, 175t, *176*
  monitoring during, 180
  techniques for, 178–179
  ventilator settings for, 179–180
Dynamic hyperinflation
  in asthma, 288
  weaning outcome and, 344–346, *345*

Eccentric cam and piston mechanism, for microprocessor-controlled generators, 24–25
ECCO$_2$R. *See* Extracorporeal CO$_2$ removal (ECCO$_2$R)
ECMO. *See* Extracorporeal membrane oxygenation (ECMO)
Embolism, air, ventilatory management techniques for, 315
Emphysema, interstitial, pulmonary, 51
End inspiratory lung volume, airway pressure versus, in acute lung injury, 264–265
End-expiratory pressure, cardiovascular effects of, 149–150
Endobronchial intubation, for differential lung ventilation, 175–178, *177*
Endotracheal intubation
  complications of, 193
    traumatic, 296–297
  jet tubes and, 225
  posttraumatic, indications for, 303–304, 304t

End-tidal carbon dioxide, monitoring of, 40–41

EPAP (expiratory positive airway pressure), 12–13, *13*
  in neuromuscular diseases, 334

Epinephrine, for asthma, 275

Equipment load, weaning outcome and, 346

Evaluation, of ventilators, 31–32

Exhalatory pressure release, pressure support ventilation with, in acute lung injury, 267

Expiratory flow, monitoring of, 39

Expiratory positive airway pressure (EPAP), 12–13, *13*
  in neuromuscular diseases, 334

Expiratory volume, monitoring of, 39

Extracorporeal CO_2 removal ($ECCO_2R$), 208, *209,* 236–242, *237, 238*
  in acute lung injury, 267–268
  in adult respiratory distress syndrome, 243t, 243–244
    logistic and personnel problems with, 244
    rationale for, 243
  clinical management for, 240–241
  complications of, 241t, 241–242
  inclusion criteria for study of, 236–237
  results with, 242, 242t
  technique for, 237–240, *239*
    anticoagulation and, 240
    artificial lungs and, 239
    cannulation and, 237–238
    pumps and, 239–240

Extracorporeal membrane oxygenation (ECMO), 233–236
  in acute lung injury, 267
  in adult respiratory distress syndrome, 243t, 243–244
    logistic and personnel problems with, 244
    rationale for, 243
  clinical management for, 235
  complications of, 235–236
  inclusion criteria for study of, 234, 234t
  results with, 236
  technique for, 234–235
    anticoagulation and, 235
    cannulation and circuit and, 234–235

Extravascular lung water, continuous positive airway pressure and positive end-expiratory pressure and, 151

Extrinsic PEEP, for asthma, 280–281

Fat embolism syndrome, ventilatory management techniques for, 315–316

Fentanyl, for asthma, 283, 284t, 285

Flail chest
  lung mechanics and gas exchange and, 307
  ventilatory management techniques for, 313–314

Flow controlled, volume-cycled ventilation, initial ventilator settings and, 93–94, *94*

Flow generators
  constant and nonconstant, 24–25
  microprocessor-controlled, 25–31, 26t, *27*

Flow synchrony, 158–159

Flow-cycled mechanical inhalation, 23–24

Fluids
  for asthma, 282
  retention of, with end-expiratory pressure, 150

Fracture fixation, timing of, 316

Gas entrainment, injection systems using, 226

Gas exchange
  with continuous positive airway pressure and positive end-expiratory pressure, 142
  in trauma patients. *See* Posttraumatic ventilation, lung mechanics and gas exchange and

Gas flow systems, continuous, in neuromuscular diseases, 333

Gastrointestinal bleeding, in ventilator-dependent patients, 297

Gastrointestinal function, positive-pressure ventilation effects on, 83

Glycopyrrolate, for asthma, 275t, 275–276

Gravity-dependent pressure valves, 119, *120*

Gravity-independent pressure valves, 119–120, *121*

Guillain-Barré syndrome, 332

Haloperidol, for asthma, 283, 284t, 285

Head injury, 323–326, *324*
  lung mechanics and gas exchange and, 305–306
  ventilatory management techniques for, 311–313, 312t

Heart failure
  in chronic obstructive pulmonary disease, 298

Heart failure (*Continued*)
  congestive, end-expiratory pressure in, 149–150
Helium, for asthma, 278
Hemodynamics, continuous positive airway pressure effects on, 63–64
Hemolysis, extracorporeal CO_2 removal and, 241
Hemorrhagic shock, lung mechanics and gas exchange and, 305
Hemothorax, following chest trauma, lung mechanics and gas exchange and, 306
Hepatic function, positive-pressure ventilation effects on, 80–82
  decreased cardiac output and, 81
  increased bile duct pressure and, 82
  increased hepatic vascular resistance and, 81–82
High frequency jet ventilation (HFJV), 221
  circuits for, *222,* 223–224
  clinical indications for, 228–231
    in anesthesia, 229–230
    in critical care, 230–231
  humidification and warming of gases for, 224
  lung volume and pressures and, 226–227, *228*
High frequency positive pressure ventilation (HFPPV), 221
  clinical indications for, 228–231
    in anesthesia, 229–230
    in critical care, 230–231
  lung volume and pressures and, 226
High frequency ventilation (HFV), 221–232.
    See also specific types of high frequency ventilation
  in acute lung injury, 266
  advantages and disadvantages of, 369
  clinical indications for, 228–231
    in anesthesia, 229–230
    in critical care, 230–231
  contraindications to, 232
  effects on cardiovascular system, 67
  lung volume and pressures and, 226–228, *227–229*
  technical aspects of, 221–226
    circuits for high frequency jet ventilation and, *222,* 223–224
    humidification and warming of gases and, 224
    injection modes and, 225–226

Home ventilation, chronic, for chronic obstructive pulmonary disease, 294
Humidification, of gases, for high frequency jet ventilation, 224
Hydrostatic pressure valves, 119
Hypercapnia
  permissive, in acute lung injury, 266
  weaning outcome and. *See* Weaning, in hypercapnic respiratory failure
Hyperinflation
  dynamic
    in asthma, 288
    weaning outcome and, 344–346, *345*
  physiologic limit to, 49–50
Hyperoxia, alveolar, in acute lung injury, 255
Hyperventilation
  for head injury, 311
    excessive, avoidance of, 323–324
  physiologic limit to, 49–50
Hypervolemia, cardiac output in, 63
Hypoperfusion, exacerbation by mechanical ventilation, 45–46
Hypotension, exacerbation by mechanical ventilation, 45–46
Hypoventilation, controlled, for asthma, 282–283
Hypovolemia
  cardiac output in, 63
  systolic pressure in, *69,* 69–70
Hypovolemic shock
  lung mechanics and gas exchange and, 305
  ventilatory management techniques for, 308–309
Hypoxemia
  initial ventilator settings and, 91–92
  positive pressure ventilation in, 195
  weaning outcome and, 340

I/E (inspiratory:expiratory) time ratio, 366
  for airway pressure release ventilation, 187–188
  initial ventilator settings and, 95–97, *96*
  techniques to increase, 166, *167,* 168, *168*
IMV. *See* Intermittent mandatory ventilation (IMV)
Infants, newborn
  intermittent mandatory ventilation for, historical background of, 123–125, *124–126*
  with respiratory distress syndrome, 54

Infection
  as chronic obstructive pulmonary disease
    precipitant, 290
  in ventilator-dependent patients, 297
Infection, Nosocomial, pneumonia,
    endotracheal intubation and, 193
Inhalation anesthetics, for asthma, 278–279
Initial ventilator settings, 89–101
  alarms and, 99, 101
  fractional inspired oxygen concentration
    and, 89–92
  inspiratory flow rate and inspiratory:
    expiratory ratio and, 95–97, *96*
  inspiratory pause and, 97–99, *98*
  tidal volume and respiratory rate and, *92,*
    92–95, *94*
  ventilation mode and, 99, *100*
Injector cannulas, for high frequency
    ventilation, 225
Inspiratory flow rate, initial ventilator settings
    and, 95–97, *96*
Inspiratory flow wave patterns, 24–25, *25*
Inspiratory pause, initial ventilator settings and,
    97–99, *98*
Inspiratory positive airway pressure (IPAP), in
    neuromuscular diseases, 334
Inspiratory pressure, maximal, weaning
    outcome and, prediction of, 349
Inspiratory time, 95
Inspiratory:expiratory (I/E) time ratio, 366
  for airway pressure release ventilation,
    187–188
  initial ventilator settings and, 95–97, *96*
  techniques to increase, 166, *167,* 168, *168*
Inspired oxygen concentrations, in acute lung
    injury, 254–255
Intermittent mandatory ventilation (IMV), 3,
    10–11, *11,* 123–136
  advantages and disadvantages of, 367–368
  clinical applications of, 128–136, 129t,
    130t
    advantages with, 128–134
    disadvantages with, 134–136
  effects on cardiovascular system, 65–66
  historical background of, 123–127
    in adults, 125–127, *127*–*129*
    in neonates, 123–125, *124*–*126*
Intermittent positive-pressure breathing (IPPB),
    195–196, 198–199

Intermittent-flow expiratory ventilation,
    216–217, *217*
Interstitial emphysema, pulmonary, 51
Intrabronchial catheters, 225–226
Intracranial pressure
  control of, 312–313
    pharmacologic, 324–325
  increased, patients at risk for, 304
Intratracheal catheters, 225–226
Intratracheal gas insufflation, 215–217
  clinical applications of, 215–217, *217*
Intratracheal pulmonary ventilation, 215
Intrinsic positive end-expiratory pressure,
    weaning outcome and, 344–346,
    345
Inverse ratio ventilation (IRV), 165–172
  administration method for, 168–169
  advantages and disadvantages of, 368
  controversy regarding, 171–172
  effects on cardiovascular system, 67–68
  inspiratory/expiratory ratio and, techniques
    for increasing, 166, *167,* 168, *168*
  pitfalls and complications of, 170–171
IPAP (inspiratory positive airway pressure), in
    neuromuscular diseases, 334
IPPB (intermittent positive-pressure breathing),
    195–196, 198–199
Ipratropium bromide, for asthma, 275t,
    275–276
IRV. *See* Inverse ratio ventilation (IRV)

Jet endotracheal tubes, 225

Left-sided heart failure, in chronic obstructive
    pulmonary disease, 298
Lorazepam, for asthma, 283, 284t, 285
Low flow extracorporen chronic obstructive
    pulmonary disease, 298
Lorazepam, for asthma, 283, 284t, 285
Low flow extracorporeal removal of carbon
    dioxide (ECCO$_2$R). *See*
    Extracorporeal CO$_2$ removal
    (ECCO$_2$R)
Lung(s)
  artificial, extracorporeal CO$_2$ removal and,
    239
  injury of. *See* Acute lung injury (ALI); Adult
    respiratory distress syndrome
    (ARDS)

Lung compliance
  decreased
    in acute lung injury, work of breathing
      and, 256–257, *257–262*
    in adult respiratory distress syndrome,
      256–257, *257–262*
    airway pressure release ventilation and,
      189–190, 190t
    in respiratory failure with elevated peak
      airway pressure, high frequency
      ventilation for, 231
  normal, airway pressure release ventilation
    and, 188–189, 189t
Lung injury. *See also* Acute lung injury (ALI);
    Adult respiratory distress
    syndrome (ARDS)
  mechanical ventilation-induced, prevention
    of, 53–54
Lung mechanics, in trauma patients. *See*
    Posttraumatic ventilation, lung
    mechanics and gas exchange and
Lung water, extravascular, continuous positive
    airway pressure and positive end-
    expiratory pressure and, 151

Macrophages, in acute lung injury, 252
Magnesium sulfate, for asthma, 278
Mandatory minute volume, 12
Marrow embolism syndrome, ventilatory
    management techniques for,
    315–316
Mask ventilation, during weaning, 354
Maxillofacial trauma, ventilatory management
    techniques for, 310–311
Maximal inspiratory pressure, weaning
    outcome and, prediction of, 349
MDI (metered dose inhalers), 274, 281–282
Memory, for microprocessor-controlled
    generators, 39
Metaproterenol, for asthma, 275, 275t
Metered dose inhalers (MDI), 274, 281–282
Methylprednisolone
  for asthma, 277, 277t
  for chronic obstructive pulmonary disease,
    291
Microprocessor-controlled generators, 25–31,
    26t, *27*
  clinical application of, 31
  closed-loop control systems for, 28–29
  memory for, 39
  open-loop control systems for, 28

Microvascular permeability, following
    mechanical ventilation, 52
Midazolam, for asthma, 283, 284t, 285
Minimal excursionary ventilation, in acute lung
    injury, 265–268
Minute ventilation, weaning outcome and,
    prediction of, 349
Minute ventilation load, weaning outcome
    and, 346–347
Monitoring
  of airway pressure, with high frequency
    ventilation, 226–228, *227–229*
  of circulation, 45–47
  during differential lung ventilation, 180
  of end-tidal carbon dioxide, 40–41
  of expiratory flow, 39
  of expiratory volume, 39
  of oxygen supply, 45
  of oxygenation, 42–45
  of transcutaneous carbon dioxide, 41
  during ventilatory support, 35–47
    in asthma, 285–286, *287*
    of circulation, 45–47
    of ventilation, 35–42
      airway pressure and, 37–49
      arterial blood gas analysis and, 42,
        Monitoring during ventilatory
        support of oxygenation, 42–45
      end-tidal carbon dioxide and, 40–41
      expiratory volume and flow and, 39
      respiratory movements and, 37
      transcutaneous carbon dioxide and, 41
Multiorgan failure, extracorporeal CO_2
    removal and, 242
Muscle(s). *See* Neuromuscular diseases;
    Respiratory muscles
Muscle relaxation. *See also* Neuromuscular
    blocking agents
  reduction of need for, intermittent
    mandatory ventilation and
    synchronized intermittent
    mandatory ventilation for, 130
Myasthenia gravis, 331–332
Myopathy, in asthma, 289–290

Neonates
  intermittent mandatory ventilation for,
    historical background of,
    123–125, *124–126*
  with respiratory distress syndrome, 54

Neural conduction, weaning outcome and, 342–343
Neurologic injuries, 317–336
  artificial airways with, 319–323
    airway obstruction and, 319–320
    airway protection and, 320
    bronchial hygiene and, 320–321
    tracheostomy and, 321–322
  brain death and, 334–336
  brain injury, 323–326, *324*
  mechanical ventilation with, 322–323
  neuromuscular diseases and, 331–334, *333*
  respiratory function and, 317, *318,* 319
  spinal cord injury, 326t, 326–329, 327t, *330,* 331
Neuromuscular blocking agents
  for asthma, 285
  effects of, 325
Neuromuscular diseases, 331–334, *333*
  weaning outcome and, 343
Neutrophils, in acute lung injury, 252
New ventilatory modes, 4–5
Newborns
  intermittent mandatory ventilation for, historical background of, 123–125, *124–126*
  with respiratory distress syndrome, 54
Noninvasive ventilation, 193–202
  for chronic obstructive pulmonary disease, 293–294
  clinical results with, 200–201
  complications of, 201–202
  frequency of delivery of, 196
  mechanisms of action of, 198
  patient-ventilator interface and, 199
  perithoracic, 194
  positive pressure, 195–198
  ventilatory mode for, 198–199
Nosocomial infection
  pneumonia, endotracheal intubation and, 193
  in ventilator-dependent patients, 297
Nutrition, in chronic obstructive pulmonary disease, 292

Obstructive sleep apnea, 319–320
Open-loop control systems, for microprocessor-controlled generators, 28
Operating algorithms, for microprocessor-controlled generators, 29, *30*

Organ donation, brain death and, 335
Orthopedic injuries, ventilatory management techniques for, 315–316
Oxidative phosphorylation, 89–92
Oxygen
  supply of, monitoring of, 45
  tracheal insufflation of, 208
Oxygen radicals, in acute lung injury, 253–254
Oxygen therapy, 365
  in acute lung injury, 255–256
  for asthma, 278
  for chronic obstructive pulmonary disease, 291–292
Oxygenation
  in acute lung injury, 254–256
  monitoring of, 42–45
  weaning outcome and, prediction of, 348
Oxyhemoglobin
  arterial blood concentration of, 43
  mixed-venous saturation of, 43–44

Paralysis, for asthma, 285
Partial ventilatory support, 362
Patient transport, of critically ill patients, 304
Patient-triggered control ventilation, *9,* 10
Patient-triggered (initiated) mechanical ventilation, 8, *9,* 10
Patient-ventilatory interface
  noninvasive ventilation and, 199
  synchrony and, 157–159, *158*
Peak inflation pressure (PIP), 7–8
  prevention of mechanical ventilation-induced lung injury and, 53–54
PEEP. *See* Positive end-expiratory pressure (PEEP)
Perithoracic ventilation, 194
Permissive hypercapnia, in acute lung injury, 266
Phosphorylation, oxidative, 89–92
Phrenic nerve pacing, 328–329, *330,* 331
Physiologic continuous positive airway pressure, 152
Physiologic positive end-expiratory pressure, 152
PIP (peak inflation pressure), 7–8
  prevention of mechanical ventilation-induced lung injury and, 53–54
Platelet activating factor, in acute lung injury, 253

Pleural pressure, measurement of, 58–59, *59,*
    60
Pneumonia, nosocomial, endotracheal
    intubation and, 193
Pneumotachograph, *113,* 113–114, *114*
Pneumothorax, 51
    following chest trauma, lung mechanics and
        gas exchange and, 306
Positive airway pressure
    in acute lung injury, 261, 263
    bi-level, in neuromuscular diseases, 334
Positive end-expiratory pressure (PEEP), 3
    advantages and disadvantages of, 369–370
    auto-PEEP
        in airway obstruction, 105–107, *106*
        in asthma, 288–289
        in chronic obstructive pulmonary disease,
            295–296, *296*
    effects on cardiovascular system, 66–67
    extrinsic, for asthma, 280–281
    intrinsic, weaning outcome and, 344–346,
        345
    paradoxical response to, as indication for
        differential lung ventilation, 174
    physiologic, 152
    physiologic considerations with, 142–151
        respiratory gas exchange, 142
        respiratory system mechanics, *143,*
            143–151, *145, 146*
    selective, for differential lung ventilation,
        178
    technical considerations with, 139–142,
        140, 141
    titration of, 152–153
    during weaning, 353–354
Positive-pressure ventilation (PPV), 75–83,
        195–198
    effect on gastrointestinal function, 83
    effects on hepatic function, 80–82
        decreased cardiac output and, 81
        increased bile duct pressure and, 82
        increased hepatic vascular resistance and,
            81–82
    effects on renal function, 75–80, *76*
        antidiuretic hormone and, 78
        atrial natriuretic factor and, 79–80
        autonomic innervation and, 77–78
        decreased cardiac output and, 76–77
        increased venous pressure and, 77
        redistribution of renal blood flow and, 77
        renin-angiotensin-aldosterone and, 78–79

high frequency, 221
    physiologic effects of, 196–198, *197*
    in spinal cord injury, 327–328
    ventilatory modes for, 195–196
Posttraumatic ventilation, 303–316
    in chest trauma, 313–315
    in head injury, 311–313, 312t
    indications for, 303–304, 304t
    lung mechanics and gas exchange and,
        304–308
        blunt chest trauma and, 306–307
        head injury and, 305–306
        shock and, 305
        spinal cord injuries and, 307–308, *308*
    in maxillofacial trauma, 310–311
    with orthopedic injuries, 315–316
    in shock, hypovolemic, 308–309
    in spinal cord injury, 309–310
PPV. *See* Positive-pressure ventilation (PPV)
Prednisone, for asthma, 277, 277t
Preload, effects of mechanical ventilation on,
        61, *62*
Pressure preset (targeted) ventilation, 103–104
    volume targeted ventilation versus, 104–108
Pressure support ventilation (PSV), 16–18, *17,*
        21, 155–162, *156,* 156t
    advantages and disadvantages of, 368
    clinical applications of, 159–162, 160t, *161*
    effects on cardiovascular system, 67
    exhalatory pressure release with, in acute
        lung injury, 267
    physiologic effects of, 155–159
        patient-ventilatory synchrony and,
            157–159, *158*
        on ventilatory muscle function, 155–157,
            157
    for weaning, 353
Pressure valves, 119–121
    gravity-dependent, 119, *120*
    gravity-independent, 119–120, *121*
    hydrostatic, 119
Pressure-controlled inverse ratio ventilation. *See*
        Inverse ratio ventilation (IRV)
Pressure-cycled ventilation, 22–23, 24t
    initial ventilator settings and, 93–94, *94*
Pressure-limited, time-cycled mechanical
        ventilation, 19, 21, *21*
Propofol, for asthma, 283, 284t, 285
Proportional assist ventilation, during weaning,
        354

Protective reflexes, 320
PSV. *See* Pressure support ventilation (PSV)
Pulmonary compliance. *See* Lung compliance
Pulmonary disease, 46
Pulmonary function, effects of mechanical
    ventilation on, 49–55, *50, 51*
Pulmonary interstitial emphysema, 51
Pulmonary parenchyma, cell lines of, 51–52
Pulmonary thromboembolism, in chronic
    obstructive pulmonary disease,
    297–298
Pulmonary vascular resistance, in acute lung
    injury, 268
Pulse oximetry, 43
Pumps, for extracorporeal CO_2 removal,
    239–240

Random access memory (RAM), for
    microprocessor-controlled
    generators, 29
Read only memory (ROM), for
    microprocessor-controlled
    generators, 29
Reflexes, protective, 320
Relaxation volume, 146–147
Renal function, positive-pressure ventilation
    and. *See* Positive-pressure
    ventilation (PPV), effects on renal
    function
Renin-angiotensin-aldosterone, positive-
    pressure ventilation and, 78–79
Respiratory alkalosis, avoidance of, intermittent
    mandatory ventilation and
    synchronized intermittent
    mandatory ventilation for,
    128–130
Respiratory center, decreased output of,
    weaning outcome and, 341–342
Respiratory distress syndrome, in neonates, 54
Respiratory failure
    with circulatory shock, high frequency
        ventilation for, 230
    with elevated peak airway pressure and
        reduced respiratory compliance,
        high frequency ventilation for,
        231
    lung management in, 54–55
    nature of, 361–363

Respiratory mechanics
    continuous positive airway pressure and
        positive end-expiratory pressure
        and, *143,* 143–151, *145, 146*
    weaning outcome and, 343–344
Respiratory movements, detection and, 37
Respiratory muscles
    atrophy and discoordination of, prevention
        with intermittent mandatory
        ventilation and synchronized
        intermittent mandatory
        ventilation, 134
    fatigue of, with intermittent mandatory
        ventilation and synchronized
        intermittent mandatory
        ventilation, 135
    pressure support ventilation effects on
        function of, 155–157, *157*
    unloading of
        in acute lung injury, 258–260
        pressure support ventilation for, 18
Respiratory quotient, 347
Respiratory rate, 365
    initial ventilator settings and, 92–95, *94*
Respiratory Systolic Variation Test, 71–72
Rib fractures
    lung mechanics and gas exchange and, 306
    ventilatory management techniques for, 314
Right-sided heart failure, in chronic obstructive
    pulmonary disease, 298
Risk factors, for acute lung injury, 251
ROM (read only memory), for microprocessor-
    controlled generators, 29

Safety, of ventilators, 31–32
Sedation
    for asthma, 283, 284t, 285
    reduction of need for, intermittent
        mandatory ventilation and
        synchronized intermittent
        mandatory ventilation for, 130
Selective PEEP, for differential lung
    ventilation, 178
Shock
    circulatory, respiratory failure with, high
        frequency ventilation for, 230
    hypovolemic
        lung mechanics and gas exchange and,
        305
        ventilatory management techniques for,
        308–309

SIMV. *See* Synchronized intermittent mandatory ventilation (SIMV)
Sleep apnea, 319–320
Sodium bicarbonate, for asthma, 283
Spinal cord injuries, 326–329, 327t, *330,* 331
  classification of, 326, 326t
  lung mechanics and gas exchange and, 307–308, *308*
  ventilatory management techniques for, 309–310
Spontaneous breathing trials, prediction of weaning outcome and, 351
Spontaneous ventilation, effects on cardiovascular system, 64–65
Steroids
  for asthma, 276–277, 277t
  for chronic obstructive pulmonary disease, 291
Supraventricular tachyarrhythmia, in chronic obstructive pulmonary disease, 298
Surgery
  intermittent mandatory ventilation during, 125–126
  intermittent mandatory ventilation following, 126–127, *127–129*
Synchronized intermittent mandatory ventilation (SIMV), 11–12, 127, *129*
  clinical applications of, 128–136, 129t, 130t
    advantages with, 128–134
    disadvantages with, 134–136
  effects on cardiovascular system, 65–66
  for weaning, 352–353
Systolic pressure, effects of mechanical ventilation on, *68–71,* 68–72

Tachyarrhythmia, in chronic obstructive pulmonary disease, 298
Tachypnea, in adult respiratory distress syndrome, 107–108
Tension pneumothorax, following chest trauma, lung mechanics and gas exchange and, 306
Terbutaline, for asthma, 275
TGI (tracheal gas insufflation)
  apneic diffusion oxygenation, 208
  for chronic obstructive pulmonary disease, 294

Theophylline, for asthma, 276
Tidal volume
  for airway pressure release ventilation, 186–187
  initial ventilator settings and, *92,* 92–95, *94*
Tidal volumes, 364–365
Time-cycled mechanical inhalation, 18–19, *20,* 20t
  pressure-limited, 19, 21, *21*
T-piece breathing, intermittent, 352
Tracheal gas insufflation (TGI)
  apneic diffusion oxygenation, 208
  for chronic obstructive pulmonary disease, 294
Tracheal insufflation of oxygen (TRIO), 208
Tracheal intubation, impossibility of, high frequency ventilation and, 230
Tracheal lesions, high frequency ventilation for, 231
Tracheostomy, with neurologic injuries, 321–322
Transcutaneous carbon dioxide, monitoring of, 41
Transport, of critically ill patients, 304
Traumatic injuries. *See also* Barotrauma; Neurologic injuries; Posttraumatic ventilation
  endotracheal intubation and, 296–297
Trigger synchrony, 158, *158*
TRIO (tracheal insufflation of oxygen), 208
TRIS, for asthma, 283
Tube trauma, 296–297

Urinary output, with end-expiratory pressure, 150

Vascular resistance
  hepatic, increase with positive-pressure ventilation, 81–82
  pulmonary, in acute lung injury, 268
Venous pressure, increase with positive-pressure ventilation, 77
Venous return, continuous positive airway pressure and positive end-expiratory pressure and, 147–149, *148,* 150–151
Venous thromboembolism, in chronic obstructive pulmonary disease, 297–298

Ventilation
  in acute lung injury, 256–268
    inspiratory muscle load reduction and,
      258–260
    mechanical ventilatory techniques for,
      263–265
    minimal excursionary ventilation in,
      265–268
    positive airway pressure in, 261, 263
    respiratory system compliance reduction
      and work of breathing and,
      256–257, *257–262*
  monitoring of, 35–42
Ventilation mode, initial ventilator settings
  and, 99, *100*
Ventilation-perfusion index (VQI), 44–45
Ventilation/perfusion matching, with
      intermittent mandatory ventilation
      and synchronized intermittent
      mandatory ventilation, 132–133
Ventilation/perfusion ratio, in acute lung
      injury, 254–255
Ventilator, weaning outcome and, 346
Ventilator settings
  for asthma, 280–281, *281*
  for differential lung ventilation, 179–180
  for head injury, 311–312
  initial. *See* Initial ventilator settings
Ventilatory challenge, in brain dead patients,
      335
Ventilatory parameters, for airway pressure
      release ventilation, 186–188
Ventilatory support principles, 359–371
  airway pressure and, 365–366
  effects of support on other organ systems,
      363–364
  inspiratory/expiratory ratio and, 366
  nature of respiratory failure and, 361–363
  need for support and, 360–361
  respiratory rate and, 365
  supplemental oxygen therapy and, 365
  tidal volume and, 364–365
Ventricular failure, high frequency ventilation
      for, 230–231
Ventricular tachyarrhythmia, in chronic
      obstructive pulmonary disease,
      298

Vocalization, restoring, following spinal cord
      injury, 328
Volume targeted ventilation, pressure preset
      (targeted) ventilation versus,
      104–108
Volume-cycled mechanical inhalation, 21–22,
      22t, *23*
Volume-cycled ventilation, flow controlled,
      initial ventilator settings and,
      93–94, *94*
VQI (ventilation-perfusion index), 44–45

Warming, of gases, for high frequency jet
      ventilation, 224
Weaning, 339–356
  from airway pressure release ventilation,
      190–191
  approach to, 354–356, 355t
  in asthma, 286, 288
  in chronic obstructive pulmonary disease,
      294–295
  determinants of outcome of, 339–347, 340t
  in hypercapnic respiratory failure, 340–347,
      341
    dynamic hyperinflation and intrinsic
      PEEP and, 344–346, *345*
    minute ventilation load and, 346–347
    muscular disorders and, 343
    neural conduction and, 342–343
    respiratory center output decrease and,
      341–342
    respiratory mechanics and, 343–344
    ventilator and equipment load and, 346
  in hypoxemic respiratory failure, 340
  from intermittent mandatory ventilation and
      synchronized intermittent
      mandatory ventilation, 133t,
      133–134
  methods for, 351–354
    intermittent T-piece breathing, 352
    mask ventilation, 354
    positive end-expiratory pressure or
      continuous positive airway
      pressure and, 353–354
    pressure support ventilation, 353
    proportional assist ventilation, 354
    synchronized intermittent mandatory
      ventilation, 352–353
  predicting outcome of, 347–351, 348t

Weaning (*Continued*)
    airway occlusion pressure and, 350
    breathing pattern and, 348–349
    derived indices and, 350–351
    maximal inspiratory pressure and, 349
    minute ventilation and, 349
    oxygenation and, 348
    spontaneous breathing trials and, 351
    pressure support ventilation for, 160t, *161,*
      161–162
    prolongation of, with intermittent
      mandatory ventilation and

    synchronized intermittent
      mandatory ventilation,
      135–136
Work of breathing, 111–116, *113–115*
    imposed, 13, *14,* 15–16
    increase in, with intermittent mandatory
      ventilation and synchronized
      intermittent mandatory
      ventilation, 135
    pulmonary compliance reduction and, in
      acute lung injury, 256–257,
      257–262